Therapeutic Modalities
for Athletic Trainers

Therapeutic Modalities for Athletic Trainers

Chad Starkey, PhD, ATC
Assistant Professor
Athletic Training Curriculum Director
Northeastern University
Bouvé College of Pharmacy and Health Sciences
Department of Physical Therapy
Boston, Massachusetts

F. A. DAVIS COMPANY • Philadelphia

F. A. Davis Company
1915 Arch Street
Philadelphia, PA 19103

Printed in the United States of America

Last digit indicates print number: 10 9 8 7 6 5 4 3 2

Senior Allied Health Editor: Jean-François Vilain
Senior Allied Health Developmental Editor: Ralph Zickgraf
Production Editor: Gail Shapiro
Cover Design By: Steven Ross Morrone

As new scientific information becomes available through basic and clinical research, recommended treatments and drug therapies undergo changes. The author(s) and publisher have done everything possible to make this book accurate, up to date, and in accord with accepted standards at the time of publication. The authors, editors, and publisher are not responsible for errors or omissions or for consequences from application of the book, and make no warranty, expressed or implied, in regard to the contents of the book. Any practice described in this book should be applied by the reader in accordance with professional standards of care used in regard to the unique circumstances that may apply in each situation. The reader is advised always to check product information (package inserts) for changes and new information regarding dose and contraindications before administering any drug. Caution is especially urged with using new or infrequently ordered drugs.

Library of Congress Cataloging-in-Publication Data

Starkey, Chad, 1959–
     Therapeutic modalities for athletic trainers / Chad Starkey.
         p.   cm.
     Includes bibliographical references and index.
     ISBN 0-8036-8099-6
     1. Sports medicine.   2. Athletic trainers.   3. Athletes—Rehabilitation.
  4. Sports—Accidents and injuries—Treatment.   I. Title.
     [DNLM: 1. Athletic Injuries—therapy.   QT 260 S8445t 1993]
  RC1210.S785   1993
  617.1′027—dc20
  DNLM/DLC
  for Library of Congress   93-4151
                                                                                                                          CIP

Epigraph on page v reprinted from "King Horse" by Costello © 1979 Plangent Visions Music Limited, with permission.

A statement of resiliency more than despair:
    "I never want to hear that song you dedicated tonight.
    Because, you see, I heard that song so long before we met,
    That it means so much more than it might."

Preface

· ·

This is an introductory text designed to fill the void between the baseline knowledge of undergraduate student athletic trainers and the information presented in existing therapeutic modality texts. Its scope and content are written in a style that will accommodate a wide range of students with varying educational backgrounds. The presentation of these modalities has a strong slant toward their application, but not at the expense of theory and research. Traditional application techniques are supported or refuted based on current literature.

The aim was to write this text to the students in a manner that facilitates their comprehension of the material. The information in this text is presented in a sequential manner. Each chapter begins with the "basics" and progresses to higher levels of information. Terms that may be new to the student are defined on the same page for quick reference and the text also includes a complete glossary. Chapters conclude with a short quiz to measure the student's learning.

The focal point of this text is Chapter 1, which presents the body's physiological and psychological response to trauma. Each subsequent chapter relates how individual modalities affect the injury response process. Chapter 2 discusses the basic physics involved in the transfer of energy.

Specific modalities are categorized by the manner in which they deliver their energy to the body. Chapter 3 presents thermal agents and the diathermies. Chapter 4 covers the principles, effects, and application of electricity. Chapter 5 deals with mechanical agents. Each modality is prefaced by an introductory section that is followed by the specific effects that the energy has on the injury response process. The unit then progresses to the modalities' instrumentation, set-up, and application, and concludes with the indications, contraindications, and precautions of its use.

Chapter 6 introduces clinical decision making through the use of the problem solving approach and is supplemented through the use of case studies. The text concludes with a chapter addressing organizational and administrative concerns in the use of therapeutic modalities.

Chad Starkey

Acknowledgments

· ·

This work would have been impossible without the direct and indirect help and support of a number of individuals. A great deal of thanks and appreciation goes to the reviewers of the original manuscript:

> Thomas Abdenour, ATC
> Sara Brown, ATC
> William Buckley, PhD, ATC
> Charles Rozanski, ATC
> Scott Ward, PT
> Peter Zulia, PT, ATC

Further assistance was provided by Jeff Ryan, PT, ATC who not only wrote Chapter 6, but also diligently reviewed the remaining chapters. Nathaniel E. P. Ehrlich, attorney and certified athletic trainer, provided a great deal of input and revisions for Chapter 7. Professor Makoto Tsuchiya, ATC, and Jodie Humphrey provided many of the photographs used in this text.

I would like to thank the O.P.G. for providing me the facilities that were frequently used during the more cerebral portions of my writing. In an era when the word "trust" carries negative connotations and "faith" is tightly budgeted, I recognize the positive impact that a former certified athletic trainer at West Virginia University, Glen Johnson, MD, made when he placed faith in me and trusted me when I needed it most. Dr. Johnson, your impact has been long-standing. I would also like to thank Joe O'Toole for being my friend and Paul Grace for helping me keep my sanity through this project. Lastly, an extreme amount of appreciation goes to "an animated French editor," Jean-François Vilain, who showed belief in me and in this endeavor (Thanks, Clouzeaux).

Contributor

· ·

Jeff Ryan, PT, ATC
Director of Rehabilitation
Temple University
Department of Orthopedics and Sports Medicine
Adjunct Professor, Temple University
Undergraduate Athletic Training Curriculum
Philadelphia, Pennsylvania

Contents

· ·

The Injury Response Process

· ·

This section is designed to expose the student to the body's physical and psychological reaction to stress and injury. It also introduces the terms and concepts used throughout this text.

Why does a text dealing with therapeutic modalities focus its initial attention on the cell? To understand the purpose and effects of therapeutic modalities, we must first gain a basic knowledge of the body's response to injury. We will see that when therapeutic modalities are applied to living tissue, we are more than simply treating an ankle or a knee. We are applying a *stress* to the cells that will regulate their function.

No modality can accelerate the healing of an injury. The body heals an injury at its own rate. However, by treating an injury with thermal, electrical, or mechanical energy, the athletic trainer is attempting to provide the best environment for healing to take place. Thus we do not speed the healing of an injury but rather, prevent the healing process from being hindered by regulating the environment and the function of the cells. As an illustration of this concept, take a cut finger. If we allow dirt and grime to enter the cut, an *infection* may occur which would delay the healing process by hindering the normal physiological response. If we clean the area, apply an antibiotic, and cover the cut with a dressing, healing occurs relatively unhindered.

Stress: A force which disrupts the normal homeostasis of a system.
Infection: A disease state produced by the invasion of a contaminating organism.

1

Stresses Placed On the Cell

Any type of force placed on the cell may be regarded as a stress. This stress may be received in physical, chemical, or emotional forms. The athlete's daily routine involves many types of stressors: the cardiovascular benefits associated with conditioning, the physical contact associated with sports such as football, the repeated pounding of the feet when running, as well as the emotional elation or anguish related to the outcome of an athletic contest. Regardless of its nature, if stress is applied at a sufficient magnitude, the body will undergo several physiological changes at both the cellular and *systemic* levels.

When a stress is placed on a cell, it will react in one of three ways:

- It will adapt to the stress.
- It will become injured, but recover.
- It will die.

Despite the negative connotation, all stresses do not have negative effects on the body. Indeed, researchers have noted that to be without stress is to be without life.[1] Both positive and negative stressors are commonplace in athletics. Contact sports, by their very nature, deliver *acute*, traumatic forces to the body. Athletes in sports such as baseball, tennis, and track are exposed to repetitive stresses whose trauma accumulates and results in an overuse injury.

The athlete's cardiovascular conditioning program, *acclimatization*, strength training, and the actual practice of the sport are considered to be positive stressors. These activities prepare the athletes for the forces they will be exposed to during their activity.

THE GENERAL ADAPTATION SYNDROME (GAS)

The way in which humans respond to stress has been the topic of many studies since the early 1900s. It was one of these early researchers, Hans Selye, who observed that hospitalized patients, no matter what their underlying *pathology*, shared a common set of symptoms. These symptoms included diffuse aches and pains in the joints, loss of muscular strength, loss of appetite, and an elevated body temperature. These striking similarities led him to conclude that the body's systems had a common mechanism for coping with stress.

This phenomenon was termed the **general adaptation syndrome** (GAS) by Selye, who outlined the following phases of stress response:[1]

- Alarm reaction
- Stage of resistance
- Stage of exhaustion

The **alarm stage,** best exemplified by the "flight or fight response," is the

---

Systemic: Affecting the body as a whole.
Acute: Of short onset. The period after an injury when the local inflammatory response is still active.
Acclimatization: The process of becoming physiologically adapted to an environment.
Pathology: Deviations from the normal that characterize disease or injury.

body's initial reaction to a change in *homeostasis.* The body's systems spring to life, mobilizing their resources to thwart the effects of the stressor by readying its defensive systems. Increased blood supplies are routed to those areas needing the resources by elevating the heart rate, the cardiac stroke volume, and the force of *myocardial* contractions. The blood supply to nonessential areas is decreased by *vasoconstriction* of the superficial and abdominal arteries. *Cortisol* is released into the bloodstream, stimulating many "animalistic" responses. Proteins are broken down into *amino acids* in preparation for long fasting periods in order to provide a potential energy source in the event that injury does occur.

Following the alarm stage there is a plateau in the body's adaptation to the stress, the **resistance stage.** The body continues to adapt to the stressor by using its homeostatic resources to maintain its integrity. This is the longest phase of GAS, lasting many days, months, or years. During this stage of stress response, the individual achieves physiological resistance or, as it is commonly referred to in athletics, "physical fitness."[2]

When the body can no longer withstand the stresses, it reaches the **exhaustion stage.** At this point, one of the body's systems cannot tolerate the stress and therefore fails. This exhaustion may manifest itself in the form of traumatic injuries, overuse injuries or, in the most severe case, cardiac failure. This stage may also be referred to as the point of distress, where the stressors being placed on the body produce a negative effect.

GAS AND ITS RELATIONSHIP TO ATHLETICS

It should now be apparent that an athlete experiences stresses that may be either beneficial or harmful to the body. Harmful stresses may take the form of an acute injury, such as a *sprain, strain,* or fracture. These injuries are characterized by the body's being overwhelmed by too much force in too short a time (macrotrauma). Distresses may also result from repeated, relatively low intensity forces, as exemplified by stress fractures or *chronic* inflammatory conditions (microtrauma). It is these types of harmful stresses that athletic trainers spend the majority of their time preventing, treating, and rehabilitating.

The amount of stress applied to the body must be of sufficient intensity and duration in order for the body to display resistance development. Therefore, if the stimulus is too intense, or of too great a duration, the body reacts negatively to the stress, and injury occurs. In the context of athletics, little (if any) physiological resistance will occur if an athlete trains at an insufficient inten-

---

Homeostasis: State of equilibrium in the body and its systems which provides a stable internal environment.

Myocardial: Pertaining to the middle layer of the heart walls.

Vasoconstriction: Reduction in a blood vessel's diameter. This results in a decrease in blood flow.

Cortisol: A cortisonelike substance produced in the body.

Amino Acids: Building blocks of protein.

Sprain: A stretching or tearing of ligaments.

Strain: A stretching or tearing of tendons or muscles.

Chronic: Continuing for a long period; with injury, extending past the primary hemorrhage and inflammation cycle.

Box 1–1 WOLFF'S LAW
Bones remodel and adapt to the forces placed on them by increasing their strength along the lines of mechanical stress. Based on changes in bones' intrinsic electrical current, the osteoblastic and osteoclastic activity changes in response to the presence or absence of functional stress. Bone will be removed from sites of little or no stress and will be formed along the sites of new stress.
Most commonly, these stresses are caused by compressive forces associated with running, throwing, and so on. However, the removal of these stresses can also result in the bone's remodeling itself. If a limb is immobilized, the daily stresses placed on its bones are removed. As a result, the body adapts to the lack of stress by removing bone.

sity. Conversely, if the intensity of the workout is too great, the body is placed in the stage of exhaustion, and injury will occur.

The body has certain mechanisms to balance the effects of positive and negative stressors. As stated by Wolff's law, bone adapts to the forces placed on it (Box 1–1). This remodeling may be exemplified by the deposition of *collagen* fibers and inorganic salts in response to a prolonged presence of stressors. This adaptation is based on the balance between the activities of *osteoblasts* and *osteoclasts*. For example, the repeated physical stresses associated with running increase the rate of osteoblastic activity along the lines of stress, resulting in new areas of structural strength. If this stress is applied too rapidly, osteoclastic activity outweighs osteoblastic activity and a stress fracture results. In contrast, a femur which is immobilized for 20 days can lose up to 30 percent of its mineral deposits, causing it to become porous and fragile.[2]

The principles presented in the general adaptation syndrome and Wolff's law are also applicable to the utilization of therapeutic modalities. If the magnitude of the modality is too low, little or no benefit is gained. Likewise, if the magnitude of the modality is too great—or applied at the wrong point in the healing process—further injury will occur.

Types of Tissues Found in the Body

The body is comprised of four different types of tissues, each with its own inherent ability to reproduce in response to stress. The reformation of these tissues is dependent on their cellular structures (Table 1–1). When an injury does occur, its scope and severity are generally in direct proportion to the number and type of cells that have been damaged.

Collagen: A protein-based connective tissue.
Osteoblast: A cell concerned with the formation of new bone.
Osteoclast: A cell that absorbs and removes unwanted bone.

Table 1–1 **TYPES OF CELLS FOUND IN THE BODY**

Type	Where Found	Ability to Regenerate
Labile cells	Skin, intestinal tract, blood	Good
Stabile cells	Bone	Some
Permanent cells	Peripheral nervous system, muscle	Some
	Central nervous system	None

EPITHELIAL TISSUES

Epithelial tissues form the outer surface of the body and line the body cavities and intestines. This type of tissue is able to secrete and absorb substances and has the distinction of being devoid of blood vessels. Epithelial tissue has a high potential to regenerate; this is fortunate because it is the type of tissue most commonly injured.

MUSCULAR TISSUES

Muscular tissues possess the ability to actively shorten and passively lengthen and are classified by the function they serve. **Smooth muscle**, which is not under voluntary control, is associated with the hollow organs of the body. **Cardiac muscle** is responsible for the pumping of blood. **Skeletal muscle** is responsible for the movement of the body's joints. Muscular tissues possess little or no ability to regenerate duplicates of lost cells.

Skeletal muscle fiber is classified by the intensity and duration of the contraction it can produce. **Type I** (slow-twitch) fibers produce a low-intensity contraction, but since they use the *aerobic* energy system, the contractions can be sustained for a long period of time. Being slow to fatigue, these fibers are prevalent in postural muscles. **Type II** (fast-twitch) fibers primarily use the *anaerobic* energy system and produce a high-intensity, short-duration contraction. Capable of generating a high amount of force in a short time, these fibers are predominant in explosive muscle contractions. Type II fibers are subcategorized as type II-B, which are totally anaerobic and type II-A, which have traits of both type I and type II fibers.

NERVOUS TISSUES

Nervous tissues have the ability to conduct *afferent* and *efferent* impulses. Individual nerve cells, neurons, form the basic functional unit of the nervous system. Each neuron is formed by two distinct segments: **dendrites** which transmit impulses towards a cell body, and the **axon** that transmits impulses away from the cell body (Fig. 1–1). Cells damaged in the central nervous system are not replaced and their function is lost. Nerve cells damaged in the peripheral

---

Aerobic: Requiring the presence of oxygen.

Anaerobic: Able to survive in the absence of oxygen. Anaerobic systems derive their energy through the breakdown of adenosine triphosphate (ATP) into adenosine diphosphate (ADP).

Afferent: Carrying impulses toward a central structure, for example, the brain.

Efferent: Carrying impulses away from a central structure. Nerves leaving the central nervous system are efferent nerves.

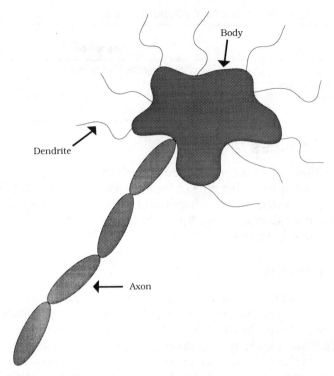

Figure 1-1. Anatomy of a Nerve. Impulses are transmitted to the body via dendrites and away from the body through the axon.

nervous system possess some ability to regenerate. Their functions may also be restored by a collateral system where intact nerves migrate towards the damaged tissues.

CONNECTIVE TISSUE

Connective tissue is the most abundant tissue type in the body, serving as a cement that supports and connects the other tissue types.[3] This tissue provides strength, support, nutrition, and defense for the other tissues. Connective tissue is found in high density in fascia, tendons, ligaments, cartilage, muscle, and bone. With the exception of meniscal cartilage, these tissues are all highly vascular.

The function of the connective tissue is dependent on the ratio of inelastic collagen fibers to elastic yellow elastin fibers. To illustrate the effect of collagen density and elasticity, consider the difference between muscle and tendon. Muscles are highly elastic because of the low proportion of collagen fibers. On the other hand, tendons have very little elasticity because 86 percent of their dry weight is collagen.[4]

The Injury Process

The body's reaction to injury may be divided into two distinct parts. The primary reaction of an injured area is the tissue destruction directly associated with the injurious force. Secondary damage occurs from cell death due to a blockage of the oxygen supply to the injured area. The damage done during the primary stage is irreversible and it is the athletic trainer's task to contain the effects and limit the amount of secondary injury.

Dead and damaged cells release their contents into the area adjacent to the injured site. The presence of these substances causes an inflammatory reaction from the body's tissues. As a result of both the primary trauma and the inflammatory mediators, *hemorrhage* and *edema* occur. This buildup of fluids results in both mechanical pressure on and chemical irritation of the nerve receptors in the area. Because of the clogging of the vasculature, further cell death results from a lack of oxygen in the surviving tissues. A subcycle occurs as a result of pain and *ischemia,* causing muscle spasm and the possibility of atrophy (Fig. 1-2).

This sequence of events, commonly referred to as the injury response cycle, the pain-spasm pain cycle, or the vicious cycle, leads to a self-perpetuating sequence of events. In order for the athlete to return to participation, this cycle must be controlled so that healing may occur.

INFLAMMATION

The natural physiological reaction to any form of injury is **inflammation,** the process that mobilizes the body's defensive systems. Although inflammation is not a pathologic condition, it represents the sum of the body's tissue reactions to cell injury or cell death.[5] This process may be triggered by such factors as chemicals, heat, mechanical trauma, or bacterial invasion. The purpose of inflammation is to control the effects of the injurious agent and return the tissue to its normal state. This process destroys, dilutes, or contains the injurious agents in an attempt to protect the area from further insult. This response occurs at two levels: (1) changes in blood flow (hemodynamic) and (2) changes in cellular functioning. The effects of inflammation are needed in the healing process. However, if the duration or intensity of the inflammation is excessive, the process becomes detrimental.

Inflammation has gained a reputation as being an unwanted, and unneeded, part of injury response. Nothing can be farther from the truth. Inflammation is an essential part of the healing process. It is when inflammation runs amuck that it becomes detrimental to healing. It is through the application of therapeutic modalities that we influence the duration and magnitude of the inflammatory response and deter the unwanted effects.

The inflammatory process may be divided into three distinct phases: (1) acute inflammation associated with the body's initial reaction to injury, (2) the subacute phase where symptoms begin to decrease (2 weeks to 1 month from onset), and (3) chronic inflammation, when the reaction persists for longer than 1 month[6] (Table 1-2).

When the body first receives a stress (in this context, "stress" refers to a

---

Hemorrhage: Bleeding from veins, arteries, or capillaries.
Edema: An excessive accumulation of serous fluids.
Ischemia: Local and temporary deficiency of blood supply due to obstruction of circulation to a part.

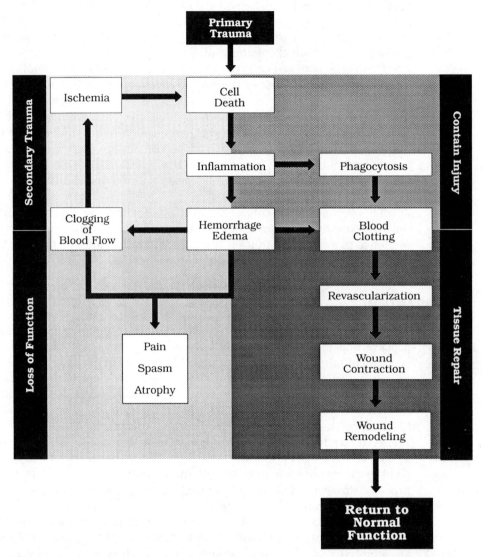

Figure 1–2. The Injury Response Process. In the case of athletic injuries, the primary trauma stems from an outside force and the physical damage inflicted is irreversible. Secondary injury occurs from a deprivation of oxygen to the tissues. This, combined with pain, spasm, and/or atrophy, leads to the tissues or body part losing their ability to function normally. The body begins its road to repair by first containing the injury and then rebuilding the damaged tissue.

Table 1–2 **STAGES OF INFLAMMATION FOLLOWING INJURY**

Stage	Process	Elapsed Time Since Injury (days)
Acute	Reaction to the injury	0–14
Subacute	Symptoms diminish	14–31
Chronic	Unwarranted inflammation	>31

traumatic injury) of sufficient magnitude, the cells undergo a primary reaction. This primary phase, also known as the reactive or inflammatory phase is characteristic of the first three or four days after the injury.

One of the body's initial responses to trauma is the vasoconstriction of local vessels to prevent blood loss in the affected area.[7] While the vessels are in the state of vasoconstriction, the *coagulation* process begins to repair the primary damage. This initial vasoconstriction is transitory and, in as little as 10 minutes after the injury, the vessels begin to dilate, increasing the volume of blood being delivered to the area.

Gaps form between the *endothelial cells* in the capillary beds, increasing their permeability to fluids and proteins. As the volume of blood being delivered to the area increases, a protein-rich *exudate* is formed. The exudate leaks into the tissue through the newly formed gaps in the capillaries, depositing *leukocytes* along the site of the injury to localize and remove any harmful substances.

Swelling occurs as a result of the presence of fluids, proteins, and cell debris in the area. As the swelling increases, vascular flow to and from the area is decreased. Inhibition of venous and *lymphatic return* causes further clogging of blood flow to the area, perpetuating the process.

Prolonged inflammation damages the connective tissue and thickens the synovial membrane. When unchecked, this condition may lead to the development of adhesions within a joint, affecting its functional range of motion. The release of cortisol, as described in the general adaptation syndrome, is effective in reducing the effects of chronic inflammation because of its cortisonelike anti-inflammatory effects.[8]

Cardinal Signs of Inflammation

The inflammation process is marked by five cardinal signs (Table 1–3). Heat and redness **(hyperemia)** are present due to the increased blood flow in the area and the increase in the rate of cell *metabolism*. **Swelling** occurs as a result of the various inflammatory agents in the area and is further promoted by the

Table 1–3 **CARDINAL SIGNS OF INFLAMMATION**

Heat
Redness
Swelling
Pain
Loss of function

Coagulation: The process of blood clotting.
Endothelial Cells: Flat cells lining the blood and lymphatic vessels, and the heart.
Exudate: Fluid that collects in a cavity and has a high concentration of cells, protein, and other solid matter.
Leukocytes: White blood cells that serve as scavengers.
Lymphatic Return: A return process similar to that of the venous network, but specializing in the removal of interstitial fluids.
Metabolism: The sum of physical and chemical reactions taking place within the body.

Table 1–4 **SELECTED INFLAMMATORY MEDIATORS**

Heparin: Inhibits coagulation by preventing the conversion of prothrombin into thrombin.

Histamine: Located in mast cells, basophils, and platelets. Its primary function is vasodilation of *arterioles* and increased vascular permeability in venules.

Kinins: A group of polypeptides that dilate arterioles, serve as strong chemotactics, and produce pain. They are primarily involved in the inflammatory process in the early stages of vascular response.

Prostaglandins: Comprised of many different types and are responsible for vasodilation and increased vascular permeability. These are synthesized locally in the injured tissues and serve to influence the duration and intensity of the inflammatory process.

Serotonin: Causes local vasodilation and increased permeability of the capillaries.

Leukotrienes: Fatty acids which cause smooth muscle contraction, increase vascular permeability, and attract neutrophils.

Necrosin: Increases the permeability of the cell membrane.

---

high concentration of proteins, *gamma globulins,* and *fibrinogen.* **Pain,** the fourth component, is caused by the release of chemical irritants in the inflamed area and increased tissue pressure. The long-term result of inflammation is the **loss of normal function.**

Mediators of Inflammation

The inflammatory process is controlled by chemicals that are released into the area. Collectively known as **mediators,** these chemicals are responsible for a wide range of cellular and vascular events (Table 1–4). Some of these chemicals are released by the damaged cells, while others are attracted to the area by *chemotaxis.* Some mediators cause a *vasodilation* of the vessels, increasing both the amount of blood, plasma proteins, and phagocytic leukocytes and the speed with which they are delivered to the area. Other mediators increase the permeability of the vessels, allowing the movement of blood proteins and blood cells out of the vessels into the surrounding tissues.

The presence of proteins changes the osmotic relationship between the blood and the adjacent tissues. During the inflammatory response, the protein content of the plasma decreases while the protein content of the *interstitial* fluid increases.[9] Water tends to follow the blood proteins out of the vessel via osmosis, resulting in edema. Edema, in turn, increases the tissue pressure, irritating the nerve receptors and blocking capillary flow.

HEMORRHAGE

In order for hemorrhage to take place, one of two prerequisites must be met: (1) the vessel must lose its continuity (be ruptured) or have a marked increase in permeability so that cells and fluids can escape, or (2) a gradient must be

---

Arteriole: A small artery leading to a capillary at its distal end.

Gamma Globulin: An infection-fighting blood protein.

Fibrinogen: A protein present in the blood plasma and essential for the clotting of blood.

Chemotaxis: Movement of living protoplasm toward or away from a chemical stimulus.

Vasodilation: Increase in a blood vessel's diameter. This results in an increase in blood flow.

Interstitial: Between the tissues.

present in which the pressure inside the vessel is greater than the external pressure.[10] For hemorrhage to cease, the reverse of the two conditions must be met: The vessel must be repaired and/or the pressure gradient must be equalized.

Subcutaneous hemorrhage is easily recognized by the *ecchymosis* of the skin associated with bruising. When the hemorrhage occurs deeper in the tissues, a *hematoma* may result. In the short term, hematomas serve to equalize the pressure gradient between the inside and the outside of the injured vessel. However, the long-term presence of a hematoma in a muscle may result in a restriction in range of motion. Although hematomas are effective in reducing the amount of blood loss from a damaged vessel, a prolonged hematoma will prove detrimental to the repair process by further stimulating the inflammatory response.

It should be noted that even in the best possible scenario, the immediate treatment provided by the athletic trainer does not affect primary hemorrhaging. By the time the injured athlete is removed from competition, the shoe, sock, and pads are removed, the initial evaluation is performed, and ice is applied, several minutes have passed. In most instances, this time is sufficient for the coagulation process to seal the injured vasculature.[7] Application of cold treatments in this time frame help to limit the amount of secondary hypoxic injury and decrease pain.

EDEMA

Edema is the buildup of excessive fluid in the *intracellular* space as a result of the imbalance between the pressures inside and outside the cell membrane, or of an obstruction to lymphatic and venous return. This collection of fluids causes the tissues to expand. The amount of edema that accumulates in the injured area is proportional to: (1) the severity of the injury (the number and type of cells damaged), (2) changes in vascular permeability, (3) the amount of primary and secondary hemorrhaging, and (4) the presence of chemical inflammatory mediators. Although interrelated, these factors function independently to cause the release of proteins which attract fluids to the injured area.[9]

The movement of fluids across the capillary membrane is contingent on three basic forces:[11] the **capillary filtration pressure** that forces the contents from the capillary outward to the tissues; the **tissue hydrostatic pressure** that moves fluids from the tissues into the capillaries; and the **hydrostatic pressure,** which is the blood pressure within the capillary. The hydrostatic pressure is independently altered by changes in the position of the limb.

The formation and removal of edema is based on the relationship between these pressures. Capillary permeability increases following injury, making it easier for fluids and solid matter to leave the vessels (Fig. 1–3). If the capillary filtration pressure exceeds the tissue hydrostatic pressure, fluids are forced out of the capillaries into the tissues, and edema results. Likewise, if the tissue

---

Subcutaneous: Beneath the skin.
Ecchymosis: A blue-black discoloration of the skin caused by movement of blood into the tissues. In the latter stages, the color may appear as a greenish-brown or yellow.
Hematoma: A mass of blood confined to a limited area, resulting from the subcutaneous leakage of blood.
Intracellular: Within the membrane of a cell.

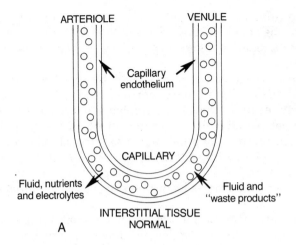

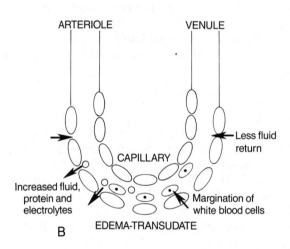

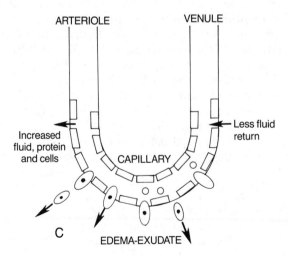

Figure 1–3. The Formation of Edema. (A) The normal pressures inside and outside of the vessel causes an outward flow of fluids and nutrients at the arteriole end and an absorption of wastes at the venule end. (B) The Transudate Stage. Following an injury, inflammatory mediators cause the arterioles to dilate. The increased capillary filtration pressure moves proteins and fluids into the tissues. (C) The Exudate Stage. Increased inflammation forces neutrophils and other blood cells out to the tissues, resulting in a thick, edematous fluid formation. (From Michlovitz,[3] p 7, with permission).

hydrostatic pressure exceeds the capillary filtration pressure, fluids are forced back into the vessels and may then be removed from the area.

The expansion of tissues causes further hypoxic injury by clogging the vascular pathways. This prevents not only the delivery of fresh blood and oxygen to the injured structures, but also inhibits venous and lymphatic return from the site. In addition, the pressure caused by the fluid buildup will produce mechanical pain by stimulating mechanical nerve receptors in the area, and chemical pain by depriving the tissues of oxygen. Lymphatic flow is disrupted by edema when the tissues become so expanded that the flap valves between the endothelial cells in the capillaries become separated. This parting of the valves renders them ineffective, thus allowing the fluids to "slosh" back into the injured area.

Edema is not only a sign that an injury has occurred, but it is also a contributing factor in the injury cycle. The edema clogs the vascular and cellular spaces, preventing oxygen from reaching the tissues and causing further cell death. The healing process itself is slowed by delayed cellular regeneration and improper collagen formation.[12] Collagen deposition is increased in the edematous area and, when uncontrolled, leads to *fibrosis* and joint contractures. These factors lead to a decrease in joint range of motion, loss of normal function, and eventually, atrophy in the afflicted body part.

One of the athletic trainer's goals during the treatment and rehabilitation phase is to reduce the amount of edema that is formed and remove it from the injury site. Removal of edema can occur through increased venous return, increased lymphatic flow, or increased blood circulation. The only mechanism for removing protein from the interstitial space is through the lymphatic system.[13]

Venous and/or Lymphatic Return

Swelling and edema are only reduced by transporting the fluid and solid wastes away from the area through the venous and lymphatic system. Since the mechanisms of these systems are similar, the function of the venous return system will be used to describe the process.

In contrast to its influence on arterial blood flow, blood pressure has little effect on the flow within the venous return system. The pumping action of the heart exerts a pressure of approximately 15 mm Hg on the venous system.[10] Once the blood passes through the capillaries, the body must rely on other mechanisms to return blood to the heart. During **skeletal muscle contraction,** the veins are compressed, reducing their diameter. Because of the function of one-way valves, the blood is forced to move out of the extremity towards the heart. As the force of the contraction is reduced, the one-way valves close, preventing the blood from moving back to its original position (Fig. 1–4). Although voluntary muscle contractions provide the most efficient method of increasing venous return, electrically induced contractions, passive motion, and massage can also increase venous flow.

The **respiratory process** serves to enhance venous return during both inspiration and expiration. When we take a breath of air, the diaphragm descends

---

Fibrosis: An abnormally large formation of inelastic fibrous tissue.

(A)   (B)   (C)

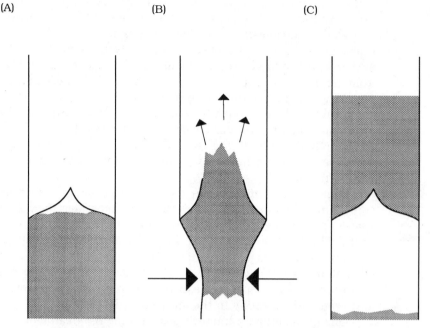

Figure 1–4. Function of One-Way Valves in Veins. (A) The position of fluids within the vein when the muscle is relaxed. (B) As the muscle contracts, pressure causes the distal portion of the vein to collapse, opening the one-way valves and forcing blood towards the heart. (C) As the muscle relaxes, the valves close preventing blood from moving back into the area.

and places pressure on the abdominal organs. This pressure is then placed on the veins, partially compressing them and forcing the blood towards the heart. During expiration, a negative pressure gradient is created between the thorax and the abdomen, causing a siphonlike effect which pulls the blood up the venous system.

Lastly, **gravity** serves to return the blood to the heart. The fluids within the venous return system are affected by gravity. Placing the extremity in a *dependent position* increases the hydrostatic pressure within the peripheral blood vessels and forces fluids into the tissues. When an extremity is placed in a nondependent position (elevated), the venous return system becomes a passive process in which there is a natural downward flow of the fluids in the vessels. The effectiveness of gravity in returning blood to the heart is based on the angle of the extremity relative to the ground, the diameter of the veins, and the *viscosity* of the blood.

The maximal effect of gravity on venous return occurs when the limb is perpendicular (90 degrees) to the earth and least effective when the limb is horizontal (Fig. 1–5). The effect that the limb's position has on gravity influencing venous return can be calculated using trigonometric sine function: The sine of 90 degrees is 1 (100% effective), the sine of 45 degrees is 0.71 (71% effective), and the sine of 0 degrees is 0 (0% effective).

The resistance to blood flow is inversely proportional to the diameter of

---

Dependent Position: An arrangement where the body part is placed lower than the heart, increasing the intravascular pressure.
Viscosity: The resistance of a fluid to flow.

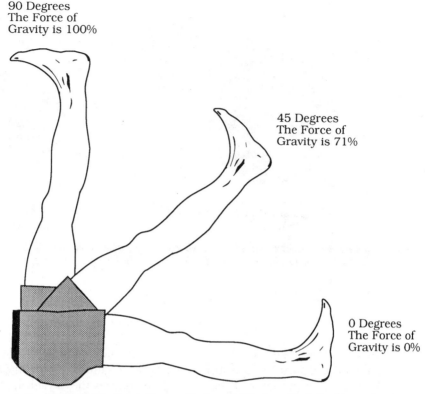

90 Degrees
The Force of
Gravity is 100%

45 Degrees
The Force of
Gravity is 71%

0 Degrees
The Force of
Gravity is 0%

Figure 1–5. Effect of Gravity on Venous Drainage at Various Limb Positions. Gravity is most effective when the limb is at 90° and least effective when the limb is parallel to the ground. A compromise between comfort and function is found when the limb is elevated at a 45° angle.

the vessel. As the cross-sectional size of the vessel decreases, the resistance to flow increases as the fourth power of the radius (radius × radius × radius × radius)[10] (Fig. 1–6). Consequently, small changes in the vessel's diameter result in great changes in its resistance to flow. *Venules* have a smaller diameter than veins; therefore greater resistance to flow will occur closer to the capillary-venule interface. The rate of blood flow to the tissues cannot exceed the rate of exchange at this interface.

Viscosity is a fluid's resistance to flow. Normally the viscosity of blood remains constant. However, following injury, the viscosity of blood increases due to the loss of plasma into the surrounding tissues, the ratio of liquids to solids decreases. Although this change in viscosity is not large enough to affect the systemic flow of blood, it may be sufficient to clog the area adjacent to the injury.

HYPOXIA

In the primary stage of injury, cell death is a result of physical trauma. Following this, further cell death is a result of ischemia, a decreased oxygen supply to the area. Once an injury occurs, several vascular changes take place that block

---

Venule: A small vein exiting from a capillary.

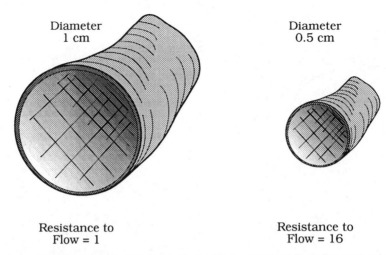

Diameter
1 cm

Diameter
0.5 cm

Resistance to
Flow = 1

Resistance to
Flow = 16

Figure 1–6. Vessel's Diameter Relative to its Resistance to Blood Flow. Decreasing the diameter of a vessel by one-half will increase the resistance to blood flow 16 times.

the supply of fresh blood and result in ischemia. As a result of swelling in the interstitial space (via the primary reaction), capillaries in the adjacent areas rupture. This perpetuates the cycle by obstructing the oxygen supply and killing additional cells. This cell death continues to block more vascular structures, blocking even more blood and oxygen from being delivered to the site.

This phenomenon, known as **secondary hypoxic injury,** may be limited by decreasing the amount of blockage and decreasing the need for oxygen in the area. The blockage of the vasculature may be reduced by limiting the amount of fluids that collect in the area via the use of compression and elevation. The need for oxygen may be reduced by decreasing the rate of cellular metabolism through the use of cold application (see Chapter 3: Effects of Immediate Treatment, p. 60).

MUSCLE SPASM

Muscle spasm, the involuntary shortening of muscle fibers, is regarded as the body's intrinsic mechanism for splinting and protecting the injured area.[14] Spasm may result from direct trauma or a decreased oxygen supply.

Muscle spasm causes pain by stimulating mechanical and chemical pain receptors. The tension produced by the shortened fibers stimulates mechanical pain fibers. Chemical pain fibers are irritated by the effects of a decreased oxygen supply. If the muscle spasm persists, irritation of the associated ligaments and tendons occurs.[15] As a result, the amount of muscle spasm increases in an attempt to protect the structures. This becomes a self-perpetuating cycle that is continued by pain, decreased oxygen supply, and a decreased amount of positive stress (in the form of movement).

ATROPHY

When a muscle is immobilized or has lost its nerve supply, its fibers become progressively smaller and its *actin* and *myosin* contents are decreased. Disuse atrophy results when a body part is immobilized either by an external splint or when the individual consciously or unconsciously refuses to use the extremity because of pain. *Denervation* atrophy occurs when there is no intact nerve supply to the muscle group. In either case, the resultant changes are similar.

Muscle fibers begin to show physiological changes as little as 24 hours after they are immobilized. The size and functioning of the cells decrease in response to a lack of physical stress. Accordingly, the synthesis of protein, energy production, and contractility of the tissues begin to dwindle to the point of **degeneration,** where the muscle's ability to generate force decreases.[16] Slow-twitch (type I) fibers are the first to show clinical and laboratory signs of atrophy.[17]

The injury response process accelerates the rate of atrophy. Edema and inflammation stimulate *Golgi tendon organs*, increasing the rate at which atrophy occurs (Box 1–2). As a muscle atrophies, the blood supply to the remaining fibers decreases and the innervation of the muscle is hindered.[18] The continuing process of atrophy leads to reflex inhibition, where the effusion and painful impulses create an inhibitory loop that essentially causes the athlete to "forget" how to contract the muscle.

Rest is a double-edged sword in the treatment and rehabilitation of athletic injuries. Immobilization is necessary to protect the injured structures, but the lack of physical stress can inhibit proper remodeling of the tissues.[19] The atro-

---

| Box (1–2) | **MISGUIDED INTENTIONS** |

Golgi tendon organs (GTO) function closely with **muscle spindles** in monitoring the amount of tension placed on a muscle and its tendon. Located within the muscle belly, projections from the spindle twine around individual muscle fibers. When the muscle contracts, the spindles monitor the rate and magnitude of tension produced.

Golgi tendon organs divide into many branches with the highest density being located at the muscle–tendon junction. When the muscle contracts, it places varying amounts of force on the tendon. The GTOs monitor the amount of strain placed on the tendon in order to prevent damage resulting from too much tension. If the rate of stimulation of GTOs or muscle spindles becomes too great, a nerve impulse is generated that inhibits the muscle contraction.

During the process of injury response these nerves can be mechanically stimulated by pressure resulting from muscle spasm and/or edema, or they can be chemically stimulated by inflammatory mediators. **Regardless of the nature of the stimulation an inhibitory influence is placed on the muscle. If this process is allowed to perpetuate, atrophy of the muscle group occurs.**

Actin: A contractile muscle protein.
Myosin: Noncontractile muscle protein.
Denervation: Lack of proper nerve supply to, for example, an area or muscle group.
Golgi Tendon Organ: A sensory nerve ending found in tendons and aponeuroses.

phy process may be deterred by several methods. Muscles which are immobilized in a lengthened position are more resistant to atrophy than those immobilized in a shortened position.[20] However, depending on the body part, the structures involved, and the type of injury, it is not always practical to immobilize the muscle in a lengthened position. Isometric exercise and/or electrical muscle stimulation have also been shown to be effective in delaying the atrophy process (see Chapter 4: Electrical Modalities, p. 130).

The Healing Process

The body's return to normal function begins with the inflammatory process. This encourages the removal of debris and toxic substances from the injured area and protects the tissues from further damage. *Phagocytosis*, the body's cellular defense system, involves ingestion of toxic organisms and other foreign particles, and their removal via the lymphatic system. These wastes, known as exudate, are commonly visible in the form of pus. During this process, scavenger cells and leukocytes devour toxic and dead tissues by trapping them with armlike appendages and engulfing them (Fig. 1–7). This entrapment occurs by

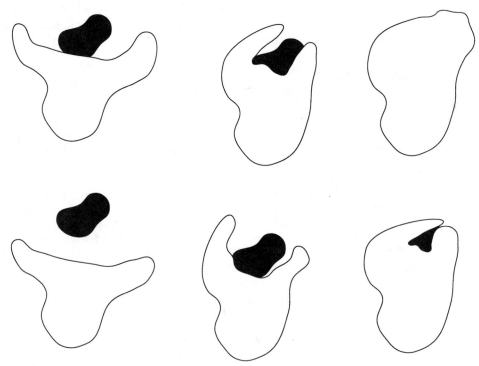

Figure 1–7. The Process of Phagocytosis. Scavenger cells randomly collide with vascular debris. Using arm-like appendages, the phagocytes surround, devour, and subsequently remove the waste.

Phagocytosis: The ingestion and digestion of bacteria and particles by phagocytes.

random chance, and the utilization of pain-free range of motion exercises may increase the level of phagocytic activity.

BLOOD CLOTTING

The repair of the vascular bodies in the injured area consists of the formation of a *platelet* plug and the transformation of *fibrinogen* into *fibrin*. This is a complex process and is only presented in this text in its basic form.

When disruption occurs in a vessel, an initial seal is formed by platelets. **Margination** occurs where the platelets and leukocytes flowing in the bloodstream begin to tumble along the walls of the vessel. Eventually, these substances adhere to collagen exposed by the trauma, through the process of **pavementing.** As platelets are unable to adhere to themselves, they must release adenosine diphosphate (ADP) that serves to "glue" one layer of platelets to the other.[6] This series of platelet depositions forms an unsteady and leaky patch over the injured site. Further events must occur to form a permanent repair.

The ruptured vessel releases an enzyme that serves as a distress signal to the body that an injury has occurred. A subsequent set of reactions, combined with the platelet deposition, results in a permanent seal being formed. *Prothrombin*, a free-floating element found in the bloodstream, reacts with the enzyme factor X, converting prothrombin into *thrombin*. The presence of thrombin in the area then stimulates fibrinogen to unwind into its individual fibrin elements (Fig. 1–8).

Single, activated fibrin filaments, fibrin monomer, are split from fibrinogen and group together to form long threads around the injured area. During this process, red and white blood cells, along with platelets, are trapped by the fibrin threads. As these threads contract, they remove the plasma and compact the platelets, forming a "patch" to repair the damaged vessel.

Inflammation serves as both an aid and a deterrent to the coagulation process. In general, the inflammatory process encourages the delivery of prothrombin to the injured area by increasing blood flow. However, one of the chemical mediators, *heparin*, hinders the coagulation process by preventing prothrombin from being converted to thrombin. A proper balance must be maintained between heparin and the other mediators. Too much heparin could completely block the coagulation of blood; too little heparin could result in unwanted blood clots.

Platelet: A free-flowing cell fragment in the bloodstream.
Fibrin: A filamentous protein formed by the action of thrombin on fibrinogen.
Prothrombin: A chemical found in the blood which reacts with an enzyme to produce thrombin.
Thrombin: An enzyme formed in the blood of a damaged area.
Heparin: An inflammatory mediator produced by the mast cells of the liver. It inhibits the clotting process by preventing the transformation of prothrombin into thrombin.

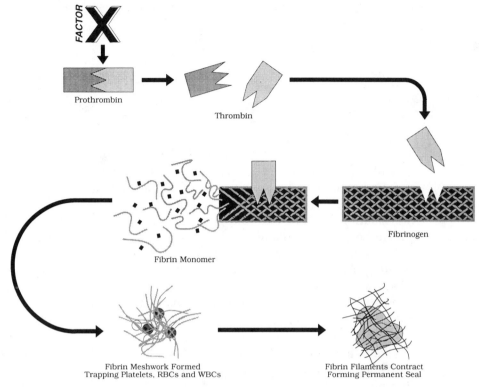

Figure 1–8. The Process of Blood Clotting. Activated by the presence of Factor X, Prothrombin is broken down into Thrombin. In turn, the presence of Thrombin causes Fibrinogen to unwind into individual Fibrin elements. The Fibrin Monomer deposits itself over the site in the damaged vessel, trapping platelets, red blood cells, and white blood cells. Following contraction of the Fibrin filaments, a permanent seal is formed.

REPAIR PHASE

Repair of an injured structure involves the interaction between two types of cells: (a) the cells belonging to the injured structure and (b) connective tissue. Inflammation is needed for tissue repair. However, too much inflammation is detrimental to the process. It is by the application of therapeutic modalities, the use of immobilization devices, exercise, anti-inflammatory medication, and so on, that athletic trainers, physical therapists, and physicians attempt to control the inflammatory process. In acute situations, inflammation may be considered to be an active process where the rate is controlled by the body's metabolism. In chronic situations, inflammation is a passive process in which the body forms new, and possibly unwanted, connective tissues.

The quality of the repair process is related to the number and type of cells that have been damaged. Labile cells (see Table 1–1), such as those found in the skin, have the greatest ability to produce a "clone" of the original tissues. In the case of skeletal muscles, the process involves the deposition of fibrous scar tissue which does not replicate the original structure.

Regeneration of tissues occurs when the new cells are of the same type as the original structure and are capable of performing the same function as the original. **Replacement** of tissues results when the damaged cells are replaced by a different type of cell. When uncontrolled, this process leads to scar tissue and an eventual decrease or loss of function.

Soft-tissue repair occurs through the proliferation of *granulation tissue* and it requires three separate but related processes:[4] Fibroblast formation, synthesis of collagen, and tissue remodeling and alignment.

Revascularization

The process of repair begins at the periphery, where *macrophages* and *polymorphs*, both of which can withstand the low-oxygen environment, produce new capillary beds and form granulation tissue. This process gradually works its way toward the center of the injured area, forming a scaffold around which new tissue will be formed.

Fibroblasts are attracted to the area indirectly by the presence of macrophages. Once in the area, fibroblasts begin laying down collagen to form a seal over the injured structure. This deposition of collagen is random, with little order in the fibrous arrangement. Stresses, in the form of gentle joint movements, may cause these fibers to arrange themselves rapidly in a more orderly fashion.[21]

Wound Contraction

Wound contraction occurs following the revascularization of the injured area. Myofibroblasts accumulate at the margins of the wound and begin to move towards the center. Possessing a high actin content, each new myofibroblast shortens to pull the ends of the damaged tissues closer together (Fig. 1–9).

As the scar tissue matures, its continuity begins to resemble that of the tissue it is replacing. With time, the strength of the scar is increased by the replacement of the old collagen with a newer, stronger type. Wound contraction should not be confused with a *contracture*, which results in the limitation of a joint's range of motion and strength. With proper remodeling of the collagen, contractures may be avoided.

Wound Remodeling

The purpose of the remodeling stage is to develop order in the previously deposited scar tissue. The presence of external stress causes the alignment of the fibers to remodel the wound. Use of early range of motion exercises has been shown to increase the tensile strength of healing ligaments.[22] Initially, the collagen is laid down in a random matrix, causing the scar to be fragile. During remodeling, the fibers form a more organized matrix, thus increasing their strength. However, scar tissue is never as functional as the tissue it replaces.[3]

Since scar tissue is inelastic, it is more similar in structure and function to ligaments and tendons than it is to muscle. Repair of muscular tissue may be enhanced through a mechanism similar to that which occurs when muscle

---

Granulation Tissue: Delicate tissue composed of fibroblasts, collagen, and capillaries formed during the revascularization phase of wound healing.

Macrophage: A cell having the ability to devour particles; a phagocyte.

Polymorph: A type of white blood cell; a granulocyte.

Contracture: A condition resulting from the loss of a tissue's ability to lengthen.

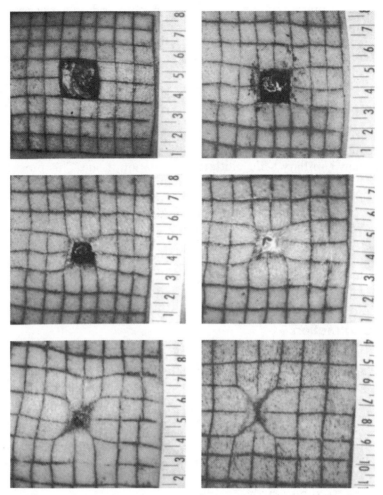

Figure 1–9. Schematic of Wound Contraction. The outer margin of the wound moves toward the center drawing the ends together. (From Fitzpatrick: Dermatology in General Medicine. McGraw-Hill, New York, NY, 1987, p. 330, with permission.)

hypertrophies in response to strength training. Muscle fiber contains **satellite cells** that remain dormant in certain muscle fibers. These cells lack the cytoplasm and proteins found in other muscle cells. Following an injury, repair of muscular tissue can occur by recruiting satellite cells as the source of nuclei for new muscle cells.[23]

Chronic Inflammation

Inflammation which persists for longer than 1 month is termed chronic. In this case, the inflammatory response is marked only by loss of function. The remain-

---

Hypertrophy: To develop an increase in bulk, for example in the cross-sectional area of muscle.

ing cardinal signs need not be present. During this phase of the inflammatory process, the body is still reacting to the presence of foreign material and/or infection.

Fibroblastic activity continues to the point where large quantities of collagen envelop the affected area forming a *granuloma*. This granuloma affects the function of the involved part, leading to a loss of full function and development of secondary reactions in associated structures. This may be demonstrated by a baseball pitcher with chronic rotator cuff inflammation: The presence of a granuloma in the supraspinatus may decrease the range of motion and strength of the joint. By continuing to pitch, the athlete is further irritating the tendon.

Pain

Of all the components of injury response, none is more inconsistent than an individual's response to pain. Pain is a diffuse entity that is very much ingrained throughout the nervous system. Sensory and motor nerves, the spinal cord, the brain stem, and the brain form a complex network of afferent and efferent pathways for transmitting, perceiving, and reacting to pain. Each element in this network has an influence on an individual's reaction to pain.

Pain serves as one of the body's defense mechanisms by providing a warning that tissues may be in jeopardy; yet it may be experienced without any physical damage to tissues.[24] The pain response is classified by sensory, behavioral, and emotional responses. When the tissues are insulted, pain impulses are sent as an alarm and warn the brain that the body's integrity is at risk. The sensory component is the brain's interpretation of these signals as pain. The emotional response may be expressed by screaming, crying, fainting, or just thinking, "%@!#, that hurts!"

When the pain is intense or unexpected, the brain immediately activates the behavioral response by sending instructions to motor nerves to remove the body part from the stimulus. An example of this would be accidentally sticking your finger with a pin. In this case, the pin activates certain nerve fibers to send signals through a peripheral nerve network that gets routed up the spinal cord. When the afferent impulses reach the brain stem a reflex loop is formed. One portion of the loop is sent back down the spinal cord to activate the muscles necessary to remove your finger from the stimulus. The other portion of the reflex continues on to the brain where the impulses are translated as pain, and you respond by saying, "Ouch!"

In the event that an individual has prior knowledge of a painful stimulus, such as receiving an injection, cognitive mechanisms can inhibit the reflex loop. As the painful stimulus increases, so does the conscious effort required to keep from trying to escape from the stimulus. The emotional component may still be in place as you grimace, make a fist, or think, "What's this jerk doing to me!"

The activation of pain fibers is caused by *noxious* input or *nociceptive*

Granuloma: A hard mass of fibrous tissue.
Noxious: Harmful, injurious.

stimulus. Pain fibers are activated by chemical irritation or mechanical deformation of nerve endings. In athletics, pain is initiated by the initial mechanical force of the injury (whether sudden or gradual in onset), and is continued by chemical irritation resulting from the inflammatory process. In subacute and chronic conditions, pain may be continued by reflex muscle spasm in a positive feedback loop[25] or through the continued presence of chemical irritation. The pain response is initiated by stimulation of **nociceptors,** the specialized nerve endings thought to respond to painful stimuli. **Mechanosensitive** pain receptors are excited by mechanical stress or damage to the tissues. **Chemosensitive** receptors are excited by various chemical substances, such as bradykinin, serotonin, *histamine*, and prostaglandins, all of which are released during the inflammatory response. Chemical irritation of nerve endings may produce a severe pain response without true tissue destruction.[5] Unlike other types of nerve receptors, nociceptors display sensitization to repeated or prolonged stimulation. During the inflammatory process, the threshold is lowered and the continued stimulation of the chemosensitive receptors perpetuates the cycle.[26]

THEORIES OF PAIN TRANSMISSION AND PERCEPTION

Physiological as well as psychological mechanisms have been proposed to account for pain's many parameters and for the factors which influence pain perception. As research continues it becomes apparent that pain transmission and interpretation cannot be described by a single model, but are products of many devices. An abbreviated history of pain transmission theories follows; it concludes with a summary of current thought regarding this process.

Specificity Theory

The first attempt to explain the transmission of pain proposed the existence of specialized receptors responding only to specific stimuli. It was postulated that the skin held four distinct types of receptors that responded to heat, cold, touch, and pain. These receptors were "wired" directly to the brain via a continuous nerve. Perception of the stimulus was therefore based on the type of receptor being activated (Fig. 1–10). Although this method of pain transmission is the easiest to conceptualize, the specificity theory fails to account for all of the components involved in the transmission and perception of pain.

Pattern Theory

In the pattern theory, there are no specialized receptors in the skin. Rather, a single nerve responds differently to each type of sensation by creating a uniquely coded impulse. The code is formed by a **spatiotemporal pattern** involving the

---

Nociceptive Stimulus: Impulse giving rise to the sensation of pain.
Histamine: A blood-thinning chemical released from damaged tissue during the inflammatory process.

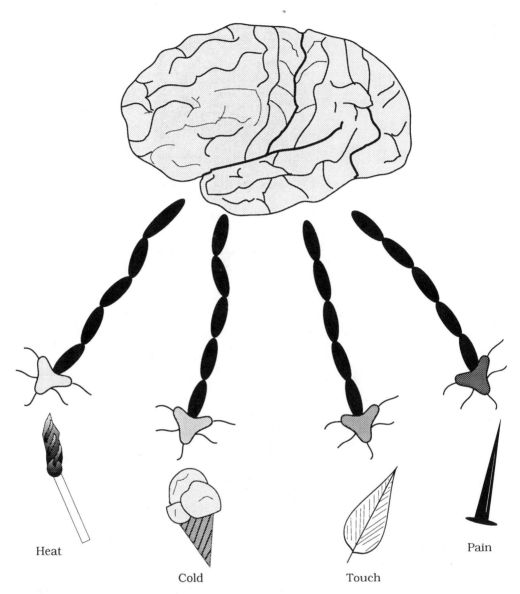

Figure 1–10. The Specificity Theory of Pain Transmission. This theory proposed that the body contained four separate types of sensory nerve endings. Depending on their type, each would only respond to heat, cold, touch, or pain.

frequency and pattern of nerve transmission. An analysis of the word's elements, "spatio" and "temporal," further defines this theory. The distance between the nerve's impulses (space) comprises the spatial coding, while the frequency of the transmission accounts for the temporal component (Fig. 1–11). An example of this type of coding can be found with most institutional phone systems: A call from inside the university has a different ring than an outside call.

While the pattern theory was closer to being neurologically correct than the specificity theory, it still had shortcomings, since examination of nerves has since indicated variation in the anatomy of free nerve endings. Additionally,

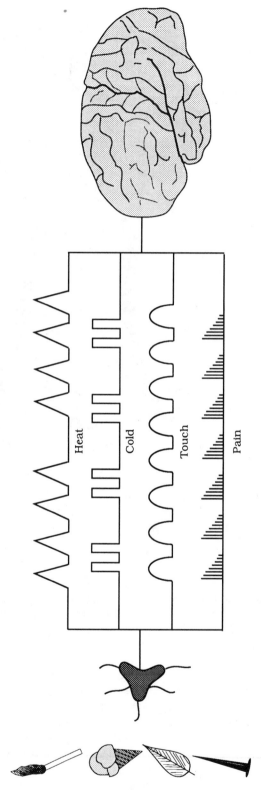

Figure 1–11. The Pattern Theory of Pain Transmission. This theory proposed that the body contained only one type of sensory nerve ending. Depending on the nature of the stimulus, the impulse would be coded using different tempos and rhythms.

this theory still failed to account for the role of the brain in the perception of pain.

Gate Control Theory

As described by Newton,[27] "The gate control theory incorporated the features of receptor specialization from the specificity theory and the spatiotemporal coding of *action potentials* from the pattern theory." This theory, proposed by Melzack and Wall in 1965, simply implies that **nonpainful stimulus can block the transmission of noxious stimulus.** If you have ever bumped your head and then rubbed the painful area, you were activating the gate control mechanism. In this example, banging your head activated the nociceptors, causing pain impulses to be sent to your brain. Rubbing the area activated sensory nerves that caused the pain sensation to be reduced.

This theory centers around a *modulation* system located in the substantia gelatinosa (SG) in the gray matter of the spinal cord. Here, two different sets of nerves, those carrying pain information and those carrying nonpain impulses, are monitored by the SG which allows the information from only one set of nerves to proceed up to the brain. Unlike the specificity and pattern theories, the gate control mechanism allows for the brain's function in altering the transmission of, perception of, and response to pain (Fig. 1–12).

The diameter and insulation of a nerve affects the speed and efficiency of the impulses it carries. As the cross-sectional size of the fiber increases, its resistance to conduction decreases. Large-diameter nerves transmit impulses faster than small-diameter nerves. Insulation is necessary to direct and concentrate the impulses. On nerves, *myelin* serves as an insulator. *Myelinated* nerves transmit impulses more rapidly than unmyelinated nerves.

Large-diameter nerves carry nonpain impulses such as touch (sensation), temperature, and proprioceptive information. These impulses travel through myelinated A-beta and A-gamma nerve fibers. Smaller diameter, unmyelinated, C-fibers and A-delta fibers transmit painful impulses. Because of the larger diameter and myelinated covering of the nerves involved, nonpainful impulses are transmitted at a faster rate than pain impulses, which are carried by the smaller, unmyelinated fibers.

These various afferent nerves enter the SG in the dorsal horn of the spinal cord. Here, the interaction between the SG and the *T cell* allows only one type of nerve impulse to be passed along for processing by the brain. The SG serves in a capacity similar to a "switch operator" in a railroad yard. Our switch operator, the SG, monitors the amount of activity occurring on both tracts and opens and closes the gate to allow the appropriate information to be passed along to the T cell. Impulses traveling on the fast, nonpain fibers increase activity in the SG. Impulses on the slower pain fibers exert an inhibitory influ-

---

Action Potential: The change in the electrical potential of a nerve or muscle fiber when stimulated.

Modulation: Regulation or adjustment.

Myelin: A fatty layering around nerves.

Myelinated: Having a fatlike outer coating (myelin). This coating serves as insulation for nerves.

T Cell: A transmission cell that connects sensory nerves to the central nervous system. Not to be confused with T cells found in the immune system.

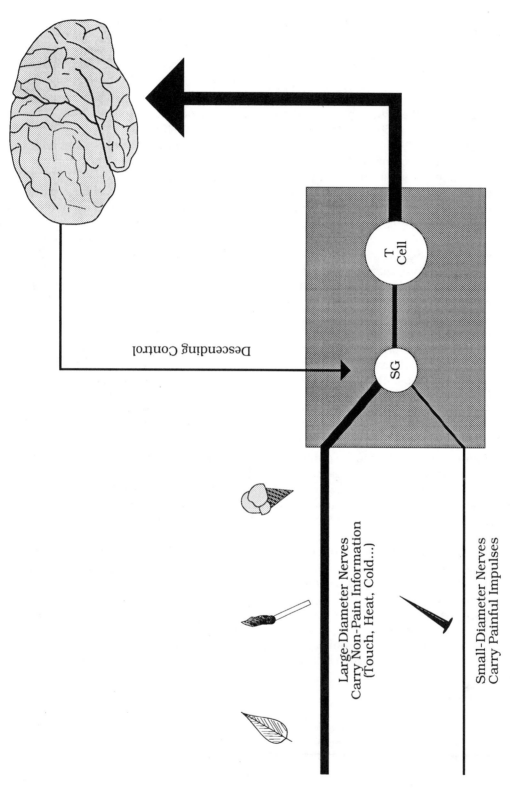

Figure 1–12. The Gate Control Theory of Pain Transmission. The substantia gelatinosa (SG) accepts input from both large (nonpain) and small (pain) diameter nerves. Based on the rate of input, the SG allows either the pain or nonpain stimulus to be passed on to the transmission cell (T Cell) and up to the brain. Since nonpain impulses travel faster than pain impulses, stimulation of nonpain fibers can override the transmission of pain. The brain allows for a descending influence on the perception of, and the reaction to, painful stimulus. This is achieved by the brain placing an inhibitory influence on both the SG and spinal cord.

ence. When the SG is active, the gate is in its "closed" position and a nonpainful stimulus is allowed to pass on to the T cell.

This passage to the T cell is part of a *convergent* system that accepts only one input. If the pain fibers are the most active, only pain impulses are allowed to pass. Likewise, if sensory fibers are the most active, the information from the pain fibers does not pass to the T cell. T cells are capable of presynaptic inhibition, preventing transfer of the chemotransmitter *substance P* by the release of enkephalin. The advantage of this method of pain reduction is that both a chemical and mechanical block are formed.

If we look back to the example of bumping your head, rubbing the abused area does not completely remove all the pain. This is because the transmission of pain involves hundreds and thousands of gates. For complete pain removal, each of the gates must be activated. If they are not all activated a decrease, rather than a complete inhibition, of pain results.

The last component of the gate theory lies in the brain's descending influences on the transmission and perception of pain. Factors influencing the transmission of pain are covered in the sections on endogenous opiates and the central biasing mechanism. Cognitive factors that affect pain perception, such as mental state, sociological factors, and past experiences, are presented in the section on influences on pain perception.

Endogenous Opiates

The body produces its own chemical pain killers in the form of beta-*endorphin* (β-endorphin) and methionine *enkephalin*. These *endogenous opiates* have an effect similar to morpine but are reported to be 10,000 times more potent.[16] Pain transmission is inhibited by blocking receptor sites found along the transmission pathway. The presence of the chemicals in these receptors prevents the noxious neurotransmitters from occupying the site.

Endorphins are naturally occurring substances which are produced in various sites in the brain and function to reduce pain perception centrally.[28] Endorphins are released into the cerebrospinal fluid in response to severe stress, physical exertion, or electrical stimulation, and their effects may last up to 4 hours.[27] Enkephalins are produced in the brain stem and pituitary gland and primarily serve to inhibit the pain-transmitting chemical substance P in the dorsal horn of the spinal cord.[18,29]

Convergent: Tending toward a common point, as when two input routes are reduced to one output route.

Substance P: A neurotransmitter thought to be responsible for the transmission of pain-producing impulses.

Endorphin: A morphinelike substance produced by the body. Endorphins are thought to increase the pain threshold by binding to receptor sites.

Enkephalin: A substance released by the body which reduces the perception of pain by bonding to pain receptor sites.

Endogenous Opiates: Pain-inhibiting substances produced in the brain. These include endorphins and enkephalins.

Central Biasing Mechanism

If all healthy individuals have the same neural mechanisms for the transmission of painful impulses, why do people deal with pain differently? If your classmates were to write a single word to describe pain or were asked what is painful and what is not, the answers would be as diverse as the people that make up the class. Ask a football player if it hurts to be tackled, and the response would more than likely be "no." Ask a member of the chess club the same question, and the answer will probably be "yes." The perception of and response to pain are greatly influenced by the brain. It is here that the differences in people's perception of pain occurs.

The relationship between the cognitive processing of information by the brain and the physiological mechanisms of pain transmission is described by the central biasing mechanism. This modulation of the pain impulse occurs along the impulse's path from the periphery to the brain. Second order neurons connect the T cell (*a first order neuron*) to the processing centers in the brain (*third order neurons*). It is at the *second order neurons* that cognitive influences are believed to either increase or decrease the perception of pain.

The individual's reaction to painful stimulus is based on three dimensions of pain. The first dimension, **sensory-discriminative,** is used to locate the site, intensity, and nature of the pain. The second dimension, **motivational-affective,** is influenced by factors such as the athlete's underlying mental state and personality type. The third dimension, **cognitive-evaluative,** is the athlete's conscious thought process regarding the pain.

Influences on Pain Perception

Several intrinsic factors influence an individual's perception of pain. For example, extroverts express pain more freely than introverts, but introverts are more sensitive to pain.[30] Cognitive-evaluative influences include the activity in which the athlete is involved, the perceived impact that the injury may have, and past experiences.

Perhaps the largest social and cultural influences on pain perception in the United States are those of sex role stereotypes. As a young child how many times did you hear, "Big boys don't cry"? Children often have engraved into their minds that boys are not supposed to cry, but it is appropriate for girls to cry. Although social consciousness has helped decrease this and other types of stereotyping, its influences are still with us.

In young athletes, pain perception may be influenced by the presence of peers. Children have been found to "tolerate" pain to a higher level when observed by their peers than when alone.[31] Likewise, athletes who are scared, dependent, or immature have lower tolerance to pain than their counterparts.[16]

Differences in the definition and expression of pain based on culture have

---

Neuron, First Order: Sensory neuron arising from a spinal nerve and having its body in a dorsal root ganglion.

Neuron, Second Order: A nerve having its body located in the spinal cord. It connects first and third order neurons.

Neuron, Third Order: A nerve having its cell body located in the thalamus and extending into the cerebral cortex.

been documented.[30] The implication of this is that people have roles cast upon them dictating when and where expression of pain is acceptable and when it is not. Furthermore, our individual bias of pain is cast upon others. If you have ever thought that an athlete was "acting like a baby" or "as tough as nails," you were comparing the athlete's reaction to pain to your own pain scale.

A person's past experience will influence the pain perception of a current injury. The experience may be recalling a previous injury that required surgery, or even the image of a similar injury on television. A fear of doctors or hospitals may cause increased anxiety because the athlete is fearful of being exposed to these stressors when an injury occurs. Likewise, if an injury is potentially career-threatening, the reaction may be increased.

There are times when certain events override the processing of pain because the brain is preoccupied with more urgent matters. Immediate processing of information not related to pain may push the processing of the pain response to the background. A good example of this would be soldiers just after a fierce battle, portrayed in the movies as:

> *I'd say ole' chap, that was a nasty one wasn't it? Too bad about*
> *your leg.*
> *My leg?*
> *Your leg. You've been hit.*
> *Oh bloody 'L. Cup of tea then?*

In this case, the soldier was so happy to make it out of combat alive, and the brain was so focused on analyzing the situation that he did not realize an injury had occurred. This same type of processing occurs in athletics. An athlete may be so focused on the competition that when an injury occurs, its magnitude may not be immediately recognized.

Based on this integrative process, the perception of pain is subjective and variable in nature. Notwithstanding, it does consist of several measurable objective parameters. When you ask an athlete how he or she feels today, the response is "better," "worse," or "the same." By doing this, you are requiring the athlete to measure the pain and compare it to the same point as yesterday. Several standardized methods are available to measure the amount of pain in relatively objective terms. Through the use of these tools, the location, intensity, and duration of the pain may be ascertained. Other methods exist that assess activities, emotions, and/or personality traits that influence the perception of pain.

PLACEBO EFFECT

Placebo, stemming from the Latin word for "I shall please," is the term used to describe pain reduction obtained through mechanisms other than those related to the physiological effects of the treatment. The placebo effect is linked to a psychological mechanism where, if the athlete *thinks* that the treatment is beneficial, a degree of pain reduction occurs.

All therapeutic modalities probably have some degree of placebo effect. This effect may be increased when the modality is applied with a sense of enthusiasm and faith. The placebo effect is so powerful, that in one instance patients who received sugar pills, but were told that they were taking a specific medication, actually displayed the side effects of the medication.[30]

The placebo effect can be exploited in the application of therapeutic modalities. Changing modalities and new approaches in the treatment of an injury can positively influence the athlete's perception and result in decreased pain.

REFERRED PAIN

Many times athletic trainers are faced with an athlete who is complaining about pain in an area where no clinical signs of injury are exhibited. This phenomena, known as referred pain, may be described as the brain's error in localizing the source of the noxious input[27] or as "displaced" pain.[32]

An explanation of the mechanisms involved in referred pain is as follows:[29] Pain fibers emerging from the injured site split into several branches within the spinal cord. Some of these branches make contact with other branches that carry only painful impulses. The rest connect with sensory nerve pathways arising from the skin. During this cross-branching, the signals become mixed-up and confused, causing the brain to misinterpret the true source of the noxious stimulus.

An example of referred pain is seen when a nerve root is pinched. Pinching of the nerve produces a burning and aching sensation that radiates away from the vertebral column. Although the actual damage has occurred close to the spinal cord, the pain perceived by the athlete is in the arm, leg, or trunk (depending on the nerve root that was impinged).

Trigger points are hypersensitive areas that form within muscle or connective tissue. The term "trigger point" was coined because pressure on these spots resulted in the "triggering" of referred pain.[32] These areas result from macrotrauma or microtrauma, postural abnormalities, or psychological stress, and send noxious impulses to the brain, which misinterprets the location and intensity of the stimulus. This type of pain does not follow normal sensory distribution patterns, such as those of the *dermatomes*, so the actual sensation is felt in an area other than the actual location of the trigger point (Appendix A).

Although referred pain may appear to be haphazard and random, it does have some logical, orderly constructs. Pain from within the abdomen and/or thorax is generally projected outward to the corresponding cutaneous dermatomes. Examples of this may be seen in the symptoms of heart attacks, and ruptured spleens or kidneys. When the trigger point lies in the extremity, pain tends to be referred distally, rather than proximally, to the true source of the pain.[32]

It is necessary for the athletic trainer to perform a careful, thorough evaluation on athletes who are suffering from symptoms of referred pain. In cases where the true cause of the pain is suspect, or if the athletic trainer is unsure of the nature of the pain, the athlete should be referred to a physician for further evaluation.

Dermatome: A segmental skin area supplied by a single nerve root.

CHRONIC PAIN

Pain extending beyond the normal course of an injury or illness is considered to be chronic. A benchmark time frame for determining chronic pain is 6 months after the injury.[27,33] Individuals suffering from chronic pain live in a world where the pain dictates their lives, and they develop a pattern of pain behavior (Table 1–5). In these cases, pain can no longer be considered merely a symptom. It is a disease in itself.[15]

Chronic pain may be considered to be a learned response where a positive feedback loop is formed in the spinal cord. This results in a mechanism where the spinal gate remains open due to an imbalance between the stimuli allowed to enter the gate. The input accepted from the large-diameter (nonpain) fibers is less than the input accepted from the small-diameter (pain) fibers.

The treatments for acute pain problems are ineffective and often *contraindicated* when applied to athletes suffering from chronic pain.[33] The goal in the treatment of chronic pain is to break the positive feedback loop and essentially "unlearn" the pain. Exercise may increase an individual's endorphin level, assisting in the reduction of chronic pain. Also, exercise may affect the athlete's perception of pain simply by distracting the attention away from the pain to the exercise.[34] The guidance of a physician, physical therapist, or athletic trainer in the treatment of chronic pain cannot be understated.

PAIN MANAGEMENT TECHNIQUES

Pain management techniques may be classified as physical, behavioral, or cognitive. Athletic trainers tend to focus their pain control programs on physical means by using therapeutic modalities.[35] A comprehensive pain management plan should encompass all three aspects.

The physical measures used to control pain include thermal, electrical,

Table 1–5 **CHARACTERISTICS OF CHRONIC PAIN**

Symptoms lasting longer than 6 months
Few objective medical findings
Medication abuse
Difficulty in sleeping
Depression
Manipulative behavior
Somatic preoccupation

Contraindicate: To make inadvisable.

and mechanical modalities, medication, and surgery. This text focuses on the use of therapeutic modalities to control the effects of both injury and pain.

Athletic trainers may utilize both behavioral and cognitive approaches to pain management by decreasing athletes' anxiety about the injury. Explaining the effects and sensations of the treatment and using soothing or distracting stimuli distracts their attention away from the pain. These first two elements require the athletic trainer to communicate with the athlete in an attempt to remove the fear of the unknown. Distracting the athlete's attention away from the pain of the injury or treatment may be accomplished by the use of stereo headphones, television, books, talking, or any other similar device.

The athletic trainer must fully understand the differences between symptomatic and curative treatments. Processes which attack only the pain associated with the injury (electrical stimulation, medication, and so on) have little effect on the injury itself. Most treatment regimes are designed to reduce the physical damage resulting from the injury, and thus truly relieve the cause of the pain.

The Role of Therapeutic Modalities

We began this chapter by noting that the use of therapeutic modalities does not actually hasten the healing process. Rather, it attempts to provide the optimal environment for healing to take place. But what is considered to be a modality? Quite simply stated, it is the application of some form of stress to the body for the purpose of eliciting an adaptive response.

The term therapeutic is essential to fully describe the principles behind the application of thermal, mechanical, or chemical energy to the body. In order to be deemed therapeutic, the stress applied to the body must be conducive to the healing process of the injury in its current state. The optimum conditions for healing require a balance between protecting the area from further distresses and returning the body segment to normal function at the earliest possible time.[7] Hence, the application of a modality at an improper point in its recovery phase will hinder, if not actually set back, the healing process.

Summary

Athletics involve a series of positive and negative stressors. When the negative stresses outweigh the positive, or the intensity of the negative stress is too great, injury occurs. The resultant damage, the primary injury, leads to a sequence of events creating a self-perpetuating cycle which causes further cell death in the form of secondary hypoxic injury.

The body reacts to this through a defensive mechanism, inflammation. Although inflammation is needed for healing, its effects must be controlled, as prolonged inflammation is detrimental to the healing process. The process of healing is characterized by revascularization, wound contracture, and remodeling.

Pain is a nebulous entity in the injury response process and in many cases may actually be more debilitating than the injury itself. By providing nonpain stimuli, the transmission of painful impulses may be blocked.

Therapeutic modalities are used to control and limit the negative effects of inflammation by providing the optimum environment for healing to occur. Each modality used in the treatment of an injury should be judged for the effect it will have on the injury response process in the current stage of healing. Applying the wrong modality at the wrong stage is not therapeutic and causes a delay in the healing process.

CHAPTER QUIZ

. . . .

1. Which of the following physiological events occurs during the alarm stage of the general adaptation syndrome?
   A. Cell death occurs.
   B. Proteins are broken down into amino acids.
   C. The cardiac stroke volume is decreased.
   D. A vasodilation occurs in nonessential muscle groups.

2. An example of an injury caused by macrotrauma is:
   A. Stress fracture
   B. Sprain
   C. Tendonitis
   D. Flat feet.

3. Stress fractures result when?
   A. Osteoclastic activity is greater than osteoblastic activity.
   B. Osteoblastic activity is greater than osteoclastic activity.
   C. Osteoclastic and osteoblastic activity are equal.
   D. The body reaches the stage of resistance.

4. Which of the following tissue types has the best potential to reproduce itself following an injury?
   A. Epithelial tissue
   B. Muscular tissue
   C. Nervous tissue
   D. Connective tissue.

5. Water leaves the cell and enters the interstitial space by following:
   A. Histamine
   B. Debris
   C. Cortisol
   D. Proteins.

6. Pain transmission travels on which of the following nerve fiber types?
   A. Large-diameter nerves
   B. A-gamma
   C. A-beta
   D. A-delta

7. Which of the following cell types is anaerobic and therefore is able to withstand a low-oxygen environment?
   A. Fibrocyte
   B. Granuloma
   C. Macrophage
   D. Anerocyte

8. Which of the following inflammatory mediators inhibits coagulation of blood?
   A. Histamine
   B. Heparin
   C. Kinins
   D. Leukotrienes

9. In the gate theory, the component that serves to monitor the activity of the incoming nerves—and subsequently opens or closes the gate—is the:
   A. T cell
   B. Central control
   C. Substantia gelatinosa
   D. Dorsal horn.

10. Which of the following is incorrect regarding the gate theory?
    A. It encompasses features of both the pattern and specificity theories.
    B. It allows for descending controls from the brain which influence the perception of pain.
    C. It is a divergent system.
    D. It is located in the dorsal horn of the spinal gray matter.

11. Which of the following structures has the poorest blood supply?
    A. Muscle
    B. Fascia
    C. Meniscal cartilage
    D. Bone

12. The rate of atrophy is accelerated through the stimulation of:
    A. Golgi tendon organs
    B. Phasic stretch receptors
    C. Actin and myosin filaments
    D. Blood flow.

13. The healing process begins with:
    A. Inflammation
    B. Coagulation
    C. Phagocytosis
    D. Repair phase.

14. All of the following aids in venous return except:
    A. Gravity
    B. Muscular contractions
    C. The sodium-potassium pump
    D. One-way valves.

15. Mechanisms for the transmission of noxious impulses are:

    A. _____

    B. _____

16. List the five cardinal signs of inflammation and indicate the events which cause them:

	Sign	Event
A.	_____	_____
B.	_____	_____
C.	_____	_____
D.	_____	_____
E.	_____	

17. The attraction of one chemical to an area due to the presence of another is termed

_____

18. Describe the mechanisms for removing blood and exudate from the injured area. How can the athletic trainer facilitate this process? What is the only mechanism available to remove proteins?

19. Describe techniques which an athletic trainer may employ to decrease an athlete's perception of pain.

REFERENCES

1. Allen, RJ: Human Stress: Its Nature and Control. Burgess Publishing, Minneapolis, 1983.
2. Fahey, TD: Athletic Training: Principles and Practice. Mayfield Publishing, Minneapolis, 1986, p 58.
3. Reed, B and Zarro, V: Inflammation and repair in the use of thermal agents. In Michlovitz, S (ed): Thermal Agents in Rehabilitation, ed 2. FA Davis, Philadelphia, 1990, pp 1–17.
4. Enwemeka, CS: Inflammation, cellularity, and fibrillogenesis in regenerating tendon: Implications for tendon rehabilitation. Phys Ther 69:816, 1989.
5. Wilkerson, GB: Inflammation in connective tissue: Etiology and management. Athletic Training 20:298, 1985.
6. Kloth, LC and Miller, KH: The inflammatory response to wounding. In Kloth, LC, McCulloch, JM, and Feedar, JA (eds): Wound Healing: Alternatives in Management. FA Davis, Philadelphia, 1990, pp 1–13.
7. Knight, KL: Cryotherapy: Theory, Technique, and Physiology. Chattanooga Corporation, Chattanooga, 1985.
8. Denegar, CR, Perrin, DH, Rogol, AD, and Rutt, R: Influence of transcutaneous electrical nerve stimulation on pain, range of motion, and serum cortisol concentration in females experiencing delayed onset muscle soreness. JOSPT 11:100, 1989.
9. Voight, ML: Reduction of post traumatic ankle edema with high-voltage pulsed galvanic stimulation. Athletic Training 19:278, 1984.
10. Vander, AJ, Sherman, JH, and Luciano, DS: Human Physiology: The Mechanisms of Body Function, ed 3. McGraw-Hill, New York, 1980.
11. Vanudevan, SV and Melvin, JL: Upper extremity edema control: Rationale of the techniques. Am J Occup Ther 33:520, 1980.
12. Halvorson, GA: Therapeutic heat and cold for athletic injuries. Physician and Sportsmedicine 18:87, 1990.
13. Kolb, P and Denegar, C: Traumatic edema and the lymphatic system. Athletic Training 18:339, 1983.
14. Kisner, C and Colby, LA: Therapeutic Exercise: Foundations and Techniques. FA Davis, Philadelphia, 1990.
15. Cailliet, R: Soft Tissue Pain and Disability. FA Davis, Philadelphia, 1977.
16. Arnheim, DD: Modern Principles of Athletic Training, ed 7. Times Mirror/Mosby College Publishing, St. Louis, 1989, pp 387–388.
17. DeVahl, J: Neuromuscular electrical stimulation (NMES) in rehabilitation. In Gersh, MR (ed): Electrotherapy in Rehabilitation. FA Davis, Philadelphia, 1992, pp 218–268.
18. Spence, AP and Mason, EB: Human Anatomy and Physiology, ed 3. Benjamin/Cummings, Menlo Park, CA, 1987, p 235.
19. Hunter-Griffin, L: Athletic Training and Sports Medicine. American Academy of Orthopaedic Surgeons, Park Ridge, IL, 1991.
20. Lieber, RL and Kelly, MJ: Factors influencing quadriceps femoris muscle torque using transcutaneous neuromuscular stimulation. Phys Ther 71:715, 1991.
21. Daly, TJ: The repair phase of wound healing—Re-epithelialization and contraction. In Kloth, LC, McCulloch, JM, and Feedar, JA (eds): Wound Healing: Alternatives in Management. FA Davis, Philadelphia, 1990, pp 14–30.
22. Lechner, CT and Dahners, LE: Healing of the medial collateral ligament in unstable rat knees. Am J Sports Med 19:508, 1991.
23. Russell, B, Dix, DJ, Haller, DL, and Jacobs-El, J: Repair of injured skeletal muscle: A molecular approach. Med Sci Sports Exerc 24:189, 1992.
24. Roeser, WM, Meeks, LW, Venis, R, and

Strickland, G: The use of transcutaneous nerve stimulation for pain control in athletic medicine. A preliminary report. Am J Sports Med 4:210, 1976.

25. Halvorson, GA: Therapeutic heat and cold for athletic injuries. Physician and Sportsmedicine 18:88, 1990.

26. Walsh, D: Nociceptive pathways—relevance to the physiotherapist. Physiotherapy 77:317, 1991.

27. Newton, RA: Contemporary views on pain and the role played by thermal agents in managing pain symptoms. In Michlovitz, S (ed): Thermal Agents in Rehabilitation, ed 2. FA Davis, Philadelphia, 1990, p 20.

28. Bechtel, TB and Fan, PT: When is TENS effective and practical for pain relief? J Musculoskel Med, 2:37, 1985.

29. Ottoson, D and Lundeberg, T: Pain Treatment by Transcutaneous Electrical Nerve Stimulation: A Practical Manual. Springer-Verlag, New York, 1988, p 15.

30. French, S: Pain: Some psychological and sociological aspects. Physiotherapy 75:255, 1989.

31. Lord, RH and Kozar, B: Pain tolerance in the presence of others: Implications for youth sports. Physician and Sportsmedicine 17:71, 1989.

32. Travell, JG and Simons, DG: Myofascial Pain and Dysfunction: The Trigger Point Manual. Williams & Wilkins, Baltimore, 1983, p 13.

33. Spengler, DM, Loeser, JD, and Murphy, TM: Orthopaedic aspects of the chronic pain syndrome. In The American Academy of Orthopaedic Surgeons Instructional Course Lectures, Vol 29, CV Mosby, St. Louis, 1980, p 101.

34. Raithel, KS: Chronic pain and exercise therapy. Physician and Sportsmedicine 17:204, 1989.

35. Singer, RN and Johnson, PJ: Strategies to cope with pain-associated with sport-related injuries. Athletic Training 22:100, 1987.

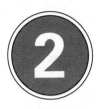

The Transmission of Energy

∙ ∙

This chapter introduces the student to the principles and effects of electromagnetic, infrared, and acoustic energy transfer. These effects are then related to the physical and physiological principles used in the application of therapeutic modalities.

The Electromagnetic Spectrum

We are constantly being bombarded by various forms of energy: The light from the sun, the heat from a fire, and the waves emitted from radio transmitters. This energy, known as **electromagnetic radiation**, is produced by virtually every element in the universe. Each of these forms of energy travels through space at the same velocity, 300 million meters per second. Each form of energy is ordered on the **electromagnetic spectrum** on the basis of its wavelength or frequency (Fig. 2–1).

This introduces the basic relationship: velocity = frequency × wavelength. For these different forms of energy to travel at the same speed, their *frequencies* must be altered. Shorter wavelengths must have a higher frequency to match the velocity of longer wavelengths. This concept may be visualized by picturing

---

Frequency: The number of times an event occurs in one second; measured in Hertz, cycles per second, or pulses per second.

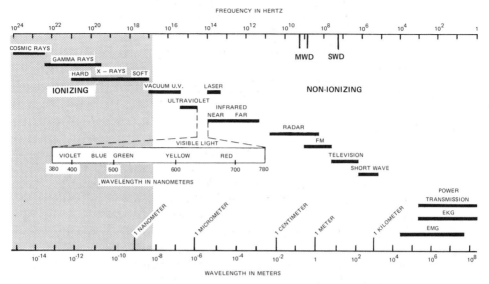

Figure 2–1. A graphical representation of the electromagnetic spectrum. (From Michlovitz, SL: Thermal Agents in Rehabilitation, ed 2. Philadelphia, FA Davis, 1990, p 46, with permission.)

two people walking side by side. One of these people is 7 feet tall and has a stride length of 3 feet. The other is 5 feet tall and has a stride length of 1.5 feet. After traveling 90 feet, the taller person has taken 30 steps; the shorter has taken 60 steps.

REGIONS OF THE ELECTROMAGNETIC SPECTRUM

It is the wavelength of the energy that uniquely defines each portion of the electromagnetic spectrum. The reference measure for wavelength is the meter (Table 2–1). Energies on the electromagnetic spectrum have common characteristics (Table 2–2). This fact notwithstanding, various regions of this spectrum also possess unique characteristics. The following sections detail these characteristics and relate how they affect healing or healthy tissue. It is important to note that not all therapeutic modalities utilize electromagnetic radiation. The most notable of these is ultrasound, which uses acoustical energy (Box 2–1). Other modalities covered in this text, such as massage, traction, and compression pumps are mechanical modalities. Each chapter in this text will provide specific information about the physics of the modality being described.

Table 2–1 **UNITS OF MEASURE FOR WAVELENGTHS RELATIVE TO THE METER (39.37 INCHES)**

Angstrom	Å	10^{-10} m
Nanometer	nm	10^{-9} m
Micrometer	μ	10^{-6} m
Millimeter	mm	10^{-3} m
Centimeter	cm	10^{-2} m
Meter	m	----
Kilometer	km	10^{3} m

Table 2–2 **PROPERTIES OF ELECTROMAGNETIC ENERGY**

Transports energy through space
No medium is required for transmission
All forms of electromagnetic energy travel through a vacuum at a constant rate, 300 million meters
  per second
Electromagnetic energy does not have mass and is composed of pure energy

Ionizing Range

Energy within the ionizing range is characterized by the relative ease able to bring about changes in atoms that result in the generation of free *electrons*, *protons*, or *neutrons*. Ionizing radiation can easily penetrate the tissues and deposit its energy within the cells. If this energy is sufficiently high, the cell loses its ability to divide, resulting in its death.

Energy within the ionizing range is used diagnostically in x-rays (below the threshold required for cell death) and therapeutically in radiation treatment for some forms of cancer (above the threshold). Because ionizing radiation is hazardous, the total dose of exposure must be tightly monitored and controlled. Energy found in this portion of the electromagnetic spectrum is not used in athletic training.

The Light Spectrum

This portion of the spectrum encompasses ultraviolet, visible, and infrared light energy. Electromagnetic radiation possessing a wavelength between 380 and 780 nm forms the spectrum of **visible "white" light.** White light is the

---

Box **2–1**	THE ACOUSTICAL SPECTRUM

The transmission of acoustical energy varies greatly from the transmission of electromagnetic energy. While electromagnetic energy is capable of being transmitted through a complete vacuum, acoustical energy requires a medium for transmission of energy, and the denser the better. Electromagnetic radiation involves the transmission of individual particles that prefer not to be hindered by a medium. The sun emits a particle of light that travels unhindered through the vast void of space. This particle will stay in motion until it strikes a differing density such as the earth or the earth's atmosphere.

In contrast to the emission of individual particles, acoustical energy is transmitted by mechanical waves (vibration) that deform the medium. Therefore, the transmission of acoustical energy is impossible in the vacuum of space. If you yell at a person across the street, your voice causes a deformation in the air. This wave travels through the air and is received by the other person's ear.

The acoustical and electromagnetic spectra do share common features. Like electromagnetic energy, acoustical energy is capable of being reflected, refracted, and absorbed.

Electron: A negatively charged atomic particle.
Proton: A positively charged atomic particle.
Neutron: An electrically neutral particle found in the center of an atom.

combination of seven colors, each representing a different wavelength on the spectrum. These seven colors, ranked from the shortest to the longest wavelength are violet, indigo, blue, green, yellow, orange, and red.

Light energy having a wavelength greater than 780 nm is termed **infrared light** or infrared energy. Since this wavelength is greater than the upper limits of what the human eye is capable of detecting, infrared energy is invisible. Any object possessing a temperature greater than *absolute zero* emits infrared energy proportional to its temperature. Hotter sources transmit more infrared energy possessing a shorter wavelength than cooler objects.

The infrared spectrum is divided into two distinct sections: The **near infrared** is that portion of the spectrum that is closest to visible light, with wavelengths ranging between 780 and 1,500 nm. The **far infrared** portion is located between 1,500 and 12,500 nm. Energy in the near infrared range is capable of producing thermal effects 5- to 10-mm deep in tissue, while far infrared energy results in more superficial heating of the skin (less than 2-mm deep).

Light with a wavelength shorter than visible light is **ultraviolet light**. Like infrared energy, ultraviolet light is undetectable by the human eye. Energy in the **near ultraviolet** range has wavelengths ranging between 290 and 380 nm, while the **far ultraviolet** range encompasses wavelengths between 180 and 290 nm. Both of these forms of ultraviolet light produce superficial chemical changes in the skin. Sunburns are an example of the effect of an overdose of ultraviolet radiation.

Many therapeutic modalities utilize energy within the light range of the electromagnetic spectrum. Ultraviolet light is used for the treatment of certain skin conditions. Depending on the relative temperatures involved, transfer of infrared energy is used to heat or cool the body's tissues. Medical lasers produce beams of energy in the ultraviolet, visible, and infrared light region that can result in either tissue destruction or therapeutic effects within the tissues.

Diathermy and Electrical Currents

Electromagnetic radiation of longer wavelengths has an intensity sufficient to cause an increase in tissue temperature. Collectively known as **diathermy**, these types of electromagnetic energies create a magnetic field that is changed into heat through the process of **conversion**. The two most common types of therapeutic diathermy are microwave and shortwave diathermy.

In the range above shortwave diathermy and extending on to infinity are electrical stimulating currents. These devices use the direct flow of electrons and ions to elicit physiological changes within the tissues. It should be noted that the physical manipulations done to the electrical current do not allow for its precise location on the electromagnetic spectrum. The exception to this is uninterrupted direct current, possessing the theoretical wavelength of infinity.

Absolute Zero: Theoretically the lowest possible temperature, equal to $-273°C$ or $-460°F$. At this point, all atomic and molecular motion ceases.

THE TRANSFER OF ENERGY

Electromagnetic radiation requires no *medium* for transmission. This enables it to be transmitted through the vacuum of space, the earth's atmosphere, or a brick wall. Energy is transmitted from an area of high concentration to an area of lower concentration by **energy carriers**.[1] Taking many forms, these carriers may be mechanical waves, *photons*, electrons, and molecules. Note that heat is not actually a form of energy; rather, it is the name given to a particular form of energy exchange.[2]

Within the range of thermal therapeutic modalities, the exchange of energy in the form of heat involves the exchange of *kinetic energy*. This transfer of energy occurs by one of four means:

Conduction involves the transfer of heat between two objects that are in physical contact with each other. A temperature gradient is required to initiate a process where kinetic energy is exchanged through the collision of molecules, moving the energy from an area of high temperature to an area of lower temperature. This concept can be illustrated by heating one end of a metal rod. The heat is gradually passed from one end of the rod to the other until the rod has an equal temperature along its length.

Some materials are better conductors of energy than others. Consider a wooden picnic table and a metal picnic table that have been sitting in direct sunlight and have the same temperature. If you placed one hand on the wooden table and the other hand on the metal table, the metal table would feel ''hotter'' more rapidly. Even though you are touching two objects with equal temperatures, the greater ability of metal to conduct heat (compared to wood) warms your hand more rapidly.

Examples of therapeutic modalities that operate by way of conduction include moist heat packs and ice application. Within the body, the transfer of energy from one tissue layer to another occurs by way of conduction.

Convection involves the transportation of heat by the movement of a medium, usually air or water. Of the three *states of matter*, gasses are the poorest conductors of heat, while liquids are good conductors, and solids, generally speaking, are better conductors. Adding motion to gasses and liquids such as circulating air or water increases their ability to transport heat.

The actual transfer of energy from the medium to the body still occurs as a result of conduction; it is the delivery of the energy that occurs by movement of the media. The circulation of the medium results in the cooling of one object and the subsequent heating of another object. Whirlpools are the most common example of therapeutic modalities that deliver their energy through convection.

Radiation is the transfer of energy without the use of a medium, and the heat gained or lost through radiation is termed **radiant energy**. Infrared energy is emitted from any object having a temperature greater than absolute zero.

Medium: A material used to promote the transfer of energy. An object—or substance—that permits the transmission of energy through it.

Photon: A unit of light energy that has zero mass, no electric charge, and an indefinite life span.

Kinetic Energy: The energy an object possesses by virtue of its motion.

States of Matter: Physical matter can take three forms: solid, liquid, and gas. Using H_2O as an example, we see the three phases as ice, water (liquid), and steam.

Divergence of the energy radiated may occur, resulting in a reduction of the energy received by an object in its path.

All thermal therapeutic modalities provide radiant energy. Infrared lamps, for example, deliver most of their energy through radiation. Even modalities that deliver their energy to the body through conduction, such as moist heat packs, lose some of their energy through radiation. This effect can be illustrated by placing your hand just above a moist heat pack. The heat you feel is being lost from the pack via radiation.

Heat loss can also occur through **evaporation**. In this case, the change from the liquid state to the gaseous state requires that thermal energy be removed from the body. The heat absorbed by the liquid cools the tissue as the liquid changes its state into gas. Vapocoolant sprays are an example of a therapeutic modality that operates through evaporation.

INFLUENCES ON THE TRANSMISSION OF ENERGY

When electromagnetic energy is transmitted through a vacuum, it travels in a straight line. When traveling through a medium, its course is influenced by changes in density. Energy striking a medium of different density may be reflected, refracted, absorbed by the material, or continue through the material unaffected by the change (Fig. 2–2).

Reflection occurs when the wave does not proceed to the next density layer. The wave strikes the object and reverses its direction away from the material (see Fig. 2–2). Reflection may be complete, as when all energy is precluded from entering the next density layer, or it may be partial. An echo is an example of reflection that involves acoustical energy.

Refraction is the bending of waves due to a change in the speed of a wave

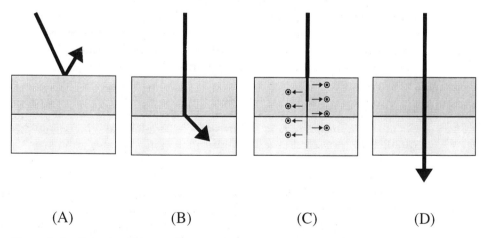

(A)   (B)   (C)   (D)

Figure 2–2. Factors Influencing the Transmission of Energy Through the Tissues. (A) Reflection of an energy wave. The energy may be fully or partially reflected by a tissue layer. (B) Refraction of an energy wave. The wave is bent as it strikes an interface between two densities. (C) Absorption of energy. Energy absorption by one layer reduces the energy available to deeper tissues. (D) Transmission of energy. Any energy that is not reflected or absorbed by a tissue layer continues to pass through the medium.

Divergence: The spreading of a beam or wave.

as it enters a medium of different density (see Fig. 2–2). When the energy leaves a dense layer and enters a less dense layer, its speed increases. When moving from a low-density to a high-density layer the energy decreases. A prism refracts light rays. As the light is bent within the prism, the velocity of the light slows to the point where each of the seven color bands becomes visible.

Absorption occurs through the medium collecting the wave and changing it into kinetic energy. The tissues may absorb part or all of the energy being delivered to the tissue (see Fig. 2–2). Any energy not reflected or absorbed by one tissue layer continues to pass through the tissue until it strikes another density layer. At this point it may again be reflected, refracted, absorbed, or passed on to the next tissue layer. Each time the wave is partially reflected, refracted, or absorbed, the remaining energy available to deeper tissue is reduced (see the law of Grotthus-Draper in the next section).

HEAT AS A PHYSICAL ENTITY

Temperatures, and the perception of them, as well as their effects, are relative. If we walk outside and the temperature is 60 degrees we will note, "It's cold," if it was 80 degrees yesterday; "It's warming up" if it was 40 degrees yesterday; or "I wish the weather would change" if the previous day's temperature was also 60 degrees. This concept also holds true for the application of thermal modalities. The classifications of "heat" and "cold" are based on the physiological response elicited by the temperature.

The basic operating principle behind any thermal modality is transfer of heat across a temperature gradient (that is, one object is warmer than the other). Heat, a form of energy, is lost from the warmer object and moved into the cooler object. The greater the temperature gradient, the more quickly energy is transferred.[3] When a moist heat pack is placed on an athlete, energy is transferred away from the pack and absorbed by the athlete's tissues. Likewise, when a cold pack is used, the heat is drawn away from the athlete's tissues and delivered to the pack.

Heat is measured in **calories**. One calorie is the amount of energy needed to raise the temperature of 1 gram of water by 1°C. When the temperature of an object is measured, it is the speed of molecular movement that is being quantified. Increased speed of molecular motion is measured as an increase in temperature.

Some objects require less energy per unit of mass to raise their temperature than others. This ability, **thermal capacity**, is measured by the number of heat units required to raise the temperature of a unit of mass by 1°C. Iron, for example, requires less energy to raise its temperature than water. If an equal mass of these two substances were to be heated with an equal amount of energy, the iron would reach the terminal temperature faster than water. Likewise, the water would cool to its original temperature faster than the iron.

An object's ability to transmit thermal energy is measured in terms of **specific heat**. The specific heat of an object is determined by the ratio of its thermal capacity to that of water, which has been given the baseline thermal capacity of 1. In comparing the specific heat of the three states of water, ice has a specific heat of 0.50, water 1.0, and steam 0.48.

Energy's Effect on the Tissues

The *efficacy* of a particular treatment is dependent on the proper choice and application of a modality. The modality must be capable of producing the desired physiological changes at the intended tissue depth. A superficial heating agent will have little positive effect on a deep-seated injury. The proper modality will not produce optimal results if it is applied incorrectly.

For physiological changes to occur the energy applied to the body must be absorbed by the tissues. Across the electromagnetic spectrum, there is little correlation between wavelength and the ability to penetrate the body's tissues.[4] Both x-rays and radio waves penetrate the tissues despite their polar positions on the spectrum. However, for infrared modalities, there is a direct relationship between wavelength and depth of penetration. Longer wavelengths in this region penetrate deeper into the tissues than do shorter wavelengths.

When energy strikes the body, the maximal effect occurs when the rays strike the tissues at a right angle (90°). The **cosine law** states that as this angle deviates away from 90°, the effective energy varies with the cosine of the angle: effective energy = energy × cosine of the angle of incidence. With radiant energy, a difference of ± 10 degrees from the right angle is considered to be within acceptable limits during treatment.[5]

The intensity of radiant energy is dependent on the distance between the source and the tissues. This relationship is defined by the **inverse square law**. The intensity of the energy striking the tissues is proportional to the square of the distance between the source of the energy and the tissues:

$$E = E_S/D^2$$

Where E = the amount of energy received by the tissue
E_S = the amount of energy produced by the source
D^2 = the square of the distance between the target and the source

Doubling the distance between the tissue and the energy will decrease the intensity at the tissue by a factor of four (Fig. 2–3).

To enable energy to affect the body, it must be absorbed by the tissues at a level sufficient to stimulate a physiological response. As we have previously seen with the general adaptation syndrome, if the amount of energy absorbed is too little, no reaction will take place and if the amount of energy is too great, damage will result. This concept applied to the application of therapeutic modalities is known as the **Arndt-Schultz principle** and is translated into clinical practice through the application of the proper modality at the proper intensity for the appropriate duration.

Any energy that penetrates the body and is not absorbed by one tissue layer is passed along to the next layer. The **law of Grotthus-Draper** describes an inverse relationship between the penetration and absorption of energy. The more energy that is absorbed by the superficial tissues, the less that remains to be transmitted to underlying tissues.

Consider, for example, the application of moist heat to the quadriceps muscle group. Some of the energy will be absorbed by the skin, decreasing the

---

Efficacy: The ability of a modality or treatment regime to produce the intended effects.

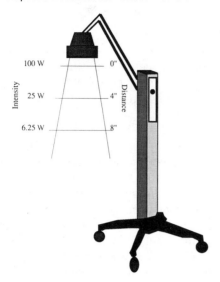

Figure 2–3. An Example of the Inverse-Square Law. Each time the distance between the source of infrared energy and the tissue is doubled, the intensity of the energy delivered to the tissue is reduced by a factor of four.

amount of energy delivered to the adipose tissue. Some of the remaining energy will be absorbed by the adipose tissue leaving only a fraction of the initial energy left to heat the muscle. This also illustrates the fact that adipose tissue can act as an insulator, inhibiting the thermal heating of muscle.

Measures

Distances, weights, and temperatures can be described on many different scales. In the United States, the English system of measure, using inches, pounds, and degrees Fahrenheit, is most commonly used. However, most published scientific research in this country uses the International System of Units (SI) measured in meters, grams, and degrees Celsius (referred to as the metric system). Additionally, the metric system is the standard system in most other countries. The purpose of this section is to provide a reference for converting back and forth between these two systems. Because this textbook has a strong emphasis on clinical application, the English system will be used in describing therapeutic temperature ranges and large measures of distance. The metric system will be used when it is a standard measure (such as describing wavelengths) or to describe measures of less than one inch.

Table 2–3 **COMPARISON BETWEEN ENGLISH AND SI MEASURES OF LENGTH***

Millimeters	Centimeters	Meters	Inches	Feet	Yards
1 mm = 1.0	0.1	0.001	0.03937	0.00328	0.0011
1 cm = 10.0	1.0	0.01	0.3937	0.03281	0.0109
1 in = 25.4	2.54	0.0254	1.0	0.0833	0.0278
1 ft = 304.8	30.48	0.3048	12.0	1.0	0.333
1 yd = 914.4	91.44	0.9144	36.0	3.0	1.0
1 m = 1000.0	100.0	1.0	39.37	3.2808	1.0936

*Source: Adapted from Thomas, CL (ed): Taber's Cyclopedic Medical Dictionary, ed 16. FA Davis, Philadelphia, 1989.

DISTANCE CONVERSION

The basis of measurement in the metric system is the meter (m), a distance of 39.37 inches. The exact distance of one meter is the wavelength associated with a specific frequency in the electromagnetic spectrum. The inch, as history goes, was derived from the length of the middle phalanx of a king's index finger. Table 2–3 illustrates the relationship between the standard units of measure of these two systems.

To convert English measures to meters, multiply the unit by the following conversion constants. To convert meters to the English system, divide by the constant.

English Measure	Constant
inches	0.0254
feet	0.3048

WEIGHT AND MASS CONVERSION

The terms "weight" and "mass" are often used synonymously, but this is incorrect. Weight refers to the effect of the Earth's gravitational force on the mass. The mass refers to the amount of matter that an object contains. As such, the true weight of an object varies from location to location. For example, your weight is greater when you are standing on the beach (sea level) than if you were standing on the top of Mount Everest. This is because the gravitation pull of the earth is greater at sea level than at higher altitudes.

Despite the variability of weight, mass does not change. This is best illustrated by astronauts who are floating weightless in space. Although they do not exhibit weight, their physical mass does not change. While mass and weight may have the same numerical value, it is important to express the unit as one of mass or one of weight: 1 gram is a unit of mass, 1 gram *weight* is a unit of weight.

The basis of the measurement of mass in the SI system is the gram or kilogram (1000 g). To convert English measures to grams, multiply by the following constants. To convert grams to English measures, divide by the constant.

English Measure	Constant
Ounces	0.0283495
Pounds	0.4535924

TEMPERATURE CONVERSION

The SI system of temperature is Celsius and the various degrees are measured in centigrade (C). The Celsius system was established so that 0°C represented the freezing point of water and 100°C represented the boiling point.

To convert Fahrenheit to centigrade:

$$\text{degrees centigrade} = (\text{degrees Fahrenheit} - 32) \times 5/9$$

To convert centigrade to Fahrenheit:

$$\text{degrees Fahrenheit} = (\text{degrees centigrade} \times 9/5) + 32$$

Summary

This chapter has described the various types of energy that can be applied to the body to elicit an involuntary response. Most of these energies are located on the electromagnetic spectrum, although ultrasound is on the acoustical spectrum and others, such as massage, are not found on any spectrum. Any applied energy must penetrate the outermost tissue layer and then subsequently be absorbed by the tissue to elicit physiological changes.

The exchange of energy occurs through the use of energy carriers. As seen in athletic training, these carriers take the form of molecules, electrons, photons, and mechanical waves. The transfer of heat involves the exchange of kinetic energy from molecule to molecule. Within the body this exchange always occurs through conduction.

When determining the effectiveness of a particular modality, four factors should be considered: (1) how deep the particular modality penetrates, (2) the ability of the injured structure to absorb the energy, (3) the conductive properties of the tissues being treated, and (4) the desired physiological responses for the particular stage of inflammation being treated.

The following chapters describe the physical characteristics of different energy transfer methods. The physical and physiological effects are related to the injury response process so that the athletic trainer can make proper judgments in determining the criteria for choosing a therapeutic modality.

CHAPTER QUIZ

. . . .

1. Of the following forms of energy, which has the highest velocity?
   A. Cosmic waves
   B. X-rays
   C. FM radio waves
   D. Shortwave diathermy
   E. They are all equal.

2. Which of the following forms of energy has the longest wavelength?
   A. Cosmic waves
   B. X-rays
   C. FM radio waves
   D. Shortwave diathermy
   E. They are all equal.

3. Which of the following forms of energy has the highest frequency?
   A. Cosmic waves
   B. X-rays
   C. FM radio waves
   D. Shortwave diathermy
   E. They are all equal.

4. This portion of the electromagnetic spectrum is characterized by the ease with which it strips atoms of electrons.
   A. Ionizing range
   B. Ultraviolet light
   C. Infrared light (near range)
   D. Infrared light (far range)
   E. Diathermy range

5. The use of a prism to separate visible light into its seven component colors is an example of:
   A. Reflection
   B. Refraction
   C. Divergence
   D. Conversion

6. The method of heat transfer that involves the cooling of one object with the subsequent heating of another object through the circulation of air or water is:
   A. Radiation
   B. Evaporation
   C. Conduction
   D. Convection

7. The measure of the number of heat units required to raise a unit of mass by 1°C is termed:
   A. Calorie
   B. Thermal capacity
   C. Specific heat
   D. Change of state

8. Using the inverse square law, a lamp producing 50 watts of power at its source would provide _____ watts of power to tissues located 5 inches from the source.
   A. 0.01
   B. 2.0
   C. 100
   D. 250
   E. 500

9. The precept that any energy which penetrates the body and is not absorbed by one tissue layer must be transmitted to the next layer is attributed to:
   A. Arndt-Schultz
   B. Brown-Thor
   C. Grotthus-Draper
   D. Thermal capacity

10. Ten degrees centigrade is equal to _____ Fahrenheit.
    A. −26.4°
    B. −12.2°
    C. 37.6°
    D. 50.0°
    E. 74.3°

REFERENCES

1. Weinberger, A and Lev, A: Temperature elevation of connective tissue by physical modalities. Critical Reviews in Physical and Rehabilitation Medicine, 3:121, 1991.
2. Sekins, KM and Emery, AF: Thermal science for physical medicine. In Lehmann, JF (ed): Therapeutic Heat and Cold, ed 4. Baltimore, Williams & Wilkins, pp 62–112, 1990.
3. Knight, KL: Cryotherapy: Theory, Technique, and Physiology. Chattanooga Corporation, Chattanooga, 1985, p 28.
4. Kloth, LC and Ziskin, MC: Diathermy and pulsed electromagnetic fields. In Michlovitz, SL (ed): Thermal Agents in Rehabilitation, ed 2. FA Davis, Philadelphia, pp 170–199, 1990.
5. Griffin, JE and Karselis, TC: Physical Agents for Physical Therapists, ed 3. Charles C Thomas, Springfield, IL, pp 229–263, 1988.

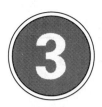

Thermal Agents

· ·

The following unit contains information regarding those modalities that rely on electromagnetic properties to elicit various responses in the body's systems. The unit is broken down into two sections, cold and heat, with specific modalities covered according to their various local effects.

Thermal agents transfer energy to or from the tissues. This transfer of energy may be based on a temperature gradient, as with ice or heat, or the conversion of electromagnetic energy, as with the diathermies. Compared to the extreme range of temperatures found on the electromagnetic spectrum there is relatively little difference between the upper and lower temperature limits of thermal treatments. Within our tissues, the 65°F that form the upper and lower limits of heat and cold modalities elicit a wide range of cellular and vascular events.

Cold Modalities

Cold is a relative state characterized by decreased molecular motion. In the application of therapeutic modalities, cold modalities range from 32°F to 65°F. The basic effects of cold will be discussed in this section, while the various methods of application are presented individually.

The application of a cold modality to the human body is known as **cryotherapy**. During the treatment, heat is removed from the body and absorbed by the cold modality. The body reacts to the treatment with a series of local and *systemic* responses. The magnitude of these effects is related to the temperature and duration of the treatment, as well as to the surface area exposed.

Table 3–1 **LOCAL EFFECTS OF COLD APPLICATION**

Vasoconstriction
Decreased rate of cell metabolism resulting in a decreased need for oxygen
Decreased cellular waste
Reduction in inflammation
Decreased pain
Decreased muscle spasm

The local effects of cold application include vasoconstriction and a decrease in metabolic rate, inflammation, and pain transmission (Table 3–1).

The application of cold to the skin activates a mechanism designed to conserve heat in the body's core. It is through this reaction that the beneficial effects of cryotherapy are obtained. A moderate correlation between skin temperature and *intra-articular* temperature has been observed ($r = 0.65$).[1] Therefore, the more the skin is cooled, the greater the cooling of underlying tissues.[2] This same principle can be applied to the application of heat modalities.

The most rapid and significant temperature changes occur in the skin and *synovium* (Fig. 3–1). The degree of this response varies among the different methods of cold application. Using implanted probes in dogs, measured intra-articular temperatures have been shown to drop 36.4°F during ice immersion, compared to a drop of 11.7°F when an ice pack was applied to a joint.[3]

If the temperature of circulating blood is decreased by 0.2°F, the *hypo-*

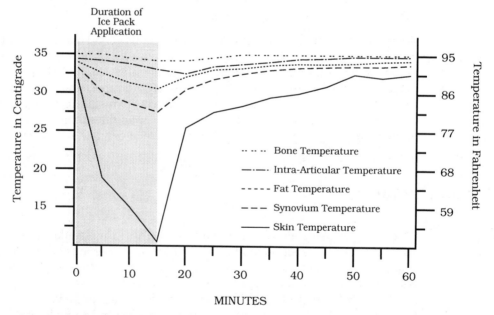

Figure 3–1. Depth of Penetration During the Application of an Ice Pack. Using implanted electrodes in a dog's knee, this figure indicates the rate, magnitude, and duration of temperature decrease in subcutaneous tissues. (From Bocobo et al,[3] p 183, with permission.)

Intra-articular: Within a joint.
Synovium: Membrane lining the capsule of a joint.

Table 3–2 **GENERAL SYSTEMIC EFFECTS OF COLD EXPOSURE**

General vasoconstriction in response to cooling of the posterior hypothalamus
Decreased respiratory and heart rates
Shivering and increased muscle tone

thalamus responds with several systemic effects (Table 3–2). A body-wide vasoconstriction occurs and the heart rate is decreased in an attempt to localize the cold. In an attempt to maintain the body's core temperature, the heart rate is reduced, limiting the rate at which cool blood is circulated. If the athlete's core temperature continues to decrease toward the point of *hypothermia*, shivering and increased muscle tone assist in keeping the body heat inward. This severe response is normal when athletes are exposed to extremely cold environments (e.g., falling into a near-frozen lake). It is NOT a common response in therapeutic cold application.

Cold modalities may be used effectively during all stages of the inflammatory response. Indications for the use of cold include acute injury or inflammation, pain, muscle spasm, and decreased range of motion (Table 3–3). Primary contraindications for the use of cold are conditions where the body is unable to cope with the temperature due to allergy, hypersensitivity, or circulatory insufficiency.

EFFECT ON THE INJURY RESPONSE CYCLE

Cellular Response

The most beneficial effect of cold application during an acute injury is to decrease the need for oxygen in the area being treated.[4,5] A cold environment decreases cellular metabolic rate, consequently decreasing the amount of oxygen required by the cells to survive. By reducing the number of cells killed by

Table 3–3 **GENERAL INDICATIONS AND CONTRAINDICATION FOR COLD TREATMENTS**

Indications
Acute injury or inflammation
Acute or chronic pain
Small, superficial first-degree burns
Postsurgical pain and edema
In conjunction with rehabilitation exercises
Spasticity accompanying central nervous system disorders
Acute or chronic muscle spasm

Contraindications
Cardiac or respiratory involvement
Uncovered open wounds
Circulatory insufficiency
Cold allergy
Anesthetic skin
Raynaud's phenomenon

Hypothalamus: The body's thermoregulatory center.
Hypothermia: Decreased core temperature.
Raynaud's Phenomenon: A reaction to cold consisting of bouts of pallor and cyanosis.

a lack of oxygen, the degree of secondary hypoxic injury is limited. Since fewer cells are damaged from secondary hypoxic injury, smaller amounts of inflammatory substances are released into the area (see Chapter 1).

Blood and Fluid Dynamics

Since cold application decreases the rate of cell metabolism and thereby reduces the need for oxygen, it would seem to follow that blood flow to the treatment area would be lessened. Despite this seemingly sound logic, the effects of cold application on blood flow have been (and still remain) a topic of much investigation.

Vasoconstriction occurs due to the stimulation of local nerve receptors; this triggers a response from the sympathetic nervous system which instructs the vessels to constrict. As the molecular motion of the blood and tissue fluids slows, their viscosity increases. The reduction in blood flow occurs too late to affect the hemorrhaging process, but it may prevent hematoma formation.[4,6]

After 5 minutes of cold application, the skin should be marked by *hyperemia*, indicating that the circulatory system is continuing to deliver warm blood, even though the skin temperature has dropped substantially. If the area displays signs of *pallor*, the circulatory system has been unable to maintain tissue temperatures within normal physiological limits. In this case the superficial vasculature has constricted to conserve heat in the underlying tissues. If the tissues become *cyanotic*, the treatment should be discontinued.[7]

An early exploration on the dynamics of blood flow during cold treatments was performed by Lewis[8] in 1930. When the fingers were immersed in cold water, alternating periods of cooling and warming were seen in the skin. Termed the **hunting response**, it appeared that the vessels underwent a series of vasoconstrictions and vasodilations in an attempt to adapt to the temperature. However, the hunting response has only been identified in selected areas of the body.[9]

Later, Knight[4] examined the reputed increase in blood flow as the result of **cold-induced vasodilation**. His work suggested that the vasodilation only lessened the amount of initial vasoconstriction. Despite the vasodilation, there was still a net vasoconstriction when compared to the vessel diameter prior to treatment (Fig. 3–2).

Recent studies using *impedance plethysmography* produced conflicting results concerning the effect of cryotherapy on blood flow. Baker and Bell[10] determined that the application of cold packs did not significantly reduce blood flow in the human calf. Furthermore, they concluded that ice massage may actually increase blood flow. Taber and associates,[9] using a protocol similar to that of Baker and Bell, but with the addition of blocking venous return, had

---

Hyperemia: A red discoloration of the skin caused by increased blood flow. The skin will turn white when pressure is applied.

Pallor: Lack of color in the skin.

Cyanosis (Cyanotic): A blue-gray discoloration of the skin caused by a lack of oxygen.

Impedance Plethysmography: A determination of blood flow based on the amount of electrical resistance in the area.

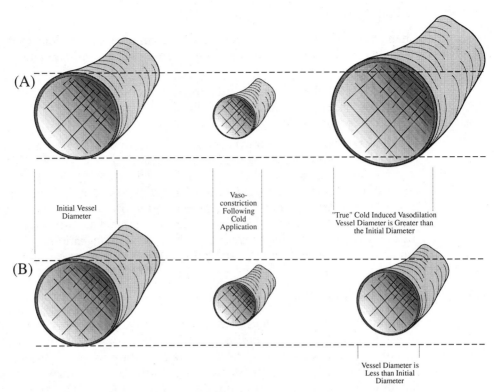

Figure 3–2. Vascular Response to Cold Application. (A) The concept of cold induced vasodilation. Following the application of cold there is an immediate vasoconstriction. This event is followed by a vasodilation resulting in a larger diameter than prior to the ice application. This event has not been substantiated. (B) Vascular reaction as suggested by Knight[4]. Following the initial vasoconstriction there is a dilation of the vessel, but its diameter is still reduced compared to the original diameter.

the opposite result. They concluded that application of a cold pack for 20 minutes produced "an immediate and sustained reduction in blood flow."

Both studies did agree, however, that reactive vasodilation did not occur during either 20-minute application period. Taber's study did note that after 13 minutes of cold application, a slight increase in blood flow was observed. This increase was transitory, and they attributed it to another mechanism such as increased heart rate or stroke volume, as the vessel diameter did not appear to change.

Evidence supporting the beneficial effects of cold in reducing the collection of edema is not as great as once thought, and the mechanisms are unclear.[10] One study reported that ankle edema after the acute phase of injury increased following cold immersion.[11] In treatment immediately after injury, it appears that compression and elevation serve to limit the formation of edema, while cold prevents further hypoxic injury (see section on the effects of immediate treatment).

Effect on Inflammation

Changes in cellular function and blood dynamics serve to control the effects of acute inflammation. Cold application suppresses the inflammatory response by

- reducing the release of inflammatory mediators[5,6]
- decreasing prostaglandin synthesis[5]
- decreasing capillary permeability[5]

Secondary edema and hemorrhage are reduced due to an inhibitory effect on the mediators and decreased capillary permeability.

As described by the injury response cycle (see Fig. 1-2), limiting the amount of inflammation inhibits the effects of the remaining components. The degree of hemorrhage and edema are reduced by limiting inflammatory mediators. Pain is decreased by lessening the mechanical pressure on nerves. As muscle spasm and edema are reduced, there is less congestion in the area, and the amount of secondary hypoxic cell death is limited.

Muscle Spasm and Function

Cold reduces muscle spasm in two ways: (a) it decreases pain by reducing the threshold of afferent nerve endings, and (b) it decreases the sensitivity of muscle spindles. A drop of 9°F in surface skin temperature reduces the sensitivity of muscle spindles. The drop in muscle spindle activity, combined with the decreased rate of afferent nerve impulses, inhibits the stretch reflex mechanism and results in decreased muscle spasm.[6,12] A short-term break in the pain-spasm pain cycle may result in long-term relief of muscle spasm.

This mechanism also affects the voluntary functioning of the body part. The decreased nerve conduction velocity, decreased sensitivity of muscle spindles, and increased fluid viscosity lead to a decrease in the ability to perform rapid muscle movements.

Pain Control

A traditional athletic training text[13] states that during cryotherapy, the athlete will experience a sequence of four sensations: cold, burning, aching, and *analgesia*. The *numbing* effect is a result of decreasing the nerve conduction velocity and increasing the threshold required to fire the nerves.[5] As cold application continues, the nerve conduction rate will drop to a point where conduction ceases.[7]

By stimulating the large-diameter neurons, cold inhibits pain transmission, acting (in terms of the gate theory) as a *counterirritant*. The sensory events associated with the application of a cold modality stimulate the large-diameter nerves to decrease the transmission and perception of pain.

Physiologically, the transmission of noxious impulses is reduced by low-

---

Analgesia: Absence of the sense of pain.
Numbness: Lack of sensation in a body part.
Counterirritant: A substance causing irritation of superficial sensory nerves so as to reduce the transmission of pain from underlying nerves.

ering the excitability of free nerve endings, resulting in an increased pain threshold. Small-diameter, myelinated nerves are the first to exhibit change in their conduction velocities. The last to respond to cold temperatures are unmyelinated, small-diameter nerves.[14] This sequence of nerve fiber activation can provide an explanation for the sequence of sensations that accompany cryotherapy.

Not all athletes experience the same sensations during cold application. Ingersoll and Mangus[15] examined the sensory component of ice immersion using the *McGill Pain Questionnaire*. Numbness (anesthesia) was not reported until 18 to 21 minutes into the application and true analgesia was never exhibited.

Cold will decrease the speed of nerve conduction by slowing communication at the *synapse*. In certain cases, this can lead to *neurapraxia* and *axonotmesis*.[16] Cold-induced nerve palsy has been reported in the treatment of injuries to the anterior compartment of the lower leg.[17,18]

Since cold disrupts muscle spasm, pain is reduced by alleviating the mechanical stimulation placed on the nerve receptors in the spasmodic area. A brief disruption in pain may serve to break the injury response cycle and allow tissue healing and repair to proceed unhindered.[5]

FROSTBITE

When frozen water is used as a means of cold application, there is little chance of frostbite occurring under normal conditions.[7,12] Picture in your mind these forms of ice application: ice bag, ice massage, and ice immersion. During the course of each of these treatments water is present. An ice bag fills with water as it melts, ice massage leaves a trail of water with each stroke, and water is the medium during an ice immersion.

The presence of water indicates that ice is melting, and therefore that the temperature of the surface of the ice is 32°F. Frostbite occurs when the skin temperature falls below freezing. When the subcutaneous temperature falls below 55°F, tissue damage occurs. During the course of a 20-minute treatment, cold modalities that have water present cause a decrease in subcutaneous tissue temperatures of 9° to 18°F, a temperature range well within the limits of safety.[12]

If the treatment is applied below the recommended temperature or if the duration of the treatment exceeds the recommended time, or if the athlete suffers from severe circulatory insufficiency, the risk of frostbite (or cold injury) increases (Box 3–1). Prolonged exposure to intense cold decreases circulation throughout the body. Blood traveling through the veins cools the incoming arterial blood and acts to increase the amount of systemic vasoconstriction and further lower the heart rate. If the treated area is highly ischemic, warm blood cannot reach the tissues.

The risk of frostbite *is* present when using reusable cold packs. These devices contain water mixed with antifreeze and are stored at temperatures

---

McGill Pain Questionnaire: One of many pain scales, this device uses a choice of words in describing the type, magnitude, and location of the pain.
Synapse: The junction where two nerves communicate.
Neurapraxia: A temporary loss of function in a peripheral nerve.
Axonotmesis: Damage to nerve tissue without physical severing of the nerve.

Box 3-1	SIGNS AND SYMPTOMS OF FROSTBITE

Even the most minor case of frostbite is accompanied by extreme pain. This pain is so severe that athletes who have normal sensory function will not allow the treatment to continue. The primary cases for concern are those where athletes have sensory and/or circulatory impairment or where reusable ice packs are applied.

The first physical sign of frostbite is the fading of the redness normally associated with cold application. This color is replaced by a waxy white sheen. If allowed to continue, the skin will blister or molt and lead to an obvious buildup of edema.

During any physical procedure, the circulation to the athlete's extremities can be checked by monitoring the flow of blood to the nail beds. Gently squeezing the nail removes the blood, making it turn white or pale. When the force is removed, the original color should return. If it fails to return, circulatory impairment should be suspected.

If frostbite is suspected, immediately remove the athlete from the source of the cold. Rewarm the body part by immersing it in water at 100°F and refer the athlete to a physician for follow-up evaluation.

---

below freezing. Since the surface temperature of the pack may be below freezing, a medium such as a wet towel must be place between the pack and the athlete when these packs are used.

THE EFFECTS OF IMMEDIATE TREATMENT

Immediate treatment—rest, ice, compression, and elevation (RICE)—serves to counteract the body's initial response to an injury. **Rest** limits the scope of the original injury by preventing further trauma. In athletes, "rest" may take the form of immobilizing the body part, the use of crutches, or other methods of avoiding additional insult to the injured tissues.

The function of **ice** application during immediate treatment is to decrease the cell's metabolism and therefore decrease the need for oxygen in the injured area. This reduces the amount of secondary hypoxic injury by enabling the tissues in the injured area to survive on the limited amount of oxygen they are receiving. Ice application may also provide a secondary benefit in the immediate treatment of an injury through the reduction of pain. Because of the other factors surrounding the injury (e.g., the severity of the injury or the athlete's emotional state), the effects of ice on limiting pain cannot be accurately predicted for every case.

Compression serves to decrease the pressure gradient between the blood vessels and tissues. This discourages further leakage from the capillary beds into the interstitial tissues while also encouraging increased lymphatic drainage. Compression wraps are best applied so that a pressure gradient is formed between the distal end of the wrap and the proximal end. This is done by applying the wrap from distal to proximal, gradually decreasing the pressure with each turn. Wraps applied with even pressure throughout their length are often counterproductive as they form a kind of tourniquet inhibiting flow both to and from the area.

Wilkerson[19] describes three methods of applying compression to an injured area:

Circumferential compression provides an even pressure around the entire circumference of the body part. The cross-sectional area remains circular, but the diameter of the body part decreases. Common forms of circumferential compression are elastic wraps and pneumatic or water-filled sleeves. This type of compression is best suited for evenly shaped body areas such as the knee or thigh.

Collateral compression produces pressure on only two sides of the body part, so that the cross-sectional area deforms elliptically. The soft tissues are compressed between the device and the bone. A common form of collateral compression is found in air-filled stirrup braces.

Focal compression, applied with U-shaped "horseshoe" pads, provides direct pressure to soft tissue surrounded by prominent bony structures (e.g., the lateral ligaments of the ankle or the acromioclavicular joint). The pad is placed over the area so that it is in contact with the injured soft tissue while avoiding the bone. A circumferential or collateral compression wrap is then used to apply pressure (Fig. 3–3).

Compression and **elevation** act to decrease the hydrostatic pressure within the capillary beds and encourage absorption of edema by the lymphatic system. This effect is greatest when the extremity is at 90 degrees to the ground; however, this position is not necessarily practical. The limb should be elevated as high as possible, while still maintaining a comfortable position. Mechanical implements such as split-leg tables can effectively raise the lower extremity to a 45-degree angle, at which point the effect of gravity is 71% of that in the vertical position (see Fig. 1–5).

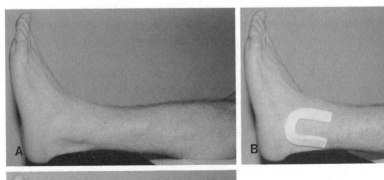
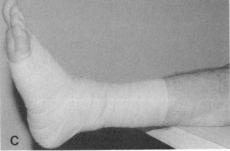

Figure 3–3. Application of Focal Compression to the Lateral Ankle Ligaments. Using a U-shaped "horseshoe," the pad is placed around the lateral malleolus, focusing the pressure on the surrounding soft tissue. The horseshoe is secured in place with an elastic wrap.

Table 3–4 **CLASSIFICATION OF HEATING AGENTS**

Superficial Heat	Deep Heat
Infrared lamps	Microwave diathermy
Moist heat packs	Shortwave diathermy
Paraffin baths	Ultrasound (Chapter 5)
Warm whirlpool and/or immersion	

CRYOKINETICS

As its name implies, cryokinetics involves the use of cold in conjunction with movement ("cryo" = cold + "kinetic" = motion). Cryokinetics is used to improve motion by eliminating or reducing the element of pain. Early, safe, pain-free motion through the normal range results in a more pronounced macrophage reaction, quicker hematoma resolution, increased vascular growth, faster regeneration of muscle and scar tissue, and increased tensile strength of healed muscle.[4]

Cryokinetics may be initiated in cases where the underlying soft tissue and bone are intact and it is pain that is limiting the amount of functional movement. Although cryokinetics is useful in increasing range of motion, care must be taken to prevent the masking of pain.

Heat Modalities

Heat, the increase in molecular vibration and cellular metabolic rate, is commonly classified into three major categories based on its source: (1) chemical action associated with cell metabolism, (2) electrical or magnetic currents as those found in diathermy devices, and (3) mechanical action as found with ultrasound (Ultrasound is presented in Chapter 5). The application of therapeutic heat to the body is referred to as **thermotherapy**, and the methods of heating are classified as being superficial or deep (Table 3–4).

The effects of heat on metabolic rate, blood and fluid dynamics, and inflammation are generally opposite to those of cold (Table 3–5). Both heat and cold application decrease pain and muscle spasm by altering the threshold of nerve endings. Systemically, local heat application results in increased body temperature, pulse rate, and respiratory rate, and a decreased blood pressure (Table

Table 3–5 **LOCAL EFFECTS OF HEAT APPLICATION**

Vasodilation
Increased rate of cell metabolism
Increased delivery of leukocytes
Increased capillary permeability
Increased venous and lymphatic drainage
Edema formation
Removal of metabolic wastes
Increased elasticity of ligaments, capsules, and muscle
Analgesia and sedation of nerves
Decreased muscle tone
Decreased muscle spasm
Perspiration
Increased nerve conduction velocity

Table 3–6 **SOME SYSTEMIC EFFECTS OF HEAT EXPOSURE**

Increased body temperature
Increased pulse rate
Increased respiratory rate
Decreased blood pressure

3–6). The use of heat is indicated in the subacute and chronic inflammatory stages of injury (Table 3–7).

Since the effects of heat application are essentially opposite to those of cold, its use in the treatment of acute injuries is to be avoided. Applying heat to an active inflammatory cycle will increase the rate of cell metabolism and accelerate the amount of hypoxic injury that occurs (Table 3–7).

EFFECT ON THE INJURY RESPONSE CYCLE

Cellular Response

The rate of cell metabolism increases in response to the rise in tissue temperature. For each increase of 18°F in skin temperature, the cell's metabolic rate increases by a factor of two to three.[20] As the cell's metabolic rate increases, so does its demand for oxygen and nutrients. As with all living organisms that consume energy, the amount of waste excreted from the cell increases as its activity increases.

There is a reciprocal relationship between tissue temperature and the rate of cell metabolism. Not only will increased temperature cause an increase in cellular metabolic rate, but an increase in cellular metabolic rate will also cause tissue temperature to rise. As with all heat applications, increased cellular metabolic rate will cause arteriolar dilation, and increased capillary flow and blood pressure. This supports the therapeutic properties of exercise.

Blood and Fluid Dynamics

The body responds to the rise in tissue temperature by dilating local blood vessels, the amount of vasodilation being greater in superficial vessels than in

Table 3–7 **GENERAL INDICATIONS AND CONTRAINDICATIONS FOR HEAT TREATMENTS**

Indications
Subacute or chronic inflammatory conditions
Reduction of subacute or chronic pain
Subacute or chronic muscle spasm
Decreased range of motion
Hematoma resolution
Reduction of joint contractures

Contraindications
Acute injuries
Impaired circulation
Poor thermal regulation
Anesthetic areas

the deeper vessels. Increased capillary flow results in an increased supply of oxygen, nutrients, and antibodies to the affected area.

The amount of edema is increased, but the capability of removing it is greater. Increased capillary pressure forces edema and harmful *metabolites* from the injured area. Increased capillary permeability aids in the reabsorption of edema and the dissolution of hematomas. These wastes then drain into the venous and lymphatic systems. If venous and lymphatic return are not encouraged, further edema forms.

Effect on Inflammation

The local application of heat serves to accelerate inflammation. Soft-tissue repair is facilitated through an accelerated metabolic rate and increased blood supply. Blood flow must be increased to encourage the removal of cellular debris and to increase delivery of the nutrients necessary for the healing of tissues.[21] Increased oxygen delivery stimulates the breakdown and removal of tissue debris and inflammatory metabolites. Nutrients are delivered to the area to fuel the cells, and there is also an increase in the delivery of leukocytes, encouraging phagocytosis.

Muscle Spasm

Increased temperature reduces the primary and secondary muscle spindles' sensitivity to stretch, decreasing the amount of muscle spasm present (see Box 1–2, page 17). Spasm is further alleviated by increasing blood flow and reducing local muscle metabolites.[1]

Range of motion is subsequently improved by increasing the extensibility of collagen. This effect alone is not sufficient to decrease contractures. Tension, in the form of gentle stretching, is necessary to elongate muscle and capsular tissues.

Pain Control

Pain transmission is stimulated by mechanical deformation and/or chemical irritation of nerve endings. In acute injuries, the primary cause of pain is the mechanical damage done to the tissue in the area. In the subacute and chronic stage of injury, chemical pain is caused by ischemia and irritation from certain chemical mediators. Mechanical pain is caused by increased tissue pressure (swelling) and the tension placed on nerves by muscle spasm. Increasing circulation to the area decreases congestion, allowing for oxygen to be delivered to the suffocating cells. Increased circulation (blood flow to and away from the area) assists in washing out the pain-producing chemicals in the area.

Mechanical pain is decreased by reducing the pressure on the nerves, thus lessening the pain-spasm pain cycle. By encouraging venous and lymphatic return through the use of elevation and muscle contraction, the swelling is removed, decreasing interstitial pressure.

An increase in temperature leads to a state of analgesia and sedation in

---

Metabolite: A by-product of metabolism.

the injured area by acting on free nerve endings. Nerve fibers are stimulated, blocking the transmission of pain with a counterirritant effect. This effect appears to last only as long as the stimulus of heat is applied and when heat is removed, the pain symptoms quickly return.[16]

DISSIPATION OF HEAT IN THE TREATED AREA

When therapeutic heat is applied to the body there is a rapid rise in skin temperature. This rise is due to the fact that energy is being absorbed faster than it can be removed by the cool blood delivered to the area. After approximately 10 to 15 minutes of exposure, the temperature gradient begins to even out. At this point the body is able to counteract the energy being applied by supplying an adequate amount of blood to cool the area. It is at this point that the athlete may claim that the modality has cooled down when, in fact, its intensity is unchanged (Fig. 3–4).

When a maximal vasodilation has occurred and the intensity of the treatment stays constant (or increases), the vessels begin to constrict. This phenomena, known as **rebound vasoconstriction**, occurs approximately 20 minutes into the treatment.[7] This is the body's attempt to save underlying tissues by

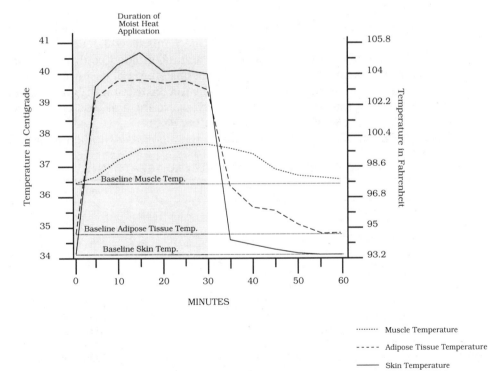

Figure 3–4. Depth of Penetration and Duration of Superficial Heating. During the application of superficial heat (moist heat pack), the skin temperature has the most significant temperature increase. Muscular temperature has the lowest temperature increase, but the increased temperature has the longest lasting effects. (Adapted from Abramson, DI, et al: Changes in Blood Flow, Oxygen Uptake, and Tissue Temperatures Produced by the Topical Application of Wet Heat. Arch Phys Med Rehabil, 42:305, 1961).

sacrificing the superficial layer. If the intensity of treatment is too great, or if the duration of exposure is too long, burns will result.

Mottling of the skin is a warning sign that tissue temperatures are rising to a dangerously high level. In this case the athlete's skin is marked by ghost-white areas and beet-red splotches. When mottling occurs, the treatment should be discontinued immediately.

The likelihood of rebound vasoconstriction occurring is greater in treatments where the temperature and intensity are kept constant. Modalities such as infrared lamps and paraffin immersion baths maintain a constant intensity throughout the treatment. With modalities such as moist heat packs, the intensity of the treatment decreases with time because the modality loses heat during the application.

Contrast and Comparison of Heat and Cold Applications

Cold modalities are more penetrating and their effects last longer than those of heat modalities. Heat causes a vasodilation that delivers cool blood to the area while the warmer blood is transported away. In contrast, cold application causes a vasoconstriction, resulting in a decreased amount of blood arriving to warm the area. This allows deeper tissues to be affected more by cold than by heat (Table 3–8).

Following the removal of the modality, the effects of cold are longer lasting than heat. This is a result of the same mechanisms which account for the depth of penetration. Following heat treatment, cool blood continues to flow to the area, decreasing the temperature. In contrast, the cool tissue temperature resulting from cold application causes the vasoconstriction of blood vessels, and a decrease in the amount of blood delivered to the area, so that a longer time is needed for rewarming than for recooling.[22]

The application of cold reduces the amounts of inflammatory mediators

Table 3–8 **COMPARISON OF HEAT AND COLD TREATMENTS**

Effect	Cold	Heat
Depth of penetration	5 cm	2 cm (superficial agents) 2–5 cm (deep-heating agents)
Duration of effects	Hours	Begins to dissipate following removal of the modality
Blood flow	Decreased (Vasoconstriction)	Increased (Vasodilation)
Rate of cell metabolism	Decreased	Increased
Oxygen consumption	Decreased	Increased
Cell wastes	Decreased	Increased
Fluid viscosity	Increased	Decreased
Capillary permeability	Decreased	Increased
Inflammation	Decreased	Increased
Pain	Decreased	Decreased
Muscle spasm	Decreased by reducing the sensitivity of muscle spindles and by decreasing pain	Decreased by reducing ischemia and pain
Muscle contraction velocity	Decreased by reducing nerve conduction velocity and increasing fluid viscosity	Increased

and cell by-products released into the area. These cellular wastes, including **lactic acid** and nitrogen, are insulting to the tissues, and increase the amount of tissue damage and pain.

When to Use Heat Versus Cold

One of the most asked questions by student athletic trainers is, "How do you know when to use heat and when to use cold?" There are no clear-cut answers to this question. Many texts and articles give definitive time frames, such as, "Use ice for the first 24 hours and heat for the next 48." Unfortunately, statements like this are incorrect and unjustified.

One of the first points made in this text was that the body heals an injury at its own rate. Not only does this rate vary from person to person, but it may vary from injury to injury with the same person. Factors such as the physical and psychological state of the athlete, as well as the type and proportion of tissue damaged, all factor into the time frame required for healing.

The decision-making process is similar to the steps involved when a pipe ruptures in the basement of a house. Before bailing out the water and cleaning up the mess, you have to stop the leak. Likewise, before encouraging an increase in the rate of cell metabolism in an injured area, the active process of inflammation must be calmed down.

Cold application is indicated (1) when the inflammatory reaction is in its acute stages, (2) prior to range of motion exercises, and (3) following physical activity. Heat application is indicated (1) when the inflammatory reaction is in its subacute or chronic stages, (2) to encourage tissue healing, (3) to reduce edema and ecchymosis, (4) to assist range of motion prior to physical activity (e.g., participation in the sport), and (5) to fight infection.

A distinction should be made between using cold modalities for range of motion exercises and using heat modalities prior to competition. As you will recall, cold increases fluid viscosity and decreases the ability to perform rapid movements. During the participation in a sport, the athlete relies on the ability to move the extremities in a rapid, powerful manner. Heat is used for its ability to allow this type of movement. Ice is indicated following the activity to prevent the inflammatory process from being reactivated.

The decision about when to use heat and cold should not be based on any predetermined time frame. This decision should be based on the desired physiological responses at any one point in time. When the desired goal is to limit or reduce the amount of inflammation, cold should be used. When the inflammatory response has subsided to the point where tissue healing begins, heat is applied. When in doubt, use cold.

Although to a lesser degree, the athlete's preference of modalities may be considered. Some athletes prefer the use of cold modalities, but more commonly, the use of heat is preferred. The change from cold to heat is, in the minds of many athletes, a milestone signaling that their healing process is progressing.

Summary

The physiological effects of heat or cold application are the result of the body's attempt to adjust to the temperature. Several considerations must be made to determine which temperature must be used in the treatment of athletic injuries. Immediate treatment of injuries involves the use of ice, compression, elevation, and rest, a procedure that serves to limit the scope of the original injury. While the inflammatory process is in its active state, or the tissues are ischemic, cold application is used primarily to decrease the amount of secondary hypoxic injury by reducing the cells' need for oxygen. Additional benefits are gained through cold application in the form of pain relief and decreased muscle spasm.

Heat application may be initiated when the inflammation process is in a more passive mode. The increased temperature accelerates the rate at which blood and nutrients are delivered to the injured tissues. The increased capillary pressure forces edema and metabolites from the area, and their removal from the area is augmented by increased capillary permeability. By decreasing the amount of mechanical pressure placed on nerve endings and supplying oxygen to the tissues, pain is reduced.

Clinical Application of Cold Modalities

ICE PACKS

Ice packs are found in three forms: (1) plastic bags filled with crushed or flaked ice, (2) reusable cold gel packs, and (3) chemical (or "instant") cold packs where the sensation of cold is produced by a chemical reaction. Each method of cold application has its own advantages and disadvantages.

Without question, **ice bags** are the most commonly used modality in athletic training. They are easy, efficient, and safe to use. The requirements are only plastic bags and either flaked or cubed ice. Some athletic trainers substitute plastic bags with reusable rubber bags (English ice bags). A drawback of this method of cold application is that ice machines are expensive and their cost may be prohibitive in some situations.

Reusable cold packs contain a gel consisting of *silica*, water, and a form of antifreeze sealed in a plastic pouch. When not in use, these packs are stored in a cooling unit. Although a convenient method for cold application in the athletic training room, their effectiveness is diminished when they are stored in an ice chest for long periods of time.

In the case of reusable cold packs the athletic trainer should be aware of the possibility of frostbite. Since this method of cold application does not involve the true use of ice (i.e., frozen water), it may lower the skin below the freezing point. To prevent frostbite, a medium such as one layer of wet toweling or a wet elastic wrap, should be placed between the pack and the skin. The liquid medium will help moderate the cold, yet still provide an effective treatment.

Care must be taken to avoid overinsulating the area. One or two layers of

---

Silica: A finely ground form of sand capable of holding water.

dry toweling will serve as good protection against frostbite. Care must also be taken to avoid adding so much insulation that the effects of cold will not reach the skin.

Instant cold packs contain two chemicals that are separated from each other by a plastic barrier. When the seal between them is ruptured, they are allowed to mix causing a chemical reaction, which produces cold. The degree of cold produced and the short duration of the reaction give them a workable life of only a few minutes. Instant cold packs are convenient in that they may be stored in the athletic trainer's kit for emergency use. These packs may be used only once and must be properly disposed of after use.

When mixed, the chemicals contained in instant cold packs are extremely caustic to the skin. If a pack should develop a leak, discard it immediately and rinse the athlete's skin with running water. For this reason, do not use instant cold packs on the athlete's face.

Effect on the Injury Response Cycle

The application of ice packs decreases tissue temperature, resulting in a decrease in cellular metabolic rate. Muscle spasm is diminished by lowering the transmission rate of nerve impulses and increasing the pain threshold. The decreased release of inflammatory mediators occurs as a result of the reduced rate of cell metabolism and reduced blood flow.

In acute injuries, the most beneficial effect of cold application is to reduce the need for oxygen. More cells are able to survive in the oxygen-starved environment because of their decreased metabolic rate. When coupled with compression and elevation, the edema in the area is reduced. These factors serve to limit the scope of the original injury and reduce the amount of secondary hypoxic injury.

Setup and Application

Ice Bags

1. Fill the bag with enough ice to last for the duration of the treatment, but avoid overfilling. If the bag becomes too full, it cannot be molded to the body part.
2. Many body parts will require more than one bag to fully cover the area.
3. In acute injuries, or when compression is desired, wet an elastic wrap and apply one layer around the injured area. (Some athletic trainers keep a tub of cold "wet wraps" in the refrigerator for this purpose.)
4. Apply the ice bags over the injured area. Secure in place with an elastic wrap.

Reusable Cold Packs

1. Select a pack large enough to cover the injured area or use multiple packs.
2. Cover the area to be treated with a wet towel or wet elastic wrap. *At no time should a fully cooled reusable cold pack be allowed to come into contact with the athlete's skin.* Equally important, do not over-insulate the area. Too much toweling may decrease the heat flow from the skin to the point of ineffectiveness.

3. Secure the pack in place with an elastic wrap.
4. Check the athlete regularly for signs of frostbite.

Instant Cold Packs

1. Shake the bag so that the contents are evenly distributed.
2. Squeeze the bag to break the inner pouch.
3. Shake the bag to thoroughly mix the contents.
4. If indicated on the instructions of the particular brand of chemical cold pack you are using, place a wet towel between the pack and the athlete's skin.
5. Secure in place with an elastic wrap.

Duration of Treatment

Treatment times range from 15 to 30 minutes and may be repeated as needed. Because of the lasting effects of cold treatments, application should be no less than 2 hours apart. In the immediate care of injuries, keep the body part wrapped and elevated between treatments.

Precautions

- Some areas, such as the acromioclavicular joint, are not practical for wet wraps. A moist towel or thin sponge may be substituted. The cold packs may then be held in place with dry wraps.
- The tension of the elastic wrap should be enough to provide adequate compression. Avoid unwanted pressure. This is especially true in cases where fractures are suspected. Check the distal extremity (fingers, toes) to assure that adequate circulation is maintained.
- Check the athlete for frostbite. Even though the chance of frostbite occurring with the use of ice bags is slim, athletes with impaired circulation are at a higher risk.
- Application of ice packs over large superficial nerves (e.g., peroneal or ulnar nerves) has been reported to cause neuropathy in isolated cases.

Indications

- Acute injury or inflammation
- Acute or chronic pain
- Postsurgical pain and edema

Contraindications

- Cardiac or respiratory involvement
- Uncovered open wounds
- Circulatory insufficiency
- Cold allergy and/or hypersensitivity
- Anesthetized skin

ICE MASSAGE

Ice massage is an appropriate method of delivering cold treatments to small, evenly shaped areas. It is most effective in cases involving muscle spasm, contusions, and other minor injuries. In many cases the athletes may treat themselves, releasing the athletic trainer to perform other tasks. This method of cold application is a convenient, practical, and time-efficient method of providing cold treatments in situations where there is not ready access to an ice machine.

Effect on the Injury Response Cycle

In addition to the effects associated with the application of ice packs, the massaging action of this treatment assists in decreasing pain and muscle spasm. The sensation of movement stimulates large-diameter nerves, inhibiting the transmission of pain, allowing for a break in the pain-spasm pain cycle.

Ice massage is not the treatment of choice for acute injuries. It has been reported that ice massage increases blood flow[10] and since no compression is available during the treatment, the amount of hemorrhage and edema may be increased. In the event that this is the only form of ice available at the time of the injury, additional steps must be taken to limit the amount of swelling. The injured body part should be wrapped with an elastic bandage and elevated to reduce edema following the treatment.

Setup and Application

1. Ice cups are made by filling paper cups three quarters full and storing them in a freezer.
2. The body part to be treated is surrounded with toweling to collect water runoff.
3. The ice is slowly massaged over the injured area in overlapping strokes or circles.
4. The paper must be continually removed to prevent it from rubbing on the skin.

Duration of Treatment

The standard treatment time is 10 to 15 minutes, or until the ice runs out. If the purpose of the ice massage is to produce numbness, the treatment may be discontinued when the athlete's skin is insensitive to your touch. These treatments may be repeated as necessary.

Precautions

- In some injuries, the pressure of the massage may be contraindicated.

Indications

- Subacute injury or inflammation
- Muscle strains

- Contusions
- Acute or chronic pain

Contraindications

- Cases in which the pressure on the injury is contraindicated
- Suspected fractures
- Uncovered open wounds
- Circulatory insufficiency
- Cold allergy and/or hypersensitivity
- Anesthetized skin

ICE IMMERSION

Ice immersion (ice slush or ice bath) involves placing the body part into a mixture of ice and water having a temperature range of 50°F to 60°F. This type of treatment is useful with those injuries involving a relatively small, irregular surface.

This is a very uncomfortable method of cold application, especially when the fingers or toes are immersed. A higher degree of pain is experienced with this treatment because of the increased surface area exposed to the cold. When the fingers or toes are immersed, they are exposed to cold across their circumference and at the distal end. Since their diameter is small, the effects of cold penetrate to the core. Another factor which may account for the increased pain experienced is stimulation of the lumina in the nailbed. This is a hypersensitive area that may be overstimulated by the presence of cold. This hypothesis may be tested on yourself by simply applying pressure with your thumbnail on the white crescent in your opposite thumbnail. When the fingers or toes are not the target of the treatment, the use of *neoprene* covering makes this treatment more tolerable.[23]

Athletes adapt to the temperature-related discomfort associated with ice immersion. As the athlete is exposed to multiple immersion treatments, the reported level of discomfort is reduced.[24]

Effects on the Injury Response Cycle

The effects of ice immersion are as described in the general effects of cold application. The intensity of cold is greater with ice immersion because of the large surface area being treated. Therefore, the resultant drop in skin and subcutaneous temperature is more pronounced than with other forms of cold application.[3] The sensory stimulation associated with ice application is enhanced. It has been reported that ankles immersed in cold water have decreased proprioceptive ability.[25] Caution should be used when ice immersion is applied prior to active exercise.

The use of ice immersion places the limb in a dependent position, increasing the hydrostatic pressure within the capillaries. This encourages the leakage of fluids into the interstitial space, resulting in increased edema. Following the

---

Neoprene: A synthetic rubber material.

treatment of acute or subacute injuries, the limb should be wrapped and elevated to encourage venous and lymphatic drainage.

Ice immersion can be used in conjunction with electrical stimulation as a form of immediate treatment. Although the effects of electrical stimulation in acute injuries are debatable (refer to Chapter 4), the limb should be wrapped and elevated following the treatment.

Setup and Application

1. Prepare a bucket, tub, or any container with cold water and ice. The temperature will be dependent on the athlete's tolerance. Generally, athletes who have had repeated exposure to this treatment can tolerate a lower temperature. Another approach is to start the athlete at a tolerable temperature and add ice as the treatment progresses.
2. The temperature of the treatment should be inversely related to the size of the body area being treated (Fig. 3–5). As the size of the area is increased, the temperature of the water is decreased.

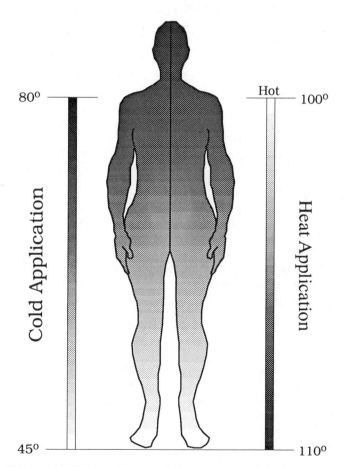

Figure 3–5. Relationship Between Treatment Temperature and the Percentage of the Body Immersed. During cold immersion, the temperature of the water increases as the percentage of the body immersed increases. During hot immersion, the temperature of the water decreases as the percentage of the body immersed increases.

3. Colder treatment temperatures may be tolerated if the fingers or toes are insulated from the water by neoprene "toe caps."

Duration of Treatment

This treatment is continued for 10 to 20 minutes. Lower treatment temperatures require a shorter duration. This treatment may be repeated as needed, with proper rewarming time allotted between treatments.

Precautions

- Ice immersion is the most uncomfortable of all the cold treatments. Beware of athletes passing out during the treatment.
- Avoid having the athlete continually immerse and withdraw the body part from the slush. During the initial minute or so, the cold will cause a burning or aching sensation. Explain to the athlete the treatment will be uncomfortable for a few minutes, but numbness will soon follow. If the limb is repeatedly removed and then reimmersed, it only increases the duration of pain.
- Since the limb is placed in a gravity dependent position, the limb should be wrapped and elevated following the treatment.

Indications

- Acute injury or inflammation
- Acute or chronic pain
- Postsurgical pain and edema

Contraindications

- Cardiac or respiratory involvement (see precautionary note, p. 55)
- Uncovered open wounds
- Circulatory insufficiency
- Cold allergy and/or hypersensitivity
- Anesthetized skin
- ABSOLUTE inability to tolerate the cold temperature

CRYOSTRETCH

The effects of cold application and passive stretching are combined in the cryostretch technique, leading to its alternate name, "spray-and-stretch." A vapocoolant spray is used to rapidly decrease the temperature of the skin and decrease pain transmission. This is combined with simultaneous passive stretching to relieve local muscle spasm. This effectively reduces the amount of pain and spasm associated with strains and trigger points. A chart of trigger point pain patterns is presented in Appendix A.

Cryostretch has traditionally been performed with ethyl chloride. When applied to the skin this agent quickly evaporates and cools the superficial tissue. Ethyl chloride possesses many inherent dangers: it is highly flammable, it acts as a general anesthetic if inhaled, and because of the severe temperature drop, it has a high potential for frostbite. Because of these risks, ethyl chloride has been replaced by fluoromethane spray, as it is less volatile and has a smaller cooling effect.[26]

Effect on the Injury Response Cycle

The effect of cold sprays is limited to that of a counterirritant. The evaporation of the coolant on the skin causes cooling in a manner that elicits a localized inflammatory response. In turn, this stimulus "masks" the previous pain by reducing the intensity and speed of pain transmission. Vapocoolant sprays have not been found to cause the cellular and vascular responses of other forms of cold application. The passive stretching assists in breaking the pain-spasm pain cycle by lengthening the muscle fibers.

Setup and Application

1. Position the athlete so that the treated muscle group being treated may be easily stretched.
2. The nozzle of the bottle should be approximately 12 inches above the skin. The spray should strike the skin at an acute angle of about 30 degrees to 45 degrees.
3. Spray the entire muscle length in a sweeping manner. The spray should be in one direction only. The speed of the sweep should allow the tissue to become covered, but not frosted.
4. Apply pressure to passively stretch the muscle group. Come to, but do not exceed, the point of pain.
5. Allow the tissue to rewarm.
6. Continue for two or three more sweeps with increasing stretch on the muscle. Allow the tissue to rewarm between each sweep.
7. Repeat until the desired amount of stretch has occurred.
8. The cryostretch treatment may be followed by a moist heat treatment or massage.[13]

Duration of Treatment

The treatment proceeds through three or four sweeps, with sufficient time for the tissue to rewarm between sprays. Treatments are given once a day.

Precautions

- Cold sprays are capable of causing frostbite if improperly used.
- If ethyl chloride is used:
  - It is extremely flammable. Avoid using it around possible sources of ignition, including smoking and electrical sparks.
  - Ethyl chloride is a local anesthetic. However, if the athlete breathes the fumes, it very quickly becomes a general anesthetic.[27]
- The use of vapocoolant sprays in the treatment of acute injuries is generally based on tradition rather than fact. While the evaporation of the liquid rapidly cools the skin and produces temporary pain relief, the other physiological effects of cold application are not achieved.

Indications

- Trigger points
- Muscle spasm
- Decreased range of motion

Contraindications

- Allergy to the spray
- Acute and/or postsurgical injury
- Open wounds
- Contraindications relating to cold applications
- Contraindications relating to passive stretching
- Use around the eyes. When treating the upper extremity, torso, or neck, protect the athlete's eyes from the spray.

COLD AND/OR HOT WHIRLPOOLS

Whirlpools are an effective method of applying heat or cold to an irregularly shaped area. Energy is transferred to or from the body by means of convection. The presence of water creates a good supportive medium for active range of motion exercises. With slow-moving exercises, the buoyancy of the limb assists motion. When exercises are performed more rapidly, the water creates a resistance to movement. The agitation and aeration of the water, provided by the turbine, provides a massaging effect resulting in sedation, analgesia, and increased circulation.

Whirlpools are characterized by the use of a turbine that regulates the water flow and the amount of air introduced into the flow (aeration). Water is introduced through an inlet on the turbine's stem where the motor forces it back into the tub causing agitation of the water (the "whirlpool" effect). Air is also introduced into the stream causing bubbles to circulate in the tank. The agitation and aeration are controlled by separate valves and can be adjusted to produce a wide range of effects (Fig. 3–6).

There is a significant relationship between the temperature of the water and the proportion of the body area being treated. In cold whirlpool treatments the temperature is increased as the body area being treated increases. In hot whirlpool treatments the temperature of the water is decreased as the total body area increases (see Fig. 3–5). In cold whirlpool treatments, the body may be placed in a state of hypothermia if too large a body area is cooled too rapidly.

When the temperature of the water is equal to or greater than the body temperature, heat loss can only occur through evaporation and respiration. If the athlete's core temperature is increased too greatly, *hyperthermia* may result. This should be remembered if the athlete is receiving a near-total body immersion. In this case, the athlete can only lose heat through the head and breathing, increasing the risk of heat stress.

Hyperthermia: Increased core temperature.

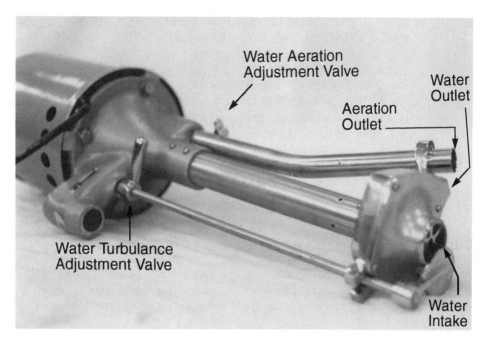

Figure 3–6. A Whirlpool Turbine. Note the position of the turbulance and aeration valves and the water intake port. The water is driven through the turbine and returned to the tub under pressure. The aeration outlet is in front of the water outlet, forcing bubbles to flow in the water.

Cold whirlpool treatments are not recommended for the care of acute injuries. Since the limb is placed in a gravity-dependent position, venous return is not promoted. The additional stimulation of the flowing water may cause an increase in edema. If this method of acute injury management is unavoidable, a compression wrap should be applied and the body part should be elevated following the treatment.

If open wounds are being treated (or if they happen to be present on the treated site) the tank should be cleaned with an appropriate disinfectant. The tank is filled with water and a disinfectant is added. Following the treatment, the tank should again be drained and cleaned. Only stainless steel tubs should be used for wound cleansing and/or debridement as tile tubs or spa-type whirlpools may harbor germs, and are much more difficult to clean properly.

Effect on the Injury Response Cycle

The effects of hot and cold whirlpools are as described in their appropriate sections. Most notably, hot whirlpools promote muscle relaxation and cold whirlpools decrease muscle spasm and muscle spasticity. An additional effect of the turbulence from the flowing water is the creation of a sedative and analgesic effect on sensory nerves.

Setup and Application

1. Instruct the athlete not to turn the whirlpool on or off, or touch any electrical connections while in the whirlpool or while the body is wet.
2. Fill the whirlpool to a depth sufficient enough to cover the area being

treated. Most turbines have a minimum depth. Be sure the amount of water is enough to run the motor safely.

3. Add a whirlpool disinfectant.
4. Adjust the temperature for the type of effect desired and the proportion of the body being treated.
5. If an extremity is being treated, position the athlete in a comfortable position using either a high chair or a whirlpool bench. If the entire body is being immersed, use a whirlpool stool or sling seat.
6. Turn the turbine on and adjust the turbulence. With subacute injuries, do not focus the turbulence directly on the affect area.
7. Athletes receiving full-body treatments, whether hot or cold, must be monitored continuously.

Duration and Frequency of Treatment

Initial whirlpool treatments are given for 5 to 10 minutes. The duration of treatments may be increased to 20 to 30 minutes as the program progresses. Treatments may be given once or twice a day.

Precautions

- The whirlpool must be connected to a ground fault interrupter (see Chapter 7).
- Instruct the athlete not to turn the whirlpool motor on or off while in the water. Ideally, the switch to the motor should be out of the athlete's reach from the whirlpool.
- Athletes who are receiving whirlpool treatments should be in view of the athletic training staff.
- Because of the discomfort associated with cold immersions, the treatment may be started at a comfortable, yet cool temperature. Decrease the temperature gradually during the treatment by adding cold water.
- The combination of increased circulation and placement of the extremity in a gravity-dependent position tends to increase edema.
- Range of motion exercises will increase blood flow in the deep muscle layers.
- Do not run the whirlpool turbine dry.
- Some athletes, especially those prone to motion sickness, may become nauseated by the flowing water.

Indications

- Subacute or chronic inflammatory conditions
- *Peripheral vascular disease*
- Peripheral nerve injuries

Peripheral Vascular Disease: Actually a syndrome describing an insufficiency of arteries and/or veins for maintaining proper circulation (also known as PVD).

Contraindications

- Acute conditions where water turbulence would further irritate the injured area or the limb is placed in a gravity-dependent position
- Fever (in hot whirlpool)
- Athletes requiring postural support during treatment
- Skin conditions in spa-type tubs. Otherwise, follow cleaning instructions noted on page 77.

CONTRAST BATHS

A contrast bath consists of alternating immersion in warm and cold water. Either stationary water or tandem whirlpools may be used for the application. This action results in a kind of vascular exercise causing a cycle of vasoconstrictions and vasodilations of the blood vessels in the area. This "pumping" action stimulates peripheral blood flow and aids in venous and lymphatic return. Contrast baths are an effective method of making the transition from cryotherapy to thermotherapy. This treatment may also increase circulation in the *contralateral* limb.[28]

Contrast baths are most commonly indicated in subacute or chronic conditions for the removal of edema and/or ecchymosis. The most effective time ratio between hot and cold has not been determined, but the most commonly used ratios are 3:1 and 4:1 (hot:cold).

The treatment may end following either the hot or cold immersion, depending on the stage of the injury, the desired effect of the treatment, and the athlete's participation plans following the treatment. When a state of vasoconstriction is desired, the treatment is terminated after a cold immersion. If vasodilation is desired, the treatment is terminated after a warm immersion. In subacute conditions, it is generally beneficial to finish the treatment with a cold immersion. In chronic conditions, the bout is most often ended following the warm immersion.

Effect on the Injury Response Cycle

The exact effects on cellular responses from contrast baths are not clear. The cellular metabolic rate increases or decreases in response to the temperature of the treatment. As a consequence, the series of vasodilations and vasoconstrictions increases circulation in both the treated and opposite extremity. The resulting influx of new blood assists in removing edema by unclogging the vasculature.

Setup and Application

1. Position the tubs as close together as possible without touching. ("Tubs" will refer to either immersion buckets or whirlpool tanks.) The athlete should be able remove the body part from one tub and immediately immerse it in the other.

Contralateral: Pertaining to the opposite side of the body. The left side is contralateral to the right.

2. Fill one tub with water in the range from 105° to 110°F and the other with water between 45°F and 60°F.
3. Position the athlete on a chair or bench in a manner requiring a minimal amount of motion from tub to tub. The athlete should have a clock or watch to time the treatment segments.
4. In most cases, heat treatments are given first.
5. Have the athlete alternate between the treatments according to the protocol being applied.
6. As with all hot or cold treatments, the athlete should be monitored.
7. The treatment ends following the hot immersion if relaxation and vasodilation are desired, or the cold immersion if vasoconstriction is desired.

Duration of Treatment

Contrast baths are given for 20 to 30 minutes and may be repeated as needed.

Precautions

- The same care taken with whirlpool treatments should be applied to contrast baths.

Indications

- Ecchymosis removal
- Edema removal
- Subacute or chronic inflammatory conditions
- Impaired circulation

Contraindications

- Acute injuries
- Hypersensitivity to cold
- Contraindications relative to whirlpool use
- Contraindications relative to cold applications
- Contraindications relative to heat applications

Clinical Application of Heat Modalities

MOIST HEAT PACKS

The moist heat pack is a canvas pouch filled with silica gel or a similar substance capable of absorbing a large number of water molecules. This pack is kept in a water-filled heating unit that is maintained at a constant temperature ranging between 160°F and 170°F.[29,30] These packs are capable of maintaining a workable temperature for 30 to 45 minutes after removal from the heating unit.

Moist heat packs are a superficial heat modality. Energy is transferred to the athlete's skin by way of conduction. Each subsequent tissue layer is heated through conduction from the overlying tissue. However, deep tissues are not generally considered to be affected by this treatment because of the large amount of superficial absorption that occurs.

The layering around the hot pack (see Setup) serves as an insulation between the pack and the skin. When the pack is placed on the athlete, there is little compression of the protective covering. This allows air pockets to form within the layering, providing additional insulation. If the hot pack is compressed, such as when the athlete is lying on it, the layering is moved together and the air is forced out of the spaces. This decreases the available insulation and increases the amount of energy being transferred, increasing the chance of burns.

Moist hot packs are suitable for use over localized areas or on areas that normally cannot be treated by immersion in water (the neck, for example). Because of the variations in size, the packs are adaptable for use over the lumbar spine (medium or large size), the cervical spine (cervical pack), the shoulder (medium size), and the knee (medium size). The effectiveness of the moist heat pack is diminished when used over irregular areas such as the ankle or fingers.

Effect on the Injury Response Cycle

The specific effects of moist heat packs are the same as described for heat in general. When compared to dry heat, moist heat is considered to be a more comfortable method of application, and may have greater benefit in reducing pain.

The application of moist heat packs results in a rapid increase in the surface temperature of the athlete's skin. As a result of vasodilation, there is an influx of blood to the area in an attempt to cool the tissues. The vasodilation, increased blood flow, and increased pulse volume associated with thermotherapy have been shown to occur only while the hot packs are in contact with the body.[10]

During the course of the treatment there is an increase of 4°F in the tissues 1 cm beneath the skin[12] and the effects may penetrate to depths of 2 cm. Moist heat leads to a relaxation of the superficial muscle layer. When treating obese individuals, the athletic trainer may find that hot packs are less effective in raising subcutaneous tissue temperature because fat tissue serves as an insulation.

Setup and Application

1. Cover the pack with a commercial terry cloth covering or fold a terry cloth towel so that there are five or six layers of towel between the pack and the athlete.
2. Place the pack on the athlete in a comfortable manner. If having the athlete lie on the pack is unavoidable, add additional toweling.
3. Check the athlete after the first 5 minutes for comfort and mottling. Adjust the toweling if needed.
4. Some clinicians will replace the hot pack every 8 to 10 minutes to maintain a maximal treatment temperature.[12] If this method of application is chosen, beware of rebound vasoconstriction.
5. Following the treatment, return the moist heat pack to the heating unit and allow it to reheat for 30 to 45 minutes before reuse.

Duration of Treatment

Moist heat packs are commonly used in treatment bouts of 20 to 30 minutes. The treatments may be repeated as needed, but sufficient time should be allowed for the skin to cool before the next treatment is given.

Precautions

- Do not allow the moist heat pack to come into direct contact with the skin as burns may result.
- If the packs are changed during the course of the treatment, additional care must be taken to prevent burns.
- Infected areas must be covered with sterile gauze or another type of material to collect seepage.

Indications

- Subacute or chronic inflammatory conditions
- Reduction of subacute or chronic pain
- Subacute or chronic muscle spasm
- Decreased range of motion
- Hematoma resolution
- Reduction of joint contractures
- Infection—When treating infection, cover the skin with sterile gauze. Following the treatment, dispose of the gauze in a biowaste container and wash the hot pack's cover according to the Universal Precautions (see Chapter 7: Bloodborne Pathogens, page 262).

Contraindications

- Acute conditions—this will increase the inflammatory response in the area.
- Peripheral vascular disease—the heat cannot be dissipated, thus increasing the chance of burns.
- Impaired circulation
- Poor thermal regulation

PARAFFIN BATH

A paraffin bath contains a mixture of wax and mineral oil in a ratio of seven parts wax to one part oil (7:1). Melted paraffin is kept at a constant temperature of 118°F to 126°F for upper extremity treatments (Fig. 3–7). Temperatures for treatments given to the lower extremity are decreased (113°F to 121°F) because the circulation is less efficient.[7] Because of its low specific heat (0.5 to 0.65), paraffin can provide approximately six times the amount of heat as water. Consequently, the paraffin feels cooler and is more tolerable than water at the same temperature (see Chapter 2: Heat as a Physical Entity, page 46).

Paraffin is a superficial agent used for delivering heat to small, irregularly shaped areas such as the hand, fingers, wrist, and foot. Although its use in sports medicine is limited, it is an effective method for delivering heat. The application of paraffin is beneficial in chronic conditions where range of motion is not an essential part of the treatment protocol, as with cases of arthritis or chronic inflammatory conditions.

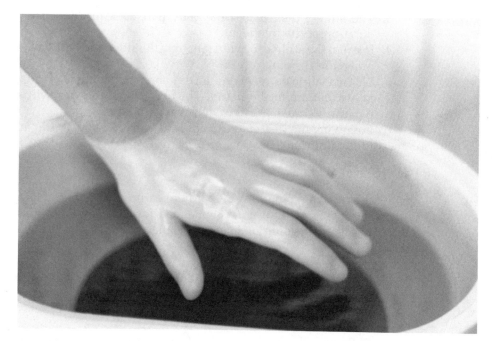

Figure 3–7. Paraffin Application. The normally translucent paraffin mixture turns a dull white color when it dries.

Effect on the Injury Response Cycle

In addition to the standard effects of heat application, paraffin increases perspiration at the treated area and serves to soften and moisturize the skin.

Setup and Application

There are several methods of paraffin application, each with its own advantages and disadvantages. The more common methods, immersion and glove, are discussed in this text. In addition to providing heat to the area, the paraffin wax may act as an insulator if it is allowed to dry on the skin. With this in mind, the athletic trainer may vary the amount of heat delivered by increasing or decreasing the wax layers. During immersion baths, the amount of insulation is increased with the number of layers added.

Preparation for Treatment

To avoid contamination of the mixture, the body part to be treated should be thoroughly cleaned and dried prior to treatment.

Immersion Bath

This is the best method for raising tissue temperature. However, the chance of burns is increased, so the athlete must be closely monitored.

1. The athlete begins by dipping the body part into the paraffin and removing it. Allow this coat to dry (it will turn a dull shade of white).
2. Dip the extremity into the wax six to twelve more times to develop the amount of insulation necessary. Allow the wax to dry between dips.

3. The athlete then places the body part back into the paraffin for the duration of the treatment.
4. Instruct the athlete to avoid touching the sides and bottom of the heating unit as burns may result.
5. Instruct athletes receiving an immersion treatment not to move the joints that are in the liquid. The cracking of the wax will allow fresh paraffin to touch the skin, increasing the risk of burns.
6. Following the treatment, scrape off the hardened paraffin and return it to the unit for reheating, or discard it.

Pack (Glove) Method

The least effective method for delivering heat to the body, the glove method, is the safest. This method is recommended for those athletes who are in the subacute stage of healing or have a vascular or nerve condition that would predispose them to burning.

1. Begin the treatment by immersing the extremity in the wax so that it becomes completely covered. Remove the body part and allow the wax to dry.
2. Continue to dip and remove the body part in the wax seven to twelve times.
3. Following the final withdrawal from the wax, cover the extremity with a plastic bag, aluminum foil, or wax paper. Then wrap and secure a terry cloth towel around the area.
4. Following the treatment, remove the towel and inner layering. Scrape off the hardened paraffin and return it to the bath for reheating, or dispose of it.

Duration of Treatment

Paraffin treatments are given for 15 to 20 minutes and may be repeated several times daily.

Precautions

- The sensation of the paraffin is misleading to the actual temperature of the treatment. The temperature of the paraffin is sufficient to cause burns, but its specific heat and thermal capacity require a longer period of time to transfer the energy (see Chapter 2).
- Avoid using paraffin with athletes who will be required to catch or throw a ball following the treatment (e.g., basketball players, wide receivers). The mineral oil in the paraffin mixture tends to make the hands slippery, making the task of catching a ball difficult.

Indications

- Subacute and chronic inflammatory conditions
- Limitation of motion following immobilization

Contraindications

- Open wounds—wax and oil would irritate the tissues.
- Skin infections—the warm, dark environment is excellent for breeding bacteria.
- Sensory loss
- Peripheral vascular disease

INFRARED LAMP

Infrared generators provide radiant energy for superficial heating of the athlete's tissues. It is considered to be a radiant modality because no medium is required to transmit the energy. There are two types of infrared generators, near infrared (luminous) and far infrared (nonluminous). The treatment energy is produced by passing an electrical current through a carbon or tungsten filament. The intensity of the treatment is controlled by adjusting the current flow through the filament, or by changing the distance between the lamp and the tissues.

Luminous generators produce some degree of visible light, placing them on the "near" end of the infrared spectrum (see Chapter 2, page 43). Since visible light is present, some of the treatment energy is reflected by the surface of the skin. Nonluminous generators do not produce visible light, placing them on the "far" end of the infrared spectrum.

Nonluminous infrared radiation is less penetrating than luminous, with effects 2 millimeters, and 5 to 10 millimeters, beneath the surface of the skin, respectively. Because nonluminous infrared is less penetrating, the skin being treated will feel warmer than with a luminous generator.

With the wide range of heating modalities available to the athletic trainer, infrared generators are not common in sports medicine settings. Infrared radiation was once thought to assist in the healing of open wounds such as turf-burns. Researchers have concluded that this practice is detrimental to the healing process as it dehydrates the tissues.[31]

Effect on the Injury Response Cycle

Infrared radiation heats the skin almost exclusively. Deeper tissues are heated by conduction to depths up to 1 cm. The primary physiological effects occur almost entirely in the superficial skin. Hyperemia occurs as a result of increased capillary flow and increased capillary pressure.

Setup and Application*

1. Warm up the lamp if necessary.
2. To prevent the concentration of heat, clean the area of any sweat, dirt, or oils, and remove any jewelry.
3. Position the athlete in a comfortable manner. Drape the body part so that only the area to be treated is exposed.

---

*Consult the user's manual of your particular modality

4. If a moist heat treatment is desired, place a damp terry cloth towel over the area.
5. Place the lamp so that the source of the heat is approximately 24 inches away from the athlete. Adjust the lamp so the energy will strike the tissues at a right angle.
6. To prevent burns, instruct the athlete not to move.
7. Check the athlete's comfort periodically. The intensity of the treatment may be adjusted by moving the lamp towards or away from the skin.
8. Instruct the athlete to summon assistance if the intensity of the treatment becomes too great.

Duration of Treatment

The treatment time is 20 to 30 minutes and may be given as needed.

Indications

- Subacute or chronic inflammatory conditions
- Skin infections
- Peripheral nerve injuries prior to electrical stimulation

Contraindications

- Acute conditions
- Peripheral vascular disease
- Areas with sensory loss or scarring
- Sunburns

SHORTWAVE DIATHERMY

Shortwave diathermy (SWD) is a deep-heating modality. The energy is similar to broadcast radio waves but has a shorter wavelength. The frequencies of 13.56, 27.12, and 40.61 Hz have been reserved for medical use by the Federal Communication Commission (FCC). One of two therapeutic diathermies, shortwave diathermy is more prevalent in the treatment of musculoskeletal injuries than its counterpart, microwave diathermy (see Box 3–2 and Fig. 3–8).

High-frequency electromagnetic energy is absorbed by the athlete's tissues and converted into heat. Shortwave diathermy creates the movement of ions by introducing an electromagnetic field having strong positive and negative poles. Free ions within this field are attracted to the pole having the opposite charge and are repelled from the pole having the like charge. Some molecules have ions that are capable of moving only within the cell membrane. This results in a *dipole* action where the ions within the membrane align themselves along the charges (Fig. 3–9).[32] The heating effect occurs as a result of friction between the moving ions and the surrounding tissues.

Structures with high water content, such as adipose tissue, blood, and muscle, are selectively heated. This heating occurs at depths of 2 to 5 cm. Local

---

Dipole: A pair of equal and opposite charges separated by a distance.

Box 3-2 **MICROWAVE DIATHERMY**

Microwave diathermy (MWD) is a deep-heating modality that converts high-frequency electromagnetic energy into heat. The FCC has reserved 915 Hz and 2450 Hz for the medical use of MWD. Although similar to shortwave diathermy, there are differences between the two.

Electrical fields are predominant with MWD, in contrast to the magnetic fields that predominate in SWD. Heating occurs by creating a dipole response within the cell membrane. The rotation of these molecules causes friction, resulting in heat production. Because of the spreading of the radio waves and absorption of the energy, superficial tissues tend to be heated more than deeper tissues.

Microwave diathermy produces biophysical effects similar to those of SWD, but the treatment is more superficial because the microwave radiation cannot penetrate the fat layer to the same extent as shortwave radiation. Since the energy is collected by the adipose tissue, the effects occur at about one third the depth of SWD effects.

The indications and contraindications for the use of MWD are similar to those for SWD. However, there can be NO metal within the treatment field (4 feet from the pads, drums, or coils). This not only includes metal on the athlete, but implanted metal (plates, screws, IUDs, etc.) as well.

The commercial availability of MWD is low in the United States. Microwave radiation possesses an inherently high risk because it tends to be reflected and scattered into the surrounding environment.

---

tissue temperature may reach 107°F, but a significant portion of the energy is dissipated by the subcutaneous fat layer. This leads to a secondary heating of the superficial muscle layer by heat conducted from the adipose tissue.[20] Shortwave diathermy is therefore less effective on athletes who have a large amount of subcutaneous fat.

Two types of SWD units are commonly found in the athletic training room: the condenser unit and the induction unit. The use of a condenser field places the athlete in the actual electrical circuit, while the use of an induction field places the athlete in the electromagnetic field produced by the equipment.

Condenser Unit

Application of shortwave diathermy by way of a condenser unit places the athlete within the actual circuit of the machine's energy. Two insulated plates are placed on either side of the site being treated. The flow of electromagnetic energy passes through the tissues, resulting in frictional heating.

Heating occurs at depths of 2.5 to 5 cm but is uneven because of differences in the resistance to energy transportation of various tissue types (Fig. 3–10). When condenser plates or pads are used, heating tends to occur in the subcutaneous tissues and the superficial muscle layer.[33]

Induction Unit

The induction method of shortwave diathermy does not place the athlete directly in the unit's circuit. Tissues are affected by radiation emitted from the electromagnetic field created by the electrode. The effects of the induction method

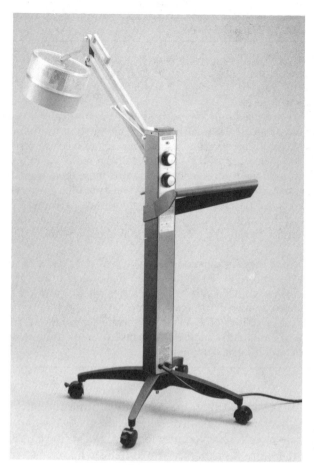

Figure 3–8. Shortwave Diathermy Induction Coil Drum. (The Auto*Therm courtesy of Mettler Electronics Corp., Anaheim, CA.)

may heat tissues up to 5 cm beneath the skin. The maximal temperature increases are found in the superficial and middle muscle layer (see Fig. 3–10).

The athlete's tissues are placed in the electromagnetic field by the use of an insulated cable electrode. The cable may be wrapped around the extremity (Fig. 3–11) or coiled flat like a pancake and placed on the athlete. Another method of shortwave induction has the cable in a self-contained drum (see Fig. 3–8).

Effect on the Injury Response Cycle

The application of SWD increases the blood flow in the deep tissues. Fibroblastic activity, collagen deposition, and new capillary growth have been reported to be stimulated by shortwave diathermy treatment.[34] Muscle spasm is reduced by the *sedation* of sensory and *motor nerves*. As with all heat applications, there is a local increase in cellular metabolic rate and in perspiration, which must be removed during the treatment.

Sedation: The result of calming nerve endings.
Motor Nerve: A nerve that provides impulses to muscles.

(A) Tissue Ions Before Application of Electromagnetic Energy

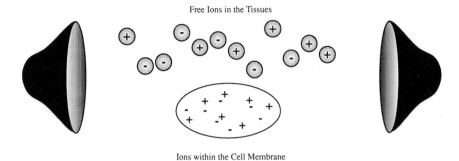

(B) Ionic Reaction to Electromagnetic Energy

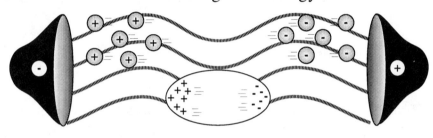

Figure 3–9. Dipole Response to an Electromagnetic Field. (A) Tissue ions before application of electromagnetic energy. (B) Ionic reaction to electromagnetic energy. The ions move towards the pole having the opposite charge.

Setup and Application*

General Preparation

1. There can be NO metal within the treatment field (4 feet from the pads, drums, or coils). This includes metal on the patient, such as jewelry, or in the patient, including plates or screws. No metal should be in the treatment table itself, such as brackets or nails. The presence of metal will collect and concentrate the energy from the treatment in the same manner that an antenna collects radio waves. Some manufacturers build metal-free tables for use with shortwave diathermy.
2. For personal safety, the athletic trainer should remove any rings, watches, bracelets, and so on.
3. Cover the area to be treated with a DRY terry cloth towel to absorb perspiration. A portion of the area to be treated must remain visible to check for burns during the treatment. Avoid any moisture buildup dur-

---

*Consult the user's manual of your particular modality.

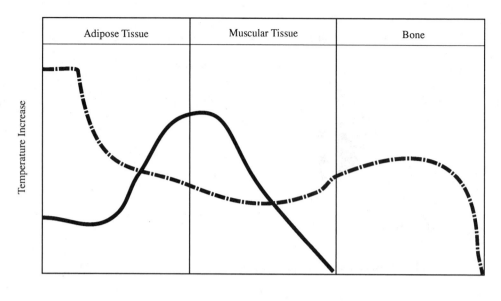

Shortwave Diathermy: Condenser Method

Shortwave Diathermy: Induction Method

Figure 3–10. Comparison of the Heating Effects of Shortwave Diathermy Delivered by the Condenser Method and Induction Method. The condenser method of application results in superficial heating of the adipose tissue layer and the bone/muscle interface. The induction method results in the muscle belly being primarily heated. (Adapted from Paetzold, J: Physical Laws Regarding the Distribution of Energy For Various Frequency Methods Applied in Heat Therapy. Ultrasonics in Biology and Medicine.)

ing the treatment as water tends to collect heat. The intensity must be turned to "zero" before drying the area.

4. Explain to the athlete that a mild warmth should be felt. Instruct the athlete to inform you if any unusual sensations are experienced.

Condenser Method

Condenser Plate Setup

1. Adjust the plates so that they are parallel to the skin, one inch above the athlete. On most units it is essential that both plates be placed at an equal distance above the tissue. This can be accomplished by using

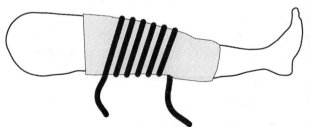

Figure 3–11. Shortwave Diathermy Application Via an Induction Cable. The cable is wrapped around the body part with equal spacing along the length. Cables that are too close together will concentrate the heat and may result in burns. Note the equal lengths running to and from the cable.

a spacer, such as a piece of wood. Place the spacer on the athlete and lower the plate until the plate and the spacer touch. Remove the spacer and repeat for the other plate. The spacer must be removed before the treatment is started.
2. Consult the user's manual for the minimum and maximum distance allowed between the condenser plates.

Condenser Pad Setup

1. Cover the area to be treated with six layers of toweling.
2. Place the condenser pads on the toweling. If the pads are used on the same side of the body, place them as far apart as possible. If they are used on opposite sides of a body part (anterior/posterior, medial/lateral) avoid having the athlete lie on the pad.
3. Secure the pads in place with sandbags or the like.

Induction Method

Cable Setup

1. Place six layers of toweling around the body part.
2. Using spacers, wrap the cable around the body part leaving a minimum of 1 inch between the coils. The leads to and from the coil should be of equal length (see Fig. 3–11).
3. Secure the cable ends so that they do not touch each other, the athlete, or the shortwave unit itself.

Coil Setup

1. Using spacers, form a coil of at least three circles approximately equal to the area being treated. There should be a minimum of 1 inch between the circles and the leads should be of equal length. Use an insulator or 1 inch of padding to separate the end of the inner coil from the coil itself (see Fig. 3–11).
2. Insulate the skin with at least six layers of toweling.
3. Place the coil on the athlete and lightly secure in place with sandbags.
4. Position the leads so they do not come into contact with each other, the athlete, or the unit.

Drum Setup

1. Position the drum approximately 0.5 to 1 inch above the toweling. There is a direct relationship between the distance of the drum from the athlete and the intensity of energy required for the treatment.

Application

1. Turn the unit on; allow to warm up if necessary.
2. Some units must be tuned to allow for maximal energy transfer. If tuning is necessary, consult the user's manual and follow the manufacturer's instructions.
3. Instruct the athlete not to move until the machine is shut off.
4. Increase the intensity until the athlete feels a mild warmth.
5. If the electrodes must be moved or if it necessary to dry the area, return the intensity to zero.

6. Regular checks must be made on the athlete. Observe the skin for signs of burns and inquire as to any unusual sensations. Adjust as necessary.
7. Following the treatment, return the intensity dial to "zero" and shut off the unit.

Duration of Treatment

At moderate intensities treatments may be given for 20 to 30 minutes and may be repeated as needed for 2 weeks. When higher treatment temperatures are used, decrease the duration of treatment and apply on alternate days.

Precautions

- Many states require a physician's prescription for the application of shortwave diathermy.
- Never allow the cables to touch each other. This may create a short circuit.
- The skin exposed to the treatment must always be covered by at least 0.5 inch of toweling.
- Do not allow perspiration to collect in the treatment field.
- Never allow the skin to come into direct contact with the heating unit or cables. Severe burns may result.
- Overheating of the athlete's tissues may cause tissue damage without any immediate signs. Deep-tissue burning can cause destruction of muscular tissue or subcutaneous fat necrosis.
- A deep, aching sensation may be a symptom of overheating the tissues.
- It is difficult to heat only localized areas. Heat formed in the treated area is dissipated by water pathways within the tissues.

Indications

- Joint inflammation (bursitis, tendinitis, synovitis). Use with caution as the deep heating may cause collagen destruction within the joint.
- Fibrositis
- Myositis
- Subacute and chronic inflammatory conditions in deep-tissue layers.
- Osteoarthritis

Contraindications

- Ischemic areas—the increased metabolic rate will increase the need for oxygen, causing further hypoxia.
- Metal implants or metals such as jewelry—the metal collects and concentrates the energy potentially causing burns.
- Perspiration and moist dressings—the water collects and concentrates the heat.
- Tendency to hemorrhage, including menstruation
- Cancer
- Fever

Necrosis: Cell death.
Osteoarthritis: Degeneration of a joint's articular surface.

- Sensory loss
- Cardiac pacemakers
- Pregnancy
- Areas of particular sensitivity:
  - *Epiphyseal plates* in children
  - The genitals
  - Sites of infection
  - The abdomen with an implanted intrauterine device (IUD)
  - The eyes and faces

Epiphyseal Plates: Growth plates of bones.

CHAPTER QUIZ

• •

1. Which of the following modalities has the greatest likelihood of frostbite?
   A. Ice immersion
   B. Reusable cold packs
   C. Ice massage
   D. Ice bag

2. Which of the following is a contraindication for the use of a paraffin bath?
   A. No range of motion
   B. Chronic conditions
   C. Pain
   D. Skin conditions

3. Which of the following modalities uses convection as its method of heat transfer?
   A. Ice bag
   B. Whirlpool
   C. Hot packs
   D. Infrared lamp

4. Which of the following is NOT a local effect of cold application?
   A. Decreased rate of cell metabolism
   B. Decreased muscle spindle activity
   C. Decreased nerve conduction velocity
   D. Decreased viscosity of fluids in the area

5. Which of the following modalities has the greatest depth of penetration?
   A. Moist heat pack
   B. Hot whirlpool
   C. Infrared lamp
   D. Ice bag

6. Which of the following is NOT a local effect of heat application?
   A. Increased rate of cell metabolism
   B. Increased elasticity of soft tissue
   C. Increased muscle tone
   D. Decreased muscle spasm

7. How does the application of cold assist in reducing secondary hypoxic injury?

8. List the components and effects of immediate treatment:

	Step	Effect
A.	_____	_____
B.	_____	_____
C.	_____	_____
D.	_____	_____

9. Why does the effect of cold application penetrate deeper and last longer than the effect of heat application?

10. Explain why the temperature of whirlpools must be altered as the surface area being treated increases.

REFERENCES

1. Weinberger, A and Lev, A: Temperature elevation of connective tissue by physical modalities. Critical Reviews in Physical and Rehabilitation Medicine 3:121, 1991.
2. Belitsky, RB, Odam, SJ, and Humbley-Kozey, C: Evaluation of the effectiveness of wet ice, dry ice, and cryogen packs in reducing skin temperature. Phys Ther 67:1080, 1987.
3. Bocobo, C, et al: The effect of ice on intra-articular temperature in the knee of the dog. Am J Phys Med Rehabil 70:181, 1991.
4. Knight, KL: Cryotherapy: Theory, Technique, and Physiology. Chattanooga Corporation, Chattanooga, 1985.
5. Wilkerson, GB: Inflammation in connective tissue: Etiology and management. Athletic Training 20:299, 1985.
6. Grana, WA, Walton, WL, and Reider, B: Cold modalities. In Drez, D (ed): Therapeutic Modalities for Sports Injuries. Year Book Medical Publishers, Chicago, 1989, pp 25–32.
7. Griffin, JE and Karselis, TC: Physical Agents for Physical Therapists, ed 3. Charles C Thomas, Springfield IL, 1988.
8. Lewis, T: Observations upon the reactions of the vessels of the human skin to cold. Heart 15:177, 1930.
9. Taber, C, et al: Measurement of reactive vasodilation during cold gel pack application to nontraumatized ankles. Phys Ther 72:294, 1992.
10. Baker, RJ and Bell, GW: The effect of therapeutic modalities on blood flow in the human calf. JOSPT 13:23, 1991.
11. Cote, DL, et al: Comparison of three treatment procedures for minimizing ankle sprain swelling. Phys Ther 68:1072, 1988.
12. Halvorson, GA: Therapeutic heat and cold for athletic injuries. Physician and Sportsmedicine 18:87, 1990.
13. Arnheim, DD: Modern Principles of Athletic Training, ed 7. CV Mosby, St. Louis, 1989.
14. Michlovitz, SL: Cryotherapy: The use of cold as a therapeutic agent. In Michlovitz, SL (ed): Thermal Agents in Rehabilitation, ed 2. FA Davis, Philadelphia, 1990, pp 63–87.
15. Ingersoll, CD and Mangus, BC: Sensations of cold reexamined: A study using the McGill Pain Questionnaire. Athletic Training 26:240, 1991.
16. Whitney, SL: Physical Agents: Heat and cold modalities. In Scully, RM and Barnes, MR (eds): Physical Therapy. JB Lippincott, Philadelphia, 1989, pp 844–875.
17. Parker, TJ, Small, NC, and Davis, PG: Case report: Cold-induced nerve palsy. Athletic Training 18:76, 1983.
18. Green, GA, Zachazewski, JE, and Jordan, SE: A case conference: Peroneal nerve palsy induced by cryotherapy. Physician and Sportsmedicine 17:63, 1989.
19. Wilkerson, GB: Treatment of the inversion ankle sprain through synchronous application of focal compression and cold. Athletic Training 26:220, 1991.
20. Cox, JS, et al: Heat modalities. In Drez, D (ed): Therapeutic Modalities for Sports Injuries. Year Book Medical Publishers, Chicago, 1989, pp 1–23.
21. Knight, KL and Londeree, BR: Comparison of blood flow in the ankle of uninjured subjects during application of heat, cold, and exercise. Med Sci Sports Exer 12:76, 1980.
22. Reed, B and Zarro, V: Inflammation and repair in the use of thermal agents. In Michlovitz, SL (ed): Thermal Agents in Rehabilitation, ed 2. FA Davis, Philadelphia, 1990, pp 3–17.
23. Nimchick, PSR and Knight, KL: Effects of wearing a toe cap or a sock on temperature and perceived pain during ice immersion. Athletic Training 18:144, 1983.

24. Ingersoll, CD, Mangus, BC, and Wolf, S: Cold-induced pain: Habituation to cold immersions (abstr). Athletic Training 25:126, 1990.
25. Gerig, BK: The Effects of Cryotherapy Upon Ankle Proprioception (abstr). Athletic Training 25:119, 1990.
26. Newton, RA: Effects of vapocoolants on passive hip flexion in healthy subjects. Phys Ther 65:1034, 1985.
27. Downer, AH: Physical Therapy Procedures: Selected Techniques, ed 3. Charles C Thomas, Springfield, IL, 1981, pp 131–133.
28. Michlovitz, SL: Biophysical principles of heating and superficial heat agents. In Michlovitz, SL: Cryotherapy: The Use of Cold as a Therapeutic Agent. In Michlovitz, SL (ed): Thermal Agents in Rehabilitation, ed 2. FA Davis, Philadelphia, 1990, pp 88–108.
29. Walsh, MT: Hydrotherapy: The use of water as a therapeutic agent. In Michlovitz, SL: Cryotherapy: The Use of Cold as a Therapeutic Agent. In Michlovitz, SL (ed): Thermal Agents in Rehabilitation, ed 2. FA Davis, Philadelphia, 1990, pp 109–133.
30. Downer, AH: Physical Therapy Procedures: Selected Techniques, ed 3. Charles C Thomas, Springfield, IL, 1981, pp 38–46.
31. Cummings, J: Role of light in wound healing. In Koth, LC, McCulloch, JM, and Feedar, JA (eds): Wound Healing: Alternatives in Management. FA Davis, Philadelphia, 1990, pp 287–301.
32. Kloth, LC and Ziskin, MC: Diathermy and pulsed electromagnetic fields. In Michlovitz, SL (ed): Thermal Agents in Rehabilitation, ed 2. FA Davis, Philadelphia, 1990, pp 170–199.
33. Fahey, TD: Athletic Training: Principles and Practice. Mayfield Publishing, Minneapolis, 1986.
34. Brown, M and Baker, RD: Effect of pulsed shortwave diathermy on skeletal muscle injury in rabbits. Phys Ther 67:208, 1987.

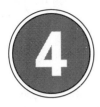

Electrical Agents

· ·

The purpose of this chapter is to describe the effects of passing an electrical current through the human body. Before this can be understood, the student must comprehend the basic principles of electricity and become familiar with the terminology. Various techniques and theories of application, and their effects on the injury response process, will be discussed in individual sections.

The effect that electricity has on the body can be difficult to comprehend. Because of the many different treatment parameters that can be modified, each type of stimulation unit produces unique effects within the tissues and produces a wide range of therapeutic responses (Table 4–1). However, all therapeutic currents have certain characteristics that remain similar. This chapter is divided into three sections. The first section introduces basic electrical principles, concepts, and terms. The second section describes the effect that an

Table 4–1 **PROPOSED THERAPEUTIC USES OF ELECTRICAL CURRENTS**

Control of acute and chronic pain
Decreasing joint contractures
Facilitating fracture healing
Facilitating muscle re-education
Facilitating tissue healing
Inhibiting spasticity
Minimizing disuse atrophy
Providing support to a joint through muscle contraction
Reducing edema
Reducing muscle spasm
Strengthening of muscle

Table 4-2 **GENERAL CONTRAINDICATIONS OF ELECTROTHERAPY**

Cardiac disability—electrical current flow may interfere with demand-type pacemakers.
Exposed metal implants such as those used for *external fixation* of fractures. This provides a path
for the current to reach inside bone.
Severe obesity. Adipose tissue may provide insulation against effective stimulation.
Areas of particular sensitivity
The carotid sinus
The esophagus
The pharynx
Skin irritation from the gel, adhesive, or current flow in athletes who wear electrodes for extended
periods of time. Altering the position of the electrodes reduces irritation.

electrical current has on the body, and the third section describes the effects of various stimulation units.

The primary precautions and contraindications for the use of electrical stimulation lie in the placement of the electrodes. Current flow through the heart, *carotid sinus*, and pharynx is to be avoided because it disrupts normal cardiovascular function. Electricity is not applied to the skull or over sites of infection or cancer because of the unknown and unpredictable effects. The general contraindications to electrical stimulation are presented in Table 4-2. Contraindications particular to specific electrical stimulators are presented in their appropriate sections.

Fundamentals of Electricity

Electricity is the force created by an imbalance in the number of electrons at two points. This force, known as electromagnetic force (EMF), potential difference, or voltage, creates a situation where electrons tend to move in an attempt to equalize the charges. The resultant flow of electrons creates an electrical current. In its simplest form, electrical current flows from the negative pole (**cathode**), an area of high electron concentration, to the positive pole (**anode**), an area of low electron concentration.

In addition to the presence of voltage, a complete circuit must be established for flow to occur. An uninterrupted circuit is said to be "closed" when a complete loop is formed allowing the current to flow to and from the source. An interrupted or incomplete path is referred to as an "open circuit." When you walk into a room and flip a switch to turn on the light, you are closing a circuit that allows the electricity to flow from its source, through the light, and back to its source. Likewise, a closed circuit is created between an athlete and an electrical stimulation device by attaching leads of opposite polarity to the body.

External Fixation: A fracture-setting technique incorporating the use of metal rods that
extend through the skin and are attached to a device outside of the body.
Carotid Sinus: An enlargement of the carotid artery near the branch of the internal carotid
artery, located distal to the inferior arch of the mandible. Receptors at this site monitor
and assist in the regulation of blood pressure.

MEASURES OF ELECTRICAL CURRENT FLOW

Electrical Charge

Electrical current results from the movement of electrons. The number of electrons required for electrical current flow is so great that it is impractical to count each one. Just as we may describe 12 objects as a dozen, or a dozen dozens as a gross, we may also describe a large number of electrons as a single unit. A **coulomb** is used to describe the charge produced by 6.25×10^{18} electrons (negative charge) or protons (positive charge), and is represented by the symbol "Q."

In the case of electrical charges, opposites attract and likes repel and this relationship is defined by **Coulomb's law**. Objects possessing opposite charges move towards each other, while those objects having similar charges repel. The strength of the attractive or repulsive forces may be amplified by increasing the magnitude of the charges or decreasing the distance between the two objects.

Voltage

Voltage, also known as the electromotive force or **potential difference** between two poles, measures the tendency for current flow to occur. Electrons placed within a field strain themselves to move to the opposite pole, thus creating the potential for work to occur (Work = Force × Distance). The **volt** is the unit of potential difference and represents the amount of work required to move 1 coulomb of charge. The energy required to move this coulomb is termed a **Joule**. Traditionally, the symbol for voltage is "E," but recently the symbol "V" has come into vogue and will symbolize voltage in this text.

The flow of electrons is not a simple passage of particles through a medium. Rather, this flow consists of the passing of electrons between atoms in a manner similar to a bucket brigade. Picture a line of people passing buckets of water. In this analogy, the people represent atoms, and the buckets of water are electrons. The first person hands his bucket to the next person. This person then passes the bucket she has in her hand to the next person and the process repeats. The flow of electrons is quite similar. Rather than a single electron passing through a wire, electrons are passed from atom to atom.

Current

The rate at which the electrical charge (measured in coulombs) flows is the amperage. More specifically, 1 ampere (A) is the current when 1 coulomb passes a single point in 1 second. Conceptually, we may make the analogy to the number of people passing through a turnstile in any given period of time. If 1 coulomb passes a point in 1 second, the rate of flow is 1 ampere. If 2 coulombs pass a point in 1 second, the rate of flow is 2 amperes.

The symbol for current flow is "I." Most electrical modalities have current flow measured in milliamperes (mA), 1/1000 of an ampere, or microamperes (μA), 1/1,000,000 of an ampere.

Resistance

All materials present some degree of opposition to the flow of electrical current. Those materials allowing current to pass with relative ease are labeled conductors; those that tend to oppose current flow, resistors. A material's resistance to the movement of electrons is measured in **ohms**. One ohm is the amount of resistance needed to develop 0.24 calories of heat when 1 ampere of current is applied for 1 second. The symbol for resistance is "R" and for ohms, "Ω" (omega).

Conductance is a measure of the ease with which current is allowed to pass. Conductance is the mathematical reciprocal of resistance and is measured by the unit **mho**; "ohm" spelled backwards.

The amount of resistance offered to any current is determined by the type of material, the length of the material, the cross-sectional area of the material, and the temperature of the circuit. These four elements together determine the total resistance to current flow. As already established, the potential difference at each end of the resistor must be great enough to overcome the resistance, or no current will flow.

Material of the Circuit

A material is classified either as a **resistor** or a **conductor** based on the number of free electrons available. As the number of free electrons in a material increases, its resistance decreases and an electrical current is more easily conducted. Likewise, if a material has few free electrons, it is a resistor. Materials having *valence shells* that are almost filled, like rubber, have few free electrons and are therefore resistors. Those having valence shells with many free electrons, such as copper, easily give up their electrons and are conductors.

Length of the Circuit

There is a proportional relationship between the length of an electrical circuit and resistance to electron flow. As the distance electrons must travel increases, the resistance to current increases. Thus, we would find that less electrical resistance is offered by a 1-inch piece of copper wire than is offered by a 1-foot length of copper wire with the same diameter.

Cross-sectional Area of the Circuit

The resistance of an electric circuit is inversely proportional to its cross-sectional area. Wider materials produce less electrical resistance than ones with a narrower cross-section. A 1-foot piece of copper wire having a diameter of 0.25 inches would offer less resistance than the same length of wire having a 0.10-inch diameter.

Temperature of the Circuit

An increase in temperature increases the amount of random movement of free electrons, making it difficult for the current to find a free path through the circuit. Current itself causes an increase in temperature as it passes through the conductor. The amount of residual heat produced is proportional to the

---

Valence Shell: An imaginary shell in which the electrons responsible for chemical reactivity orbit around the nucleus of an atom.

resistance of the medium and power of the current. Heating elements on stoves or in electric heaters take advantage of this principle.

Impedance

In an alternating current, two additional properties, **inductance** and **capacitance**, act to resist the flow of an alternating current. Collectively known as **impedance**, this form of resistance is also measured in ohms, but uses the symbol "**Z.**"

Inductance is the ability of a material to store electrical energy by means of an **electromagnetic field** and is measured by the *henry*. Variation in the magnitude and direction of electrical current creates a *flux* that induces voltage. Inductors tend to oppose electrical current flow. A transformer used to convert household current into a lower-voltage direct current is an example of an inductor. Inductance is negligible in biological systems.[1]

Capacitance is the ability of a material to store energy by means of an **electrostatic field** and provides frequency-dependent opposition to electric current flow. Created by an insulator separating two conductors, charges may be stored even after the applied voltage has been discontinued. The output of capacitors is measured in **farads** (F), microfarads (μF), or picofarads (pF). A farad stores a charge of 1 coulomb when 1 volt is applied. As we will see when frequency is discussed, the lower the capacitance of a circuit, the higher the frequency of an alternating current it will allow.[2]

Since many cell membranes act as capacitors by separating positive and negative charges between the inside and outside of the cell, capacitance is a factor in determining the effects of current flow on the body. High-frequency currents will meet less capacitive skin resistance than lower-frequency currents.

Ohm's Law

The relationship between amperage, voltage, and resistance is described by Ohm's law. Generally stated, **current (I) is directly proportional to voltage (V) and inversely proportional to resistance (R)**; that is:

$$I = V/R$$

By using Ohm's law, or a derivation of it, the amperage, voltage, or resistance in a circuit can be calculated if two of the three variables are known. In a circuit where the potential is 120 volts with 10 ohms of resistance, the amperage would be calculated as 120 volts/10 ohms, or 12 amperes. Circuits having a very high voltage can still have a very small current flow if the resistance is high. For example, applying 1,000 volts to a circuit with a resistance of 1,000,000 ohms would produce only 0.001 amperes. Likewise, low voltages can give rise to a very high current flow. Consider a 10-volt circuit with 0.01 ohms of resistance. The resultant current would be 1,000 amperes.

Henry: A measure of inductance. One henry induces an electromagnetic force of 1 volt when the current changes at a rate of 1 ampere per second.

Flux: A residual electromagnetic field created by two unlike charges.

To determine the effect that current (I) and resistance (R) have on voltage (V), we may transpose Ohm's law to give:

$$V = IR$$

In order for current to flow through a resistance, the voltage applied must be equal to or greater than the product of the amperage times the resistance. To produce a current of 12 amperes flowing through a circuit of 10 ohms, 120 volts (12 amperes × 10 ohms) would be required.

The resistance (R) found in a circuit may be calculated by again transposing the formula so that we divide the voltage (V) by the resistance (I):

$$R = V/I$$

Therefore, if we are using a device that requires 120 volts and 12 amperes, we can calculate the amount of resistance by dividing 120 volts by 12 amperes to give 10 ohms.

You will notice that in all of our equations, current is equal to 10 amperes, voltage is equal to 120 volts, and resistance is equal to 10 ohms. This illustrates the interrelationship between the variables. If we were to reduce the current to 5 amperes and increase the voltage to 200 volts, the resistance would then be 40 ohms. In any case, the voltage applied to the circuit must be greater than the resistance, or no current will flow.

Wattage

The relationship between voltage and amperage is expressed in units of wattage (P) and is used to designate the **power** of a current. Power describes the amount of work being performed in a unit of time. The voltage of the current measures the amount of work being done; amperage defines the time unit. One watt is the power produced by 1 ampere of current flowing with the force of 1 volt. With this in mind, we can then describe wattage as:

$$P = VI$$

Using our previous variables, we can calculate the power used by a device requiring 12 amperes from a 120-volt source to be 1,440 watts.

The change in wattage of an electrical circuit reflects the net change in amperage and/or voltage. If either amperage or voltage is increased or decreased the wattage changes accordingly. However, if one variable is increased and the other decreased, the wattage may increase or decrease depending on the relative magnitude of the changes in voltage and amperage.

CURRENT TYPES

Standard electrical currents are classified as being either direct currents (DC) or alternating currents (AC) depending on the course of flow. As we will later learn, there is a third classification of therapeutic current, **pulsatile currents**. The terms alternating and direct currents describe the uninterrupted flow of electrons while the term pulsatile current indicates that the electron flow is periodically interrupted. Pulsatile currents are discussed in detail in the section on classification of electrical stimulating currents.

The two primary properties of electrical flow are amplitude (intensity) and duration. The amplitude of the wave is represented by the maximal distance the impulse rises above or below the baseline. The baseline is set by the **iso-electric point**, where the electrical potential between the two poles is equal and no current flow occurs. The horizontal distance required to complete the shape represents the pulse duration. The term "pulse width" is often incorrectly substituted for pulse duration.[3] The total area within this wave form represents the amount of current the pulse contains.

Direct Currents

Direct currents are characterized by a continuous flow of electrons in one direction. The basic pattern of direct current flow is the square wave and is recognized by continuous current flow on only one side of the baseline as the electrons travel from the cathode to the anode (Fig. 4–1). The flow of an uninterrupted current may be altered into many different configurations by pulsing the flow (pulsatile current). Despite fluctuations in voltage or amperage, the current flow remains in one direction and stays on one side of the baseline (Fig. 4–2). In medical applications the term **galvanic** denotes uninterrupted direct current (see Fig. 4–1) and **monphasic** refers to pulsed unidirectional currents (see Fig. 4–2).

Perhaps the most common example of a direct current is a flashlight. The battery possesses a positive pole, which lacks electrons and a negative pole that, because of chemical reactions, has an excess of electrons. Electrons leave the negative pole of the battery and flow through a wire to the bulb. After leaving the bulb, the electrons return to the positive pole of the battery (Fig. 4–3). When the number of electrons at the negative pole equals the number at the positive pole, no further potential for current flow exists. The battery is dead.

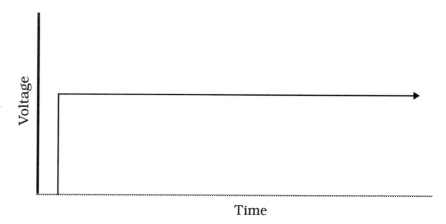

Figure 4–1. Uninterrupted Direct Current. Characterized by a constant flow of electrons in one direction from the isoelectric point.

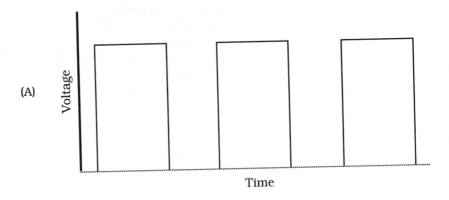

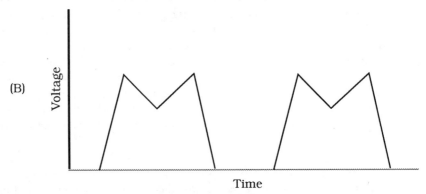

Figure 4–2. Monophasic Currents. Pulsatile current consists of discrete pulses. Like direct current, monophasic pulses are characterized by flow in one direction. (A) interrupted. (B) twin peaked monophasic.

Alternating Currents

With an alternating current, the direction and magnitude of the flow reverses, although the magnitude may not be equal in both directions. Unlike a direct current, an alternating current circuit possesses no true positive or negative pole. Electrons, rather than constantly moving in one direction, shuffle back and forth between the two electrodes as they take turns being the "positive" and "negative" poles.

Consider the flashlight example used to describe direct current flow (see Fig. 4–3). If a battery were placed on a device that allowed it to rotate between the two wires, we could more or less duplicate an AC current.[4] Electrons would flow away from terminal (A) when the cathode is in line with it. When the anode aligns with terminal (A), electrons would flow towards it (Fig. 4–4).

The basic pattern of an alternating current is the sine wave (Fig. 4–5). As with direct currents, alternating current may be altered into various configurations by interrupting the current flow with pulses to elicit the desired physiological effects (Fig. 4–6). In therapeutic modalities, bidirectional pulsed currents are referred to as biphasic currents.

The **amplitude**, or "peak value," of an AC wave is determined by measuring the maximal distance the wave rises above **or** below the baseline. In the case

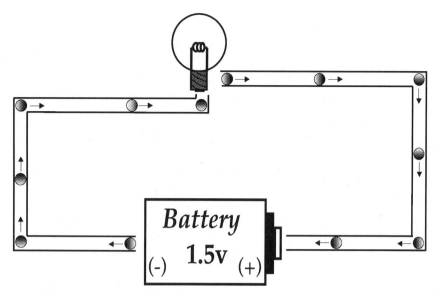

Figure 4–3. Example of a Direct Current. Electrons exit the battery through the cathode (negative pole), flow through the wire and bulb, and return to the anode (positive pole).

of the pure sine wave shown in Figure 4–7A, a peak value of 100 volts appears on either side of the baseline. The peak value refers to the wave amplitude on only one side of the baseline without regard to its duration. The **peak-to-peak value** is measured from the peak on the positive side of the baseline to the peak on the negative side. In Figure 4–7A, the peak-to-peak value would be the absolute value of the difference between the two peaks, or 200 volts. In an *asymmetric* wave form, such as the faradic wave (Fig. 4–7B), the peak value is 100 volts on the positive side of the baseline. The peak-to-peak value would be measured from the peak on the negative side (20 volts) to the peak on the positive side (100 volts), resulting in a peak-to-peak measure of 120 volts.

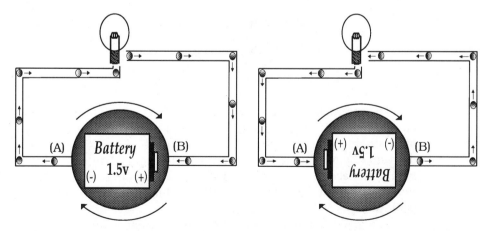

Figure 4–4. Example of an Alternating Current. Alternating currents possess no true positive or negative pole. In this type of current, electrons flow back and forth between poles (A) and (B).

Asymmetric: Lacking symmetry (e.g., two halves are of unequal size and/or shape).

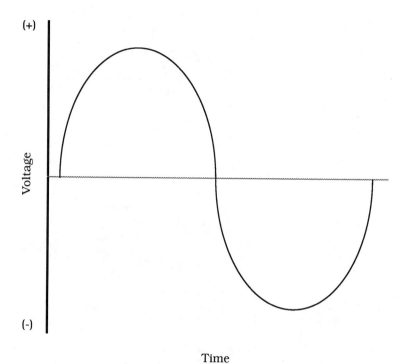

Figure 4–5. The Sine Wave. One cycle of an alternating current.

The **average current** of a wave considers one half of its complete cycle taking into account the amount of time the current is flowing. To calculate the average value of a wave, the sine values of all angles up to 180 degrees are added together and divided by the number of measurements. In the case of a perfect sine wave this value is 0.637. This figure is then multiplied by the peak value to obtain the average value:

$$\text{Average value} = \text{Mean of sines} \times \text{Peak value}$$

$$\text{Average value} = 0.637 \times 100 \text{ volts}$$

$$\text{Average value} = 63.7 \text{ volts}$$

The **root-mean-square** value (RMS) takes into account both the amplitude and duration of the pulse and describes the total amount of charge delivered by a single cycle. This figure is important because it translates the power delivered by an alternating current into the equivalent amount of power that would be needed by a direct current to produce the same amount of heat. In the case of a pure sine wave, the RMS value is calculated by multiplying the peak value by 0.707.

The cycle duration of an alternating current is measured from the originating point on the baseline to its terminating point and represents the amount of time required to complete one full cycle. The number of times that the current reverses direction in 1 second is the current's number of cycles per second and is measured in **hertz** (Hz) (Fig. 4–8). Because alternating currents are measured

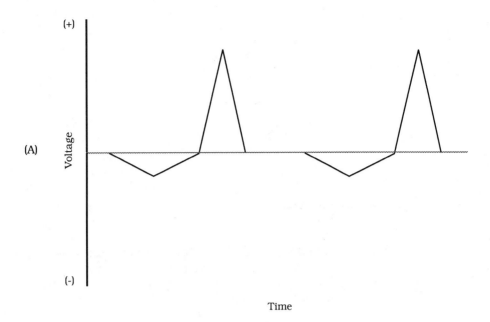

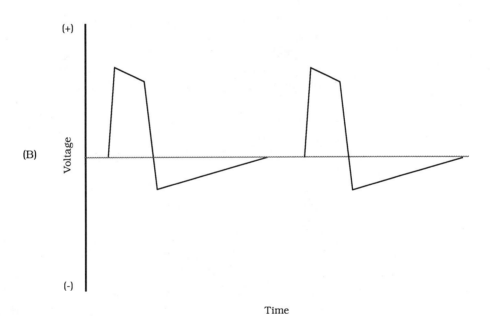

Figure 4–6. Pulsed Bidirectional Currents. An example of bidirectional pulsatile currents. (A) original faradic wave form; (B) typical transcutaneous electrical nerve stimulation wave form.

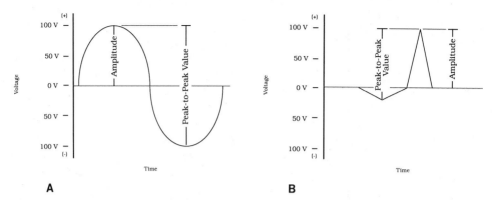

Figure 4–7. Measures of Amplitude. Peak value and peak-to-peak values for (A) symmetrical and (B) asymmetrical pulses.

in cycles per second, as the duration of the cycles increases, fewer cycles per second can occur. An alternating current of 100 Hz would change its direction of flow 100 times during 1 second. A current of 1 megahertz (MHz) would change its direction 1 million times a second.

CIRCUIT TYPES

An electrical current introduced into a conductive medium may flow along one set route (**series circuit**), through many different pathways (**parallel circuit**), or through a combination of each. Consider a string of Christmas tree lights. If the string is wired as a series circuit, when one bulb burns out, all the other lights go out as well because the current has no other path to take.

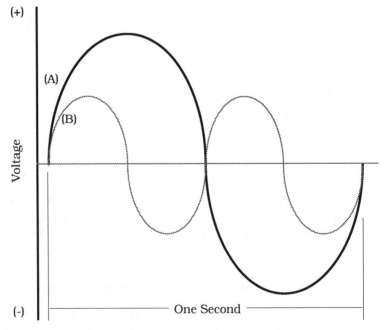

Figure 4–8. Frequency of an alternating current. Wave form (A) has a frequency of 1 Hz while wave form (B) has a frequency of 2 Hz.

In a string of lights wired in a parallel circuit, a burned-out bulb does not affect the other lights because the current still has other routes by which to reach them. Electricity operates under different constraints when traveling through series and parallel circuits, and each type of circuit has unique properties.

Series Circuit

Electrons in a series circuit have only **one pathway available for travel**. A simple series circuit can be made by connecting a wire between the two poles of a battery. In more complex series circuits, resistors are aligned "end to end" so that the current leaving one resistor will enter the next. In a series circuit, the **current remains the same** in all components along the circuit and **the total resistance is equal to the sum of the individual resistors** (Fig. 4–9).

If we know that a potential of 120 volts is applied to a circuit with 60 ohms of resistance, the amperage can be calculated by using Ohm's law. The equation for calculating the current flow through the series of resistors is

$$I = V/R_t$$

$$I = 120 \text{ volts}/60 \text{ ohms}$$

$$I = 2 \text{ amperes}$$

If each of three resistors has a different resistance (say 10 ohms, 20 ohms, and

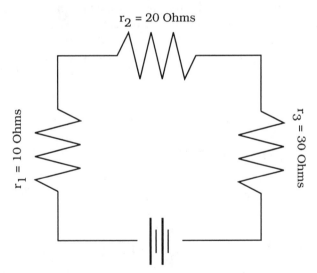

Figure 4–9. Resistance within a series circuit. The total amount of resistance to current flow is found by adding the amount of each individual resistor. The equation for calculating the total resistance of a circuit is:

$$R_t = r_1 + r_2 + r_3$$
$$R_t = 10 \text{ ohms} + 20 \text{ ohms} + 30 \text{ ohms}$$
$$R_t = 60 \text{ ohms}$$

where:

R_t = The sum of all resistors
R_n = The resistance in ohms of resistor n

30 ohms), the voltage will fluctuate between resistors. By applying a derivation of Ohm's law, $V = IR$, the voltage across each resistor may be calculated as:

$V_1 = Ir_1$ $V_2 = Ir_2$ $V_3 = Ir_3$

$V_1 = 2$ amperes $\times$ 10 ohms $V_2 = 2$ amperes $\times$ 20 ohms $V_3 = 2$ amperes $\times$ 30 ohms

$V_3 = 60$ volts

$V_1 = 20$ volts $V_2 = 40$ volts

By adding $V_1 + V_2 + V_3$, you can see that the sum of the potential across the individual resistors equals the total power applied to the circuit. The current (amperage) remains the same throughout a series circuit. It is the voltage and the resistance that vary.

Parallel Circuit

Electrons in a parallel circuit are provided with alternative pathways for travel and electrons tend to take the path of least resistance. Paths within the parallel circuit may then branch into other parallel or series circuits, but in either case, **each path has its own amperage and the voltage remains constant**. The flow in each of these pathways is inversely proportional to the resistance provided. This is quite similar to checking out of a grocery store. When we are finished shopping, we tend to get in the line with the fastest clerk rather than the slowest. In any given time frame, more people will check out through the fastest clerk, and fewer through the slowest.

To calculate the total resistance for a parallel circuit, we must keep in mind that the flow in each pathway is inversely proportional to its resistance. Since voltage is constant, this value may be canceled out and the mathematical reciprocal (1/#) of the resistance may be used (see Fig. 4–10).

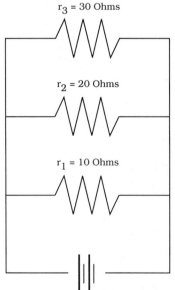

$r_3 = 30$ Ohms

$r_2 = 20$ Ohms

$r_1 = 10$ Ohms

Figure 4–10. Resistance within a parallel circuit. The flow across each resistor is inversely proportional to the resistance. The equation for calculating the total resistance of the circuit is:

$1/R_t = 1/r_1 + 1/r_2 + 1/r_3 \ldots$
$1/R_t = 1/10 + 1/20 + 1/30$
$1/R_t = 6/60 + 3/60 + 2/60$
$1/R_t = 11/60$
$1/R_t = 0.18$
$R_t = 5.56$ ohms (calculated by dividing 1 by 0.18)

Using Ohm's law, the total amperage of a circuit is calculated by:

$$I = V/R_t$$

$$I = 120 \text{ volts}/5.56 \text{ ohms}$$

$$I = 21.6 \text{ amperes}$$

The amount of current flowing across each resistor (and path) is calculated by:

$i_1 = v/r_1$	$i_2 = v/r_2$	$i_3 = v/r_3$
$i_1 = 120 \text{ volts}/10 \text{ ohms}$	$i_2 = 120 \text{ volts}/20 \text{ ohms}$	$i_3 = 120 \text{ volts}/30 \text{ ohms}$
$i_1 = 12 \text{ amperes}$	$i_2 = 6 \text{ amperes}$	$i_3 = 4 \text{ amperes}$

Where: i_n = amperage across resistor n
v = voltage applied to the circuit
r_n = resistance in ohms

Unlike series circuits, the parallel circuits have the same voltage across each path. It is the amperage and resistance that differ from path to path. Therefore, if the voltage across one path can be calculated, the voltage for the entire circuit is known.

To review: An electrical current is the flow of electrons through a medium. Electron flow is measured in coulombs per second and the voltage of the current is based on the potential difference for flow to occur. The rate of electron flow, the amperage, represents how many coulombs are being moved past a single point in 1 second. The movement of the current is always met with some degree of resistance, measured in ohms. Ohm's law describes the relationship between amperage, voltage, and resistance. The total power delivered by the current is wattage, calculated by multiplying the amperage times the voltage. Table 4–3 lists common electrical properties, their definitions, and equations describing basic laws of electricity.

Table 4–3 ELECTRICAL TERMS

Amperage (I):	The rate at which an electrical current is flowing. One ampere is equal to the rate of flow of one coulomb per second. It is analogous to the rate of flow through a pipe. $I = V/R$.
Charge (Q):	The basic unit of charge is the coulomb. It is the net charge produced by 6.25×10^{18} electrons or protons.
Coulomb's law:	Like charges repel and unlike charges attract.
Joule (J):	Basic unit of work in the International System of Units. It represents the work done by moving one coulomb of charge. One joule equals 0.74 foot-pounds of work. The conversion equation is: Joules = Coulombs × Volts.
Ohms (Ω):	Unit of electrical resistance (R). $R = V/I$.
Ohm's law:	Current is directly proportional to voltage and inversely proportional to resistance. $I = V/R$.
Voltage (V):	The potential for flow to occur. Analogous to the height of a waterfall, it indicates how much energy is available in the system. The greater the height of the waterfall, the more energy it can impart to a mill below. $V = IR$.
Watts (W):	Unit of electrical power (P). May be calculated from the relation Watts = Volts × Amperage ($P = VI$). Watts measure the ability to do work.

Electrical circuits are classified as being series or parallel. Within a series circuit, the electrons only have one path to take. The amperage remains constant, but the voltage fluctuates. Within a parallel circuit, the electrons have the option of taking more than one route, but the path of least resistance is preferred. In a parallel circuit, the amperage is varied among the paths, but the voltage remains constant.

Characteristics of Electrical Generators

Electrical modalities may be driven by either standard household current (120V AC) or by batteries (1.5V to 9V DC). Before this current is delivered to the body, it must be modified into the desired stimulation parameters.

In a simplified view, the current passes through one or more transformers to change it to the desired type (AC to DC, or DC to AC) and another to control the output current. A device, generically known as a generator, shapes the current (wave form) used by the modality. Other devices control characteristics of the electrical pulses.

Each element of the wave form has an effect on the tissues' reaction to the current flow. The following sections discuss each generator characteristic and relate how each affects the treatment.

CLASSIFICATION OF ELECTRICAL STIMULATING CURRENTS

Electrical stimulating currents are classified as being either **direct currents, alternating currents,** or **pulsed currents.**[1] The terms direct current and alternating current refer to the uninterrupted flow of electrons. Pulsed currents may flow in one direction, as in DC, or may have bidirectional movement, as in AC. However, pulsed currents are characterized by periods of no current flow (see Figs. 4–2 and 4–6).

PHASES

The building block of an electrical pulse is the **phase.** A phase is the individual section of a pulse that rises above or below the baseline for a measurable period of time. Pulses are then classified by the number and type of phases they possess.

Monophasic Currents

Pulsed direct currents are classified as monophasic because there is only one phase to a single pulse and the current flow is unidirectional. You will notice in Figure 4–11 that each pulse consists of only one component part, the phase. Despite the different shapes involved, there is only one phase, and it remains on one side of the baseline.

In this type of electrical current, amplitude is the maximal distance the wave rises above the baseline and the duration is measured as the distance required to complete one full cycle (see Fig. 4–11). You will notice that the horizontal baseline is labeled as "time," so the wavelength represents the dura-

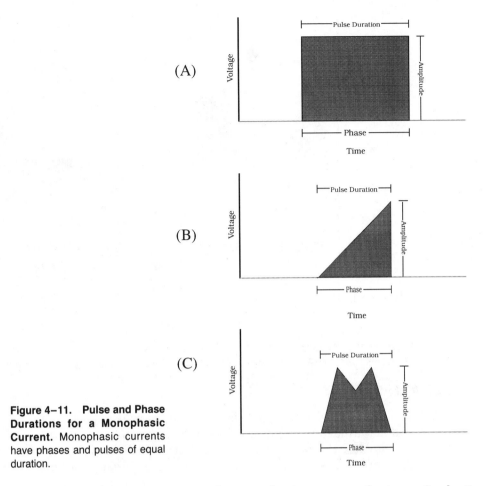

(A)

(B)

(C)

Figure 4–11. Pulse and Phase Durations for a Monophasic Current. Monophasic currents have phases and pulses of equal duration.

tion that the pulse is flowing. With monophasic currents, the terms "pulse," "phase," and "wave form" are synonymous.[5]

Biphasic Currents

Some electrical pulses, such as those presented in Figure 4–12 consist of two phases, each occurring on opposite sides of the baseline. A single AC pulse is an example of biphasic current.

The lead phase of the pulse is the first area rising above or below the baseline and the terminating phase occurs in the opposite direction. The pulse represented in Figure 4–12A is considered symmetrical because the two phases are equal in their magnitude and duration. In this case, each phase has equal, but opposite, electrical balance. Figures 4–12B and 4–12C represent asymmetrical pulses because each phase in the pulse has a different shape.

When asymmetric pulses are used, the characteristics of each phase should be considered separately. If the charge (area) of both phases are equal, the pulse is balanced; otherwise it is unbalanced. While the phases in a symmetrical pulse or balanced asymmetrical pulse cause the physiological effects of positive and negative current flow to cancel each other out, unbalanced asymmetric pulses may lead to residual physiological changes.

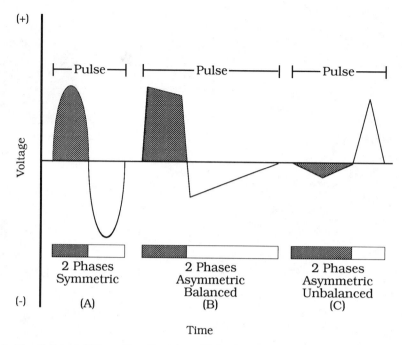

Figure 4–12. Pulse and Phase Durations for a Biphasic Current. Pulse and phase durations for (A) symmetrical biphasic, (B) balanced asymmetric biphasic, and (C) unbalanced asymmetric pulses.

PULSE ATTRIBUTES

The charge produced by an electrical generator is dependent on the duration and amplitude of the pulse. The relationship between intensity and duration of a single pulse determines the total charge delivered to the body. Increasing the amplitude and/or duration increases the total charge of the pulse.

Pulse Duration

As you will recall, the horizontal axis (or baseline) represents time. The distance that a pulse covers on the horizontal axis represents the **pulse duration**: The elapsed time from the beginning of the phase to the conclusion of the final phase, including the intrapulse interval.[1] The duration of a single pulse may be broken down into the time required for each component phase to complete its shape: the **phase duration** (see Figs. 4–11 and 4–12).

In a monophasic current, the pulse duration and phase duration are equivalent terms. In biphasic currents, the pulse duration is the sum total of the two phase durations. Note that pulse durations cannot be measured for uninterrupted direct or alternating currents.

Interpulse Interval, Intrapulse Interval, and Pulse Period

Unlike a continuous current, a pulsatile current possesses periods of time that the current is not flowing. The duration of time between the conclusion of one pulse and the initiation of the next is the **interpulse interval**. A single pulse may be interrupted by an **intrapulse interval**; however, the duration of the intrapulse interval cannot exceed the duration of the interpulse interval.[1] Jointly, the pulse duration and the pulse interval form the **pulse period**, the elapsed time between the initiation of one pulse and the start of the subsequent pulse (Fig. 4–13).

By definition, uninterrupted currents (alternating and direct currents) do not possess pulses. Therefore, pulse duration and pulse periods have no meaning for these types of currents.

Pulse Charge

A measurement of the number of electrons contained within a pulse, the **pulse charge**, is expressed in microcoulombs, as a coulomb is too large a unit to use when describing the charge produced by electrical stimulation units. Most electrotherapeutic modalities produce charges measured in microcoulombs (the charge produced by 10^{-6} electrons).

The pulse charge is a function of the amount of area within the wave form. Increasing or decreasing the amplitude or pulse duration will alter the charge of the pulse accordingly. The shape of the wave may also be altered to deliver more or less charge to the tissues per pulse.

Pulse Frequency

Any wave form repeated at regular intervals may be described in terms of its frequency or the number of events per second.[6] When a direct current is being used, the frequency is normally measured by the number of pulses per second (pps). The cycle frequency in an alternating current is measured by the number of cycles per second (cps) or Hertz (Hz) (see Fig. 4–8).

Many application protocols describe pulse frequency in terms of "low," "medium," and "high." Although the exact pulse frequency is the preferred method of describing this treatment parameter, the ranges for these terms are presented in Table 4–4.

An inverse relationship exists between the pulse frequency of an electrical current and the capacitive resistance offered by the tissues. A current having 10 pulses per second would encounter greater tissue resistance and would require an increased intensity to overcome the resistance than a current flowing at 1000 pulses per second.

Pulse Rise Time and Pulse Decay Time

Pulse rise is the amount of time needed for the pulse to reach its peak value. This value may range from *nanoseconds* (almost immediate full pulse charge) to seconds. The counterpart of pulse rise time is the pulse decay time, the amount of time required for the pulse to go from its peak back to zero (Fig. 4–14).

Nanosecond: One billionth (10^{-9}) of a second.

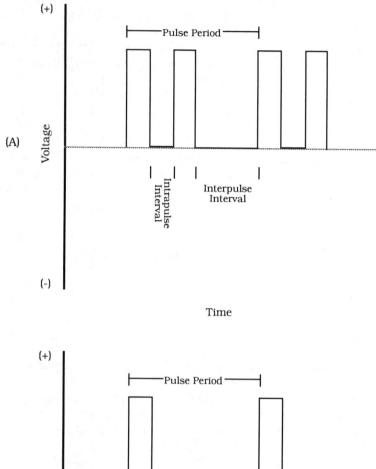

Figure 4–13. Calculation of intrapulse and interpulse intervals. (A) monophasic currents. (B) biphasic currents.

Table 4–4 **FREQUENCY RANGES COMMONLY USED IN ELECTROTHERAPY**

Descriptor	Pulses Per Second (pps)	Neuromuscular Effects
Low	<10	Individual muscle contractions
Medium	10–50	Summation of individual contractions causing increased muscle tone
High	>50	Tonic contraction

Pulse Trains

Pulse trains may be considered individual patterns of wave forms, durations, and/or frequencies that are linked together. These linked patterns repeat at regular intervals (Fig. 4–15).

The gradual rise and/or fall in amplitude of a pulse train is the **amplitude ramp**. Ramping amplitude causes a gradual increase in the force of muscular contractions by the progressive recruitment of *motor units*. As the intensity of the ramp continues to rise, more motor units are recruited into the contraction.

To the athlete, a slow rise time is appreciated because the stimulation is increased gradually and the "shock" of the current is reduced. When stimulating muscles, the gradual contraction produced by a slow rise time more closely resembles a voluntary muscle contraction. More and more fibers are recruited as the amplitude of the stimulus, or the pulse duration, increases.[7]

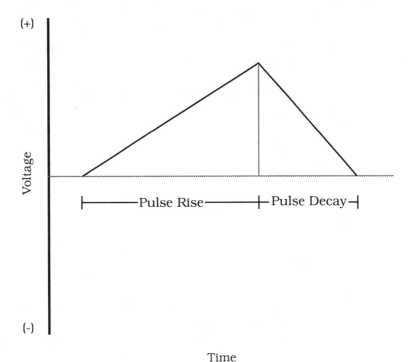

Figure 4–14. **Pulse rise and decay time of a monophasic pulse.**

Motor Unit: A group of skeletal muscle fibers that are innervated by a single motor nerve.

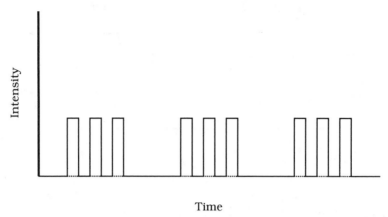

Figure 4–15. An example of pulse trains. A pattern of electrical pulses repeats at regular intervals.

CURRENT ATTRIBUTES

Average Current

The amount of current flowing per unit of time is described as the average current and is measured between two successive pulse peaks. It is reported that thermal and physiochemical changes in the tissues are based on the average current.[8] By increasing the number of pulses per second, the average current is increased and so is the perception of the stimulus. There is much more current per unit of time in high-frequency generators than with other types. A long pulse duration combined with a high average current results in an increased sensation of pain.

The average current found in most electrical stimulation units is measured in milliamperes. This measure is not meaningful for a balanced symmetrical current because the phase charges for this type of current are equal and the average current is zero.

Current Density

The physiological effects derived from electrical stimulation are related to the current density and the amount of current per unit area. The current density is inversely proportional to the size of the electrode. For example, if you are passing 300 volts through an electrode of 10 square inches, the resultant current density would be 30 volts per square inch. If the electrode's surface area is reduced by half, 300 volts are then passing through an electrode of 5 square inches, with a current density of 60 volts per square inch. If the electrode's surface area is again reduced, to a size of 1 square inch, the result is a current density of 300 volts per square inch.

As the current density increases, so does the athlete's perception of the stimulus. If the stimulus was comfortable to the athlete in our first example, it would be much more uncomfortable in the last example because the same amount of current is being delivered by one tenth of the initial surface area.

| Box | **4-1** | EXPERIMENT DEMONSTRATING VARIATIONS IN CURRENT DENSITY |

You can feel for yourself the effects of current density through the following experiment using a high-voltage pulsed stimulation unit:

- Make sure that the unit is turned off.
- Fill a plastic tub with water.
- Drop an active electrode in the tub (make sure that the rubber insulating material is facing the center of the tub) and fasten the dispersive electrode to your thigh.
- Place your hand and wrist in the water, being careful not to touch the electrode during this exercise.
- Have an assistant turn on and reset the unit. **Do not touch the unit during this experiment!** Make sure that the pulses-per-second switch is set at its highest value and the electrode alternating rate is set at "CONSTANT." The polarity may be either positive or negative.

WARNING! DO NOT ATTEMPT TO REMOVE YOUR HAND FROM THE WATER WHILE THE CURRENT IS FLOWING.

- Instruct your assistant to slowly turn up the voltage until you just begin to feel a tingling in your hand. At this point, stop turning up the voltage.
- Slowly remove your hand one quarter of the way out of the water. What does the current feel like now? (It should be slightly more intense.)
- Continue to remove your hand a little bit at a time. When the perception of the current begins to become too intense, stop withdrawing your hand, and move it back into the water, or have your assistant reduce the voltage or hit the reset switch.

Why did the current become more uncomfortable as you pulled your hand out? As you were withdrawing your hand, the current density was increasing because the surface area through which the current flowed was decreasing. So why shouldn't you completely remove your hand from the water? Think about what would happen to the current density if you did so. If you took your hand out of the water, at some point the entire current would flow through the tip of your middle finger, resulting in a very high current density.

This point should be kept in mind when treating an athlete with electrical stimulation and immersion. For this reason, always instruct the athlete not to remove the body part prior to resetting the voltage to zero.

Duty Cycle

The ratio of the amount of time the current is flowing (ON) to the amount of time without current (OFF) is known as the duty cycle. Expressed as a percentage, duty cycles are calculated by dividing the time the current is flowing by the total cycle time (the time the current is flowing + the time it is not). For example, to calculate the duty cycle of a generator producing 10 seconds of stimulation, followed by 10 seconds without current flow, the following equation would be used:

$$\text{Duty cycle (percentage)} = \frac{\text{Time current is on}}{\text{Total cycle time}} \times 100$$

$$= \frac{10 \text{ seconds (on)}}{10 \text{ seconds (on)} + 10 \text{ seconds (off)}} \times 100$$

$$= \frac{10 \text{ seconds}}{20 \text{ seconds (Total cycle time)}} \times 100$$

$$= 0.5 \times 100$$

$$= 50\% \text{ duty cycle}$$

This relationship may also be expressed as a ratio. Using the parameters from the previous examples:

$$\text{Duty cycle (ratio)} = 10{:}20$$

$$= 1{:}2$$

Duty cycles play a role in neuromuscular stimulation by preventing muscle fatigue. Muscular stimulation is started with a 25 percent duty cycle and is progressively increased as the athlete improves.[9]

The Body Circuit

The human body is a mass of tissues and fluids, each of which has a varying ability to conduct electrical currents. The electrical conductivity of a tissue is directly related to its water content. As the percentage of the water in tissue increases, its ability to transmit electricity increases.

Tissues are classified as being either **excitable** or **nonexcitable** (Table 4–5 and Box 4–2). Excitable tissues are directly influenced by the current parameters of intensity, pulse duration, and pulse frequency. Nonexcitable tissues do not directly respond to current flow, but may be influenced by the electrical fields caused by the current.

The outer layer of the skin has a low water content, making it a poor electrical conductor. Bone, tendons, fascia, and adipose tissue are also poor conductors of electrical currents because of their low water content (20% to

Table 4–5 **EXCITABLE AND NONEXCITABLE TISSUES**

Excitable Tissues	Nonexcitable Tissues
Nerve fibers	Bone
Muscle fiber	Cartilage
Blood cells	Tendons
Secretory cells	Ligaments

Electrical Agents • **121**

Box (4–2) EXCITABLE TISSUES

When an excitable tissue (nerve, muscle, etc.) remains undisturbed, its resting potential stays constant. The resulting potential acts as a stored energy source to be used in the transmission of impulses; the energy is stored as separated electrical charges on either side (inside and outside) of the cell membrane. In this sense, the membrane serves as a capacitor. The amount of depolarization required to bring these tissues to threshold is about the same for each.

A decrease (depolarization) or increase (hyperpolarization) in the cell membrane's electrical charge is required before an action potential can take place. Any stimulus, be it electrical, mechanical, chemical, thermal, or hormonal, at a sufficient magnitude, can cause a depolarization by changing the permeability of the cell, resulting in an action potential. A membrane requires approximately 0.5 msec to recover its excitability following an action potential. This "down time" following the action potential is the **absolute refractory period**. If a second impulse at the same intensity occurs within this time period, the membrane will not discharge. Following the absolute refractory period there is a **relative refractory period**, during which another depolarization can occur if the magnitude of the stimulus is increased.

30%). Conversely, muscle, nerve, and blood have a high water content (70% to 75%) and are good conductors of electrical currents. It is the membrane of the cells that provides the highest resistance to current flow. The internal organs, especially the heart, have a low resistance to electrical current flow. This is why passage of an electrical current through the heart must be avoided.

The current enters the body through a series circuit. Since the composition and texture of skin is relatively consistent, there is only one path for the flow to take. Once the current enters the tissues, it may take many different paths, forming a parallel circuit. The flow will prefer to follow the paths of least resistance, such as those formed by muscle, nerves, and blood.

The passage of current through living tissues will produce varying biophysical effects, including thermal changes, physiochemical effects, and physiological reactions. The amount of heat produced by an electrical current passing through the body is proportional to the square of the intensity, the resistance provided by the tissue, and the current flow. However, the average current produced by electrical modalities is so low that the thermal effects of the treatment are negligible.[8]

MOVEMENT OF ELECTRICAL CURRENTS THROUGH THE BODY

Most electrical stimulation is applied transcutaneously. The exceptions are electrical stimulators which have electrodes surgically implanted in the muscle or bone, such as bone growth generators. When a current is passed through the skin, it has the potential to upset the resting potential of peripheral axons. Under the cathode, a depolarization of the nerve occurs, while stimulation under the anode results in a hyperpolarization of the nerve.[10]

Once a therapeutic electrical current enters the body, the flow of electrons

---

Box 4-3   IONIC CHANGES

In its normal state, an atom has a number of electrons equal to the number of protons. Since the charges of the electrons (negative) and protons (positive) are equal, the atom has a zero (neutral) charge. Atoms which no longer have a zero net charge are known as ions. When an atom loses one or more electrons, it becomes a positive ion (cation) because the number of protons is greater than the number of electrons. Likewise, atoms that gain electrons become negatively charged ions (anions) because the number of electrons is greater than the number of protons.

Ions behave differently than their neutrally charged relatives. Since they possess an electrical charge, they are subject to electromagnetic and electro-osmotic influences. When placed in the path of a direct current, positively charged ions will migrate towards the negative pole and vice versa.

---

is replaced by the movement of *ions* (see Box 4–3). As described by Coulomb's law, ions will move away from the pole having the same charge and migrate toward the pole having the opposite charge. When an AC or pulsed biphasic current is used, the ions will move back and forth between the electrodes based on the number of cycles per second, as shown in Figure 4–4. When a DC or pulsed monophasic current is used, this migration is in one direction only.

Medical Galvanism

Galvanic stimulation involves the application of a low-voltage direct current to the body, with a known polarity under each electrode. By controlling the polarity of the electrodes, certain involuntary cellular responses may be elicited. It is important to note that true galvanism requires an uninterrupted direct current to achieve a net galvanic change under the electrodes.

Through an **electro-osmotic** process, ions are attracted to the pole possessing the opposite charge and repelled from the pole having the same charge. Positively charged sodium ions (Na^+) move towards the cathode, where they gain an electron and form an uncharged sodium atom. Through the reaction of sodium with water, proteins are liquefied, resulting in a general softening of the tissues in the area.

Physiological events under the anode are essentially opposite those occurring at the cathode. Here, tissues harden because chemical mediators force a coagulation of protein.

Short pulse duration and long interpulse interval reduce the chemical effects of pulsed high-voltage generators.[11] Symmetrical or balanced asymmetric alternating currents result in no galvanic changes since both phases have an equal but opposite charge. An imbalanced asymmetric current can result in residual chemical changes if the duration of the current is sufficient.

Ion: An atom, or group of atoms, that has a net charge other than zero.

ELECTRODES

The site where the electrodes touch the skin serves as a point of conversion between the flow of electrons used by the generator and the flow of ions within the body's tissues.[6] To form a closed circuit between the generator and the athlete's tissues, at least one electrode from each of the generator's output leads must be in contact with the athlete's skin. Properly prepared and placed electrodes increase the efficiency of the electrical current while allowing for less discomfort from the treatment (Table 4–6).

The electrodes themselves may be metal, carbon-impregnated silicon rubber, or a metallic meshed cloth. In most cases, a **medium** is required to reduce the skin's resistance and evenly distribute the current. Metal electrodes commonly use moistened sponges for this purpose. Carbon-rubber electrodes may also use moist sponges, gauze, or a conducting gel.

Conducting gels are salt-free coupling agents designed to minimize skin–electrode resistance. Their chemical properties allow for long-term use with little breakdown due to current flow or evaporation. Because of the gel's high water content, skin irritation and allergic reactions are minimized.

Electrodes used during short-term treatments are generally held in place by elastic straps. In the case of long-term treatments, the electrodes must be secured through the use of adhesive patches, although some electrodes used for this purpose are self-adhesive. Generally these types of electrodes, and their adhesives, are very durable and water resistant.

The type of electrode and the conductive medium used have been shown to affect the efficiency and comfort of electrical stimulation. Carbon-rubber electrodes deliver the greatest current with the lowest skin impedance, allowing a more comfortable stimulation.[12,13] Self-adhesive electrodes have been shown to produce the most discomfort during the treatment, with an increased burning sensation occurring under the electrode's metal connector.[13]

The site, intensity, and type of excitable tissue being stimulated is determined by a combination of electrode size and placement. In a study conducted by Leiber and Kelly,[13] a positive correlation was found between maximal isometric torque production and the size of the stimulation electrodes. However, they determined that the primary determinant of stimulation torque did not lie in stimulation parameters such as electrode size or current, but in the properties of the musculature itself. This suggests that the results of electrical stimulation, especially when the clinician is attempting to elicit muscle contractions, may vary greatly from individual to individual, regardless of the parameters used.

Table 4–6 **METHODS OF REDUCING THE SKIN'S ELECTRICAL RESISTANCE**

Moisten the electrodes with water or conductive gel, depending on the type of electrode used.
Remove dirt, oil, or flaky skin by washing with soap and water, alcohol, or acetone.
Warm the area with a moist heat pack.
Gently scrub the area with fine emery paper.
Remove excess hair.

Electrode Size

As described in the previous section, the size of the electrode inversely affects the density of the current; as the size of the electrode decreases, the current density increases. Larger electrodes have a lower impedance than smaller ones. As the electrode surface area increases, there is a greater current flow at any given voltage.[1] Smaller electrodes require less current to stimulate tissues than larger electrodes because of the high current density. By manipulating the relative sizes of the electrodes, various physiological responses may be elicited.

The size of an electrode to be used is determined relative to the size of the body area being treated and/or by the other electrodes being used. A "small" electrode used on the quadriceps could easily be a "large" electrode when it is used on the forearm. Additionally, as we will see in the next section the size of an electrode is relative to the other electrode(s) being used. The resistance to current flow (impedance) offered by the skin is reduced as the size of the electrode increases. Larger electrodes produce stronger contractions without causing pain, but the stimulation of the tissues is less specific because the current is spread over a larger area.[5]

Electrode Placement

The proximity of electrodes to one another determines which tissues are stimulated, the depth of the stimulation, and the number of parallel circuits that are formed. When the electrodes are placed close together the current flows superficially, with a relatively small number of parallel paths developed. As the distance between the electrodes is increased, the current is allowed to reach deeper into the tissues. If the distance between the two electrodes is too great, such a large number of parallel circuits are formed that the specificity of the stimulation decreases.

The orientation of the electrodes in relation to the body part must also be taken into consideration. Muscle fibers are four times more conductive when the current flows with the direction of the fibers than when it flows across them.[6]

Although each electrical circuit consists of two leads from the generator, more than one electrode can be connected to a single lead. Through bifurcation, two or more electrodes can originate from a single lead. It is not uncommon for both leads to possess two electrodes each, or for one lead to have two electrodes and the other lead to have one only.

Bipolar Technique

Bipolar application involves the use of electrodes of equal or near equal size (Fig. 4–16). Both electrodes are located in the target treatment area and since the current densities are equal, an equal amount of stimulation occurs under each electrode or set of electrodes. If the electrodes are of different sizes, the current density, and therefore the current effect, will be greater under the smaller electrode.

Monopolar Technique

Monopolar application involves the use of two types of electrodes, an **active electrode** where the treatment effect occurs and a dispersive electrode used to complete the circuit. The active electrode is placed on or near the body part

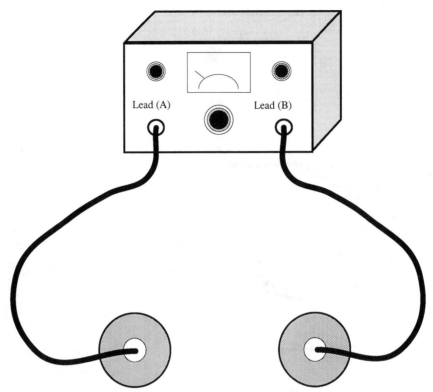

Figure 4–16. Bipolar application of electrical stimulation. The surface area of the electrodes originating from each lead is equal. This creates an equal current density and the effects of the stimulation occur equally under each set of electrode. Each lead may be split to accommodate two electrodes. So long as the electrodes are of equal size and the resulting current density is equal, the application would be bipolar.

to be treated and the **dispersive electrode** is fastened to the body at a distant location (Fig. 4–17). The high current density focuses the effect of the treatment under the smaller electrodes. As the distance between the active and dispersive electrode increases, more parallel electrical paths are formed, resulting in less specific stimulation of deep motor nerves.[5]

The surface area of the dispersive electrode is significantly larger than the total surface area of the active electrode(s). Because of the relatively low current density, little or no sensory stimulation should occur under the dispersive electrode. If the athlete does experience sensory stimulation under this electrode, the athletic trainer should reapply it at a different site, re-wet it, or use a larger electrode. Sensation under the dispersive electrode does not negate the effects of the treatment, but it is unnecessary. Motor nerve stimulation under this electrode indicates that the current densities of the electrodes are too similar. In this case, a larger dispersive electrode or a smaller active electrode should be used.

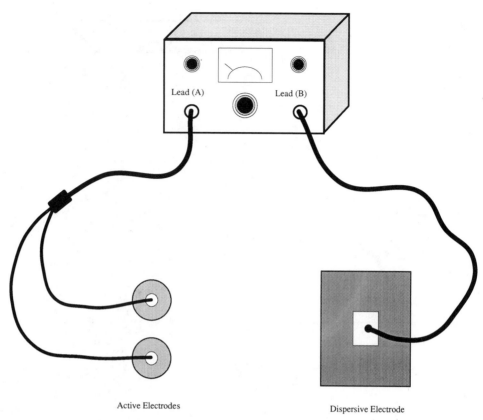

Active Electrodes

Dispersive Electrode

Figure 4–17. Monopolar application of electrical stimulation. The total area of the active electrode is significantly less than the area of the dispersive electrode. The imbalance in current density focuses the stimulation to the area under the active electrodes.

Quadripolar Technique

Quadripolar application involves the use of two sets of electrodes, each originating from its own *channel*; it may be considered the concurrent application of two bipolar stimulations. The current from each of the two channels may intersect, as is found with interferential stimulation; it then intensifies the effects of the treatment. Other quadripolar configurations include parallel placements, as are found in certain transcutaneous electrical nerve stimulation techniques, or agonist-antagonist placements used in neuromuscular electrical stimulation techniques (Fig. 4–18).

SELECTIVE STIMULATION OF NERVES

During the application of electrical stimulation, different nerve types are stimulated in an orderly, predictable manner. A nerve's response to electrical stimulation is based on three factors: (1) the relative diameter of the nerve, (2) the depth of the nerve in relation to the electrode, and (3) the duration of the pulse.

Channel (Electrical): An electrical circuit, consisting of two poles, that operates independently of other circuits.

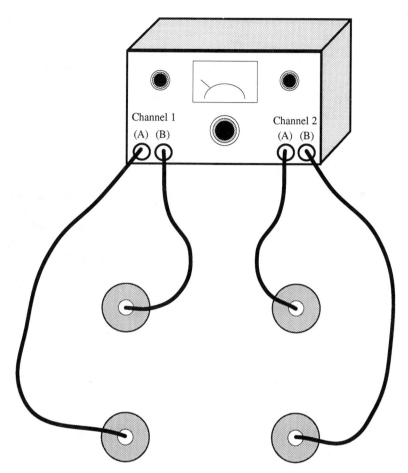

Figure 4–18. Quadripolar application of electrical stimulation. Two sets of electrodes are operating with two independent channels.

During electrical stimulation, sensory nerves are stimulated first, followed by motor nerves, and then pain fibers.

The amplitude necessary to stimulate a nerve is inversely proportional to the nerve's diameter. Nerves with larger diameters will be stimulated to threshold before nerves with smaller diameters. Because the larger cross-sectional area of the nerve provides less resistance, less current is required.

Superficial sensory nerves receive a greater amount of stimulation than do the more deeply placed motor nerves. To activate a more deeply situated motor nerve, the current must first pass through the more superficial sensory nerves. Pain fibers are more superficial than motor nerves but they are also much smaller in diameter. Their resistance to current flow is so great that motor nerves reach threshold first. This allows muscular contractions to be elicited before pain is felt. However, pain fibers may be stimulated before the deeper motor nerves. Surface stimulation of the skin will always result in the activation of sensory receptors before motor or pain nerves.[14]

Short pulse durations allow for the greatest range in stimulation intensity for excitation of the three nerve types. In this manner, there is a great range between the current required to stimulate sensory nerves, motor nerves, and pain fibers. As the pulse duration is increased, two events occur. First, less amperage is required to stimulate each nerve level. Secondly, the interval between each nerve level is decreased. Figure 4–19 depicts a typical strength–duration curve that describes the relationship between pulse duration and the threshold of excitation of the nerve types indicated. Theoretically, if the pulse duration is continued out the baseline, there would be a point where each nerve level would be stimulated almost simultaneously and at a very low intensity (Box 4–4).

Many stimulation techniques describe the intensity of the current applied with reference to the type of nerve stimulated. Sensory level stimulation describes an output that stimulates only sensory nerves. This level is found by increasing the output to the point where a slight muscle twitch is seen in the muscle. When this point is reached, the output is then decreased to the point where the muscle activity ceases. Motor level stimulation describes an intensity that produces a substantial muscle contraction without causing pain. Noxious level stimulation is current applied at an intensity that stimulates pain fibers.

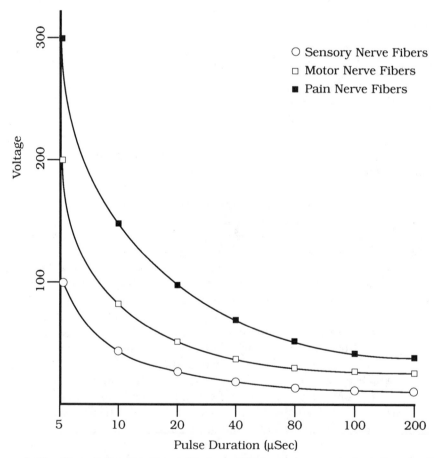

Figure 4–19. Strength-Duration Curve. Short pulse durations are more selective in the nerve fibers stimulated than longer pulse durations.

Box **EXPERIMENT DEMONSTRATING THE SELECTIVE STIMULATION OF NERVES**

If someone applies electrical stimulation to your forearm, you can see and feel for yourself how nerves are selectively stimulated. Using an electrical modality that has an adjustable pulse duration, set the duration to the lowest value. For this experiment, apply the electrodes over the muscle belly of the forearm musculature. Instruct your assistant to slowly begin increasing the intensity of the treatment and write down at what current intensity each of the following responses occur:

- As the voltage is initially turned up, you will feel "pins and needles" under the electrodes. At this intensity, only the large, superficial sensory nerves are being stimulated.
- As the intensity of the treatment is increased, muscle contractions begin to occur. At this point, the amplitude of the wave is at a level sufficient to cause the motor nerves, which are deeper and of somewhat smaller diameter than sensory nerves, to fully depolarize.
- If the intensity of the current continues to be increased, pain will be experienced. The intensity of the current is now at a level sufficient to overcome the capacitance of the nerve fibers of smaller diameter.

When the treatment becomes somewhat painful, have your assistant reduce the intensity to zero and allow your tissues a few minutes to recover from this initial bout. Increase the pulse duration to the middle setting and repeat the prior steps, again noting at what current level each response occurs. Then repeat the process with the pulse duration set at its maximal duration.

Compare your results with the sample strength-duration curve shown in Figure 4–19 by plotting your results on a similar graph. Was the interval between sensory, motor, and pain stimulation reduced as the pulse duration was increased?

CENTRAL AND PERIPHERAL NERVOUS SYSTEM INTERFERENCE

When a continuous stimulus sufficient to cause depolarization of a cell membrane remains unchanged, the resting potential of the membrane will return to its prestimulus level. This process, **accommodation**, occurs when the rate of discharge of the nerve's action potential decreases while the depolarization stimulus, in this case an electrical current, remains unchanged. Cells undergoing accommodation require a more intense stimulus to reach the threshold of depolarization.

The threshold for the initiation of an action potential varies according to the stimulation applied. Pulses which rise more slowly require a greater amount of depolarization to initiate an action potential. Nervous tissue accommodates very quickly, thus an abrupt pulse rise is needed. Muscle fibers accommodate more slowly than nerve fibers, so a gradual pulse rise may be used.[8]

The central nervous system may also play a role in decreasing the long-term sensory stimulation associated with electrical stimulation.[15] Through the process of **habituation**, the central nervous system filters out a continuous, nonmeaningful stimuli. This can be seen in everyday life: You sit down to study in the kitchen. Your roommates have gone out for the evening, so the house is quiet except for the humming of the refrigerator. After you begin studying, the sound of the refrigerator gets pushed farther and farther into the background of your consciousness. Eventually, you no longer realize that the sound is there. This stimulus stays in the background until the refrigerator stops humming. At this point you are struck by the silence of the room.

The concepts of accommodation and habituation can be demonstrated when applying an electrical modality. Increase the intensity of an electrical modality to the point where the athlete expresses slight displeasure in the comfort of the stimulus. Let the athlete experience the current flow for about 5 minutes and then ask if the intensity can be increased. More times than not, the athlete will say, "Yes." They have displayed accommodation.

Many electrotherapeutic modalities have modulation parameters to combat the effects of accommodation. The generator randomly alters the intensity, frequency, and/or duration of the pulses. This prevents the body from receiving a constant, unchanging stimulus.

Electrical Stimulation Goals and Techniques

This section presents common goals of electrical stimulation and techniques on how to achieve them. The section on clinical application in this chapter relates these goals to the different types of electrical stimulation units commonly found in the athletic training room.

ELICITATION OF MUSCULAR CONTRACTIONS

Virtually any type of electrotherapeutic modality can elicit a contraction in normal, healthy muscle, if applied at a sufficient intensity, by causing a depolarization or hyperpolarization of the motor nerve's membrane. If the magnitude of the stimulation is sufficient, an action potential will be initiated, resulting in contraction of the muscle. These contractions may be used to retard the effects of atrophy, to re-educate muscle, or to augment the strength of healthy muscle.

It is important to note that electrical stimulation of innervated muscle activates the motor nerve rather than the muscle fibers directly. Since the capacitance of motor nerves is less than that of muscular tissue, the current overcomes the resistance of the nerve first. The motor nerves are recruited into the contraction based on their size and proximity to the electrode. Large-diameter motor neurons will be recruited before smaller ones and those nerves in close proximity to the electrode respond before those more distant.

When a muscle is denervated, communication can no longer occur through the motor nerve, so the muscle fibers must be directly stimulated to evoke a contraction. In partially denervated muscle, motor nerve fibers may be selectively recruited through the use of a short pulse duration and a slowly rising wave form.[8] Denervated muscle will react to stimulation from direct current or monophasic currents possessing a long pulse duration, but not from alternating currents or pulsed currents having a short duration. This is because the current flows for a longer time in one direction when using a direct current, allowing depolarization of the muscle fiber membranes to occur.

Pulse Amplitude

As the intensity of the stimulus increases, so does the strength of the contraction. The force of the muscle contraction has been found to be linearly related to the amount of current introduced into the tissues.[16,17] The depth of penetration of the current increases as the peak current increases, thus recruiting more nerve fibers. Pain fibers are of relatively small diameter when compared to motor nerve fibers and are normally only stimulated at higher intensities; this allows for muscle recruitment without a disproportional amount of discomfort. However, it is often the pain of the stimulation that prevents maximal contractions from being achieved.

Cold treatment is often used for its anesthetic effects. Researchers have attempted to determine if the application of cold treatments prior to neuromuscular electrical stimulation would, by decreasing the discomfort associated with the stimulation, allow an increase in the torque produced by involuntary muscle contractions. One study indicated that a significant increase in torque was shown following the application of an ice massage.[18] A later study using ice packs produced no significant difference in torque production.[19] Although these studies neither support nor disprove the efficacy of cold application prior to electrically induced muscle contractions, this technique could be beneficial for those athletes who have increased sensory discomfort during the application of electrical currents.

Pulse Frequency

When the stimulation is being applied at a pulse rate of less than 15 pulses per second, there are distinguishable muscle contractions for each pulse. At this pulse rate, there is sufficient time for the mechanical process required for the muscle fibers to return their original length before the next pulse begins.

Between 15 and 25 pulses per second, the individual contractions become less and less distinguishable due to **summation**. In this case, the muscle fibers do not return to their original position before the initiation of the next pulse. As the pulse frequency increases, the amount of summation increases as a result of the greater overlap in the mechanical process of muscle contraction.[8]

Summation continues until the muscle reaches the stage of *tetany*. At this point, the muscle enters a *tonic contraction*. Increasing the frequency of the stimulation will do little to further smooth the muscle tone. It will, however, promote muscle fatigue if used for a sufficient duration. The exact number of pulses per second required to reach tetany varies between muscle groups. However, postural muscles have been found to reach tetany before nonpostural muscles.[2]

A strong tetanic contraction is required to delay atrophy or enhance strength. Low-frequency stimulation reduces fatigue, but the muscle develops 45 percent less force than it could at higher frequencies.[3] Very high frequencies have been shown to make it possible to produce tetany with greater comfort than lower frequencies.[20] High-frequency biphasic currents have also been shown to selec-

---

Tetany: Total contraction of a muscle achieved through the recruitment and contraction of all motor units.
Tonic Contraction: Prolonged contraction of a muscle.

tively fatigue type II muscle fibers, so that there is a decrease in torque production as the duration of treatment progresses.[21] This effect may be counteracted by increasing the amount of rest between treatment cycles or decreasing the pulse frequency during treatment.

Pulse Duration

To recruit motor nerves only, the use of a short pulse duration is recommended.[8] When recruiting the muscle fiber directly, a slowly rising pulse is recommended. Short pulse durations require a greater amplitude to evoke an action potential than pulses of longer durations. Pulse durations of less than 1 millisecond (msec) will not be able to stimulate denervated muscle, regardless of the current's amplitude.[2,7] The optimal pulse duration for elicitation of maximal muscle contractions has been shown to be in the range of 300 to 500 microseconds (μsec).[22]

Motor Points

Each muscle has one or more skin surface areas that are hypersensitive to electrical current flow. These motor points are discrete areas over which nerves and blood vessels enter the muscle mass. Because of their low electrical resistance, stimulation of these points will elicit a stronger contraction at lower intensities than the surrounding tissues (Box 4–5).

The exact location of motor points varies between individuals and, depending on the pathology involved, can vary for the same person over time. Motor points related to an injured area show an increased sensitivity to current flow and palpation. Appendix B presents commonly accepted motor points and is presented for reference purposes. These points must be located on each athlete by finding the point where the strongest contraction results from the lowest intensity of stimulation.

Strength Augmentation

Strength gains realized through the use of electrical stimulation are attributable to two factors.[23] First, strength gains are a response to placement of an increased functional load on the muscle. For strength gains to occur via electrical stimulation, the functional load placed on the muscle must equal a significant proportion of the torque produced by the maximal voluntary isometric contraction (MVIC). You may recognize this factor as being, in part, the basis of the *overload* principle.

The increased functional load is supplemented by the increased recruitment of **type II muscle fibers**, the second factor in strength gains. When muscles are voluntarily contracted, smaller **type I motor nerves** are recruited prior to the type II fibers. Since electrical current depolarizes larger diameter nerves first, type II fibers are brought into the contraction sooner. Several other studies

---

Overload Principle: For strength gains to occur, the body must be subjected to more stress than it is accustomed to. This is accomplished by increasing the load, frequency, or duration of the exercise.

Box  **EXPERIMENT TO IDENTIFY MOTOR POINTS**

It is relatively easy to identify motor points. For this experiment, you will need a high-voltage pulsed stimulator that has a hand-held probe (small tip), an assistant, and your posterior forearm musculature:

- Make sure the generator is turned off.
- Place the dispersive electrode on a large body mass, such as the thigh.
- Connect and activate the probe.
- Use any pulse frequency setting.
- Sit so that your forearm can rest comfortably on a table with the palm facing downward.
- Turn the unit on and reset the intensity to zero.
- Your assistant will wet the tip of the probe and place it in contact with the extensor muscle mass of your forearm.
- The voltage is then turned up until a mild sensation is felt, or until slight muscle contractions are noted.
- By slowly moving the probe over the forearm musculature, you should see individual muscles contracting. Perhaps at one point your index finger will lift off the table, at another point, your whole wrist.
- When a good contraction is established in one of the muscles (or muscle groups) you can also see the effects of varying the pulse frequency by slowly increasing and decreasing the pulse rate.

As the probe is moved around the forearm, you will see that in some areas the muscle contracts quite readily. In other places, little, if any, contraction is noted. This demonstrates the necessity for locating motor points when attempting to electrically elicit muscle contractions. You may wish to use a water-based marker and identify on yourself where the motor points are. These points can then be compared to the motor points presented in Appendix B.

One last detail. By attaching the dispersive electrode to the thigh, we have created a current path consisting of many parallel circuits. Therefore, the contractions we got were general rather than specific. To communicate more effectively with the motor points, replace the large dispersive electrode with a smaller electrode. Now attach the small dispersive electrode to the anterior musculature of the forearm and repeat the above experiment. What does this do to the contractions?

---

have supported the concept of early activation of type II fibers and noted the early fatigue of this type of muscle fiber.[21,25,26] The two elements work together so that muscle strengthening through electrical stimulation may occur at levels equaling 30 percent of the MVIC.[3,23]

It is important for athletic trainers to keep in mind that electrical stimulation is not a replacement for voluntary muscle contractions, but an adjunct technique. Although effective in increasing isometric muscle strength, electrical stimulation is less effective in increasing quadriceps torque than a biofeedback unit.[27] Strength gains obtained by electrical stimulation follow the same parameters of specificity as any other form of exercise: That is, isometric training will only improve isometric strength and will not carry over to isotonic or isokinetic strength.[28]

PAIN CONTROL

Electrical currents may be employed to reduce the amount of pain experienced by an athlete. This reduction may occur as a result of lessening the mechanical pressure placed on nerve endings, by decreasing the degree of muscle spasm or edema in the painful area. In specific pain control approaches, electrical stimulation may simply "mask" the pain or encourage the body's release of pain-controlling substances.

High-frequency, short-duration, sensory-level currents are thought to activate the gate mechanism of pain modulation. In this case, the stimulation of sensory nerves closes the gate to the transmission of pain. Low-frequency, long-duration, high-intensity stimulation is thought to stimulate the release of the body's natural opiates—β-endorphin from the pituitary gland and enkephalins from the spinal cord.

In the initial phases of pain control, electrotherapeutic treatments stimulate the dorsal horn of the spinal cord. Peripheral stimulation could relieve chronic pain if applied to the site of pain or to an area serviced by the involved peripheral nerve.

The placebo effect of electrotherapeutic modalities cannot be overlooked. Many studies and reference materials exploring the effects of electrical current flow on pain perception report that patients receiving sham treatments described a decrease in the amount of pain experienced.[29,30,31,32,33,34] This confirms that cognitive processes are involved in the pain modulation process.

WOUND HEALING

There is evidence that confirms the usefulness of electrical stimulation in the resolution of open superficial wounds, such as *dermal ulcers*.[35,36,37] Explanations for the effectiveness of tissue repair include increased circulation, increased blood clot formation, antibacterial effects, influences on the migration of cells, and the presence of an "injury potential" in damaged tissues. When tissues are damaged, an electrical potential is created between the healthy and damaged tissues.[38] This injury potential is theorized to electrically control tissue repair.

The application of a constant low-voltage direct current to injured tissues is thought to mimic the naturally occurring electrical signals used to promote healing under the positive electrode. Leukocytes tend to migrate toward the anode, resulting in increased blood clotting in the area.[35]

It should be noted that evidence supporting the use of electrical stimulation in wound healing has involved chronic conditions, with the majority of the cases being dermal ulcers. The use of electrical stimulation in the healing of acute wounds has not been investigated.

CONTROL AND REDUCTION OF EDEMA

The electrical mechanisms required for the control and reduction of edema occur at two levels. At the first level, sensory stimulation, a unit is required that delivers a direct current in order to limit the amount of acute edema formed. At the second, the motor level, elicitation of muscle contractions can be achieved by many different types of generators and is used to reduce chronic or post-traumatic edema through increased venous drainage.

Dermal Ulcer: A slow-healing, or nonhealing, break in the skin.

Sensory Level Stimulation for Edema Control

In acute trauma, negative polarity applied over, or directly around, the injury site has been found to limit the amount of edema formed in laboratory animals. This method of application is termed sensory-level because the intensity of the stimulation is kept below the motor threshold level. One proposed mechanism for this response is a reduction in capillary pressure and capillary permeability that discourages plasma proteins from entering the *extracellular* tissues.[39] Blood cells and plasma proteins are negatively charged and therefore are repelled from the treatment area. The resultant concentration gradient would then encourage fluids to follow these structures into the venous and lymphatic return systems.[40]

A frequently cited report by Michlovitz and associates[41] concluded that the application of high-voltage pulsed stimulation (HVPS) along with ice, compression, and elevation did not significantly decrease edema formation in ankle sprains, compared to those treated with the standard protocol of ice, compression, and elevation. A later study by Griffin and associates[42] reported that HVPS made a "clinically significant" but not a statistically significant reduction of chronic hand edema compared to a control group.

Motor Level Stimulation for Edema Reduction

The role of the motor level response in reducing edema formation is somewhat less controversial. In this mode, muscular contractions encourage venous and lymphatic return by squeezing the vessels and milking the fluids out of the area. Many types of electrical stimulation devices can be employed to produce an involuntary muscle contraction which forces the fluids out of the area. This technique is also referred to as muscle milking or the muscle pump.

As would be expected from what we know of the venous and lymphatic return mechanisms (see Chapter 1), the efficiency of this technique is improved when the limb is elevated so that gravity may assist in the fluid flow. Additionally, the use of an elastic wrap or tubular compressive stockings applied to the extremity assists in edema reduction.

FRACTURE HEALING

Electrical currents are employed to assist in the healing of *nonunion fractures*. Normally, fractures heal through the process of *osteogenesis*. If the fracture fails to heal properly, further repair must occur through endochondral bone formation, where the soft tissue callus must transform itself into bone.[43] Historically, nonunion fractures required the surgical grafting of bone into the site to assist the healing process. The use of electrical stimulation to aid in the healing of bone is based on the theory that bone cannot differentiate between the body's innate charges that are needed for normal bone remodeling (see

---

Extracellular: Outside the cell membrane.
Nonunion Fracture: Fracture that fails to spontaneously heal within a normal time frame.
Osteogenesis: Healing of fracture sites through the formation of callus, followed by the deposition of collagen and bone salts.

Wolff's law, Chapter 1), and those derived from outside sources, such as electrical generators.

Collectively known as bone-growth generators, these units attempt to produce electromagnetic fields that mimic the normal electrical signals produced by bone. This encourages the deposition of calcium through increased osteoblastic activity. There are many different approaches to applying bone-growth generators. Generally, those generators applied transcutaneously use alternating currents, while those having electrodes implanted in the body use direct currents.[44]

Generators with external electrodes are similar to diathermy units (see Chapter 3) in that their electrodes produce strong electromagnetic fields. These fields then create electric currents at the fracture site. When the electrodes are implanted into the tissues, the cathode is placed near the fracture site because new bone callus has been found to be electropositive.[45]

The usefulness of bone-growth generators is still debatable.[43,44] However, many facts regarding their use are apparent. These units appear to be effective only in certain nonunion fractures and are useful only for long-term treatments. Unlike most electrical stimulation techniques, stimulation by bone-growth generators needs to be constant for six months or longer in order to effect healing. They have not been found to be effective in speeding the healing of acute fractures.

The prescription of bone-growth generators is the physician's domain. However, athletic trainers should be familiar with their functions, benefits, and limitations. As this technology grows and the efficacy of this modality is established, its possibilities for use in the treatment of acute fractures increase.

IONTOPHORESIS

Iontophoresis is the delivery of medication through the skin using a low-voltage direct current. By adapting to fluctuations in tissue resistance, iontophoresis generators (iontophoresors) produce a constant voltage output by adjusting the amperage. The medication types most commonly used for iontophoresis include anesthetics, analgesics, and anti-inflammatory agents.

Based on the ionic reaction between the positive and negative poles of the generator, medication molecules travel along the lines of force created by the current. At the positive electrode, positive ions are driven through the skin; negative ions are introduced through the skin at the negative pole. This technique has been shown to deliver the medication to depths of 6 to 20 millimeters (mm) below the skin.[46]

For the application of iontophoresis, the medication is dissolved in a carrier. This mixture is then placed into a specially designed electrode that is fastened over the treatment site. The second electrode is attached to the body at a convenient nearby site. The polarity of each electrode is based on the type of charge required for delivering the medication through the skin.

The transdermal introduction of medication has advantages over the oral ingestion or injection of medication. The advantages over oral medication include: Metabolic breakdown of the medication is reduced because the liver is bypassed, the medication is not absorbed in the gastrointestinal tract, and the medication is concentrated in a localized area.[47] These advantages also hold true with injected medication, but iontophoresis is less traumatic and less painful than injected medication. Additionally, the injection of medication can result in a high concentration of the medication in a localized area and this can cause damage to the tissues.[46]

Iontophoresis is not without its disadvantages. Unreliable results are obtained with certain medications, and there may be doubt to as how much medication is actually introduced into the tissues.[48] Furthermore, many of the medications used in this technique require a physician's prescription.

Summary

Therapeutic currents are classified as being either alternating, direct, or pulsed. Alternating and direct currents are characterized by an uninterrupted flow of electrons. In pulsed currents, the flow of electrons is intermittently paused. A pulsed current may be monophasic, having a unidirectional current flow, or biphasic, having a bidirectional flow of electrons.

When a therapeutic electrical current is introduced into the body, the flow of electrons causes the movement of ions. This current enters the body through a set of electrodes that forms a closed circuit between the generator and the athlete. Within the tissues, physiological effects are related to current parameters such as amplitude, duration, and frequency. Depending on the mix of these variables, responses such as neuromuscular stimulation, pain control, control and reduction of edema, and wound healing are evoked.

Clinical Application of Electrical Modalities

This part of the chapter describes the theory, effects, and application of various forms of electrical stimulation. Although each stimulation method is presented as a distinct modality, many generators are capable of producing a wide range of electrical characteristics. For example, a generator may be adjusted to produce either a monophasic, biphasic, alternating, or direct current.

Many states require that electrical stimulation devices be applied only under the order of a physician. It is important that student athletic trainers become aware of the laws governing the use of electrical modalities in their state, as well as the policies and procedures for use at their institution. Likewise, use of these devices should be supervised by an experienced individual. This supervision is even more essential during the learning process.

Basic Guidelines for the Setup and Application of Electrotherapy

An outline of the process used in preparing the generator, electrodes, and the athlete for electrotherapy appears below. The steps involved in using the generator are later detailed for each stimulation approach.

Preparation of the Generator

1. If a portable or battery-operated unit is being used, make sure that the batteries are fully charged. If a clinical model is being used, make sure that it is properly plugged into a grounded wall socket. If the treatment

involves water immersion, the unit MUST be plugged into a ground fault interrupter circuit. The use of extension cords should be avoided.

2. Make sure that the electrode leads are not tangled. The leads should be inspected regularly for frays, broken insulation, and loose connections.

Preparation of the Electrodes

1. Clean the electrodes to remove any residual gels or skin oils.
2. If conductive sponges are used, moisten them with water. If sponges are not required, apply an even coat of conductive gel to the electrodes.
3. Connect the leads to the unit and to the electrodes.

Preparation of the Athlete

1. Determine the electrode placement technique to be used.
2. The points to be stimulated should be cleansed with alcohol to remove any body oils, lotions, dirt, and grime. Keep in mind that body hair increases resistance to electrical current flow. When possible, place the pad over areas of low hair density.
3. If a monopolar technique is being used, find a large body mass, such as the thigh or lower back to attach the dispersive electrode. If the lower back is selected for the site of the dispersive electrode, place it so that it lies on one side of the spinal column and not across it. The indentation formed by the erector muscles causes incomplete contact with the dispersive electrode and may result in sensation under this electrode. Avoid placing the dispersive electrode over the abdomen.
4. If the electrodes are not self-adhesive, use rubber and Velcro straps, elastic wraps, or sandbags to secure the electrodes in place.
5. If this is the athlete's first exposure to electrical stimulation, explain the sensations to be expected (e.g., "pins and needles" or "muscle twitch"). Be aware that some individuals are very apprehensive about electrotherapeutic treatments. The athlete should be advised against any unnecessary movements because this may break the circuit between the electrodes.

Termination of the Treatment

1. Many units will automatically stop the current flow when the treatment time has expired. If this is not the case with your unit, or if the treatment is being terminated prematurely, gradually DECREASE the INTENSITY and/or depress the STOP button.
2. Remove the electrodes from the athlete and wipe away any residual water or gel.
3. An interview should be conducted immediately upon the conclusion of the treatment to ascertain the effectiveness of the parameters used. The results should be noted in the athlete's file and adjustments made as indicated.

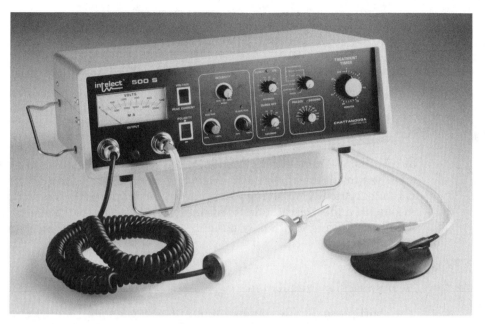

Figure 4–20. **A High Voltage Pulsed Stimulation Unit.** (The Intelect 500S courtesy of The Chattanooga Group, Hixon, TN.)

HIGH-VOLTAGE PULSED STIMULATION

High-voltage pulsed stimulation (HVPS) involves the application of a direct current to the body with a known polarity under each set of electrodes (Fig. 4–20). It should be noted that this technique is many times incorrectly referred to as high-voltage *galvanic* stimulation (see Box 4–6). High-voltage pulsed stimulation has a wide variety of uses including muscle re-education, nerve stimulation, reduction of edema, and pain control.

A typical high-voltage generator produces a twin-peaked wave form (see Fig. 4–2B) or a train of two single pulses with a pulse duration of 5 to 100 microseconds (μsec). The average current does not normally exceed 1.5 milliamperes (mA), or a pulse charge of 4 microcoulombs (Table 4–7). Because of the low pulse charge, voltages of greater than 150 volts are required to stimulate motor and sensory nerves.[3] The relatively low pulse duration allows for the activation of sensory and motor nerves without stimulating pain fibers.

The interpulse interval is much longer than the pulse duration. Because

---

Box 4–6 **CONTRADICTION AND CONFUSION ...**

The term "high-voltage pulsed galvanic stimulation" is an oxymoron similar to "jumbo shrimp" or a "perfectly straight crooked line." The contradiction arises from the use of the terms "pulsed" and "galvanic" in describing the flow of the same current. As you will recall from the discussion on direct current flow, galvanic refers to "a continuous, waveless, unidirectional current".[52] Therefore, a galvanic current cannot be pulsed. The confusion stems from the constant use of this term in the literature and in manufacturer's descriptions.

Table 4–7 **CURRENT PARAMETERS USED WITH HIGH-VOLTAGE PULSED STIMULATION**

Parameter	Range
Total current flow	1.5 mA
Pulse frequency	1–256 pps
Pulse duration	5–100 μsec
Phase duration	20–45 μsec

of this, there is time for dissipation of the residual ions attracted to the body area; as a result the amount of physiochemical reaction beneath the electrodes is limited. A study involving 30-minute applications of HVPS found no change in skin *pH* under the cathode.[49] This indicates that many of the effects attributed to polarity during HVPS may possibly be due to some other mechanism.

Biophysical Effects

Neuromuscular Stimulation

The short pulse duration found on most HVPS generators allows a moderately high intensity muscle contraction with relatively little discomfort. Mohr and associates[50] measured the contractile forces obtained by applying HVPS at pulse frequencies of 50, 80, and 120 pulses per second (all above the threshold required to reach tetany) and was able to obtain torque equal to 85 percent of the maximal voluntary contraction (MVC) using a monopolar technique. Interestingly, no difference was found in maximal torque production between the three frequencies used.

Generation of these contractile forces have not been shown to translate into increased muscular strength. An initial study by Currier and Lehman[51] in 1979 indicated that there were no differences in strength gains achieved through voluntary isometric exercise and isometric contractions assisted by HVPS. In another study, the HVPS group actually had a lower percentage pretest-posttest improvement in isometric strength than a control group which performed no type of strength training exercise.

Table 4–8 **NEUROMUSCULAR STIMULATION USING HIGH-VOLTAGE PULSED STIMULATION (HVPS)**

Parameter	Setting
Intensity	Strong, comfortable contractions
Pulse Rate	Low for individual contractions (less than 15 pps)
	Moderate for tonic contractions (35–50 pps)
Polarity	Positive (negative may be used if more comfortable)
Mode	Alternating
Electrode Placement	Bipolar—Proximal and distal to the muscle (or muscle group) to be stimulated. This method offers the most direct method of stimulating specific areas.
	Monopolar—Over motor points or muscle belly.

pH: (**p**otential of **H**ydrogen) A measure of acidity or alkalinity (bases). A neutral solution has a pH of 7. Acids have a pH of less than 7; bases greater than 7.

Table 4–9 **PAIN CONTROL USING HIGH-VOLTAGE PULSED STIMULATION (HVPS) (GATE CONTROL MECHANISM)**

Parameter	Setting
Intensity	Sensory level
Pulse Rate	100–150 pps
Polarity	Positive
Mode	Continuous
Electrode Placement	Directly over the painful site

An example of the parameters used for elicitation of muscular contractions are presented in Table 4–8. These parameters are modified to meet the goals of the specific treatment regime being implemented.

Pain Control

High-voltage pulsed stimulation may be used as an adjunct treatment in controlling acute and chronic pain through both the gate control mechanism and opiate release. The gate control mechanism of pain modulation can be activated through the application of sensory-level currents at 100 to 150 pulses per second (Table 4–9). Because of the relative lack of portability of most high-voltage generators, HVPS is not normally the modality of choice for treatments that require long-term connection to the athlete.

Generations of high-voltage pulsed stimulation are more suited pain control through opiate release because of the high intensities and short treatment times used (Table 4–10). The active electrodes used in this application should be only as large as the area being stimulated. External hand-held electrodes are often used for this method of application.

The use of the positive polarity for acute pain and of negative polarity for chronic pain has been recommended.[52] Acute pain is associated with an acid reaction that **may** be repelled by the effects of the positive polarity. In the case of chronic pain, the negative pole is used for its reputed liquefying and vasodilative properties.

Control and Reduction of Edema

Research has indicated that clot formation increases on the inside walls of the vessels under the positive electrode.[53] In an acute injury this may reduce the amount of extracellular bleeding that occurs (Table 4–11). However, this treatment approach has undergone much scrutiny.

In subacute or chronic conditions, edema may be removed through the elicitation of muscle contractions which milk the lymphatic and venous return systems and thus encourage drainage of the area (Table 4–12). This response is increased by elevating the limb.

Table 4–10 **PAIN CONTROL USING HIGH-VOLTAGE PULSED STIMULATION (HVPS) (OPIATE RELEASE MECHANISM)**

Parameter	Setting
Intensity	Motor level
Pulse Rate	1–5 pps
Polarity	Positive
Mode	Continuous
Electrode Placement	Directly over the painful site, distal to the spinal nerve root origin, trigger points, or acupuncture points

Table 4-11 **CONTROL OF EDEMA FORMATION USING HIGH-VOLTAGE PULSED STIMULATION (HVPS)**

Parameter	Setting
Intensity	Sensory level
Pulse Rate	Moderate or high
Polarity	Acute—positive
	Subacute—alternating positive and negative throughout treatment
	Chronic—negative
Mode	Continuous
Electrode Placement	Active electrodes are placed over the edematous site; or the cold water immersion method may be used.

One study compared the effectiveness of HVPS in the reduction of post-traumatic edema in rat limbs.[54] Twenty-minute treatments were applied 24, 48, and 72 hours following the initial trauma, with negative polarity being used over the injury site. This study failed to demonstrate a significant reduction of edema compared to the control group which received no stimulation. This result could be due to the low number of treatments and the time span between treatment bouts.

Other studies involved the effects of various HVPS parameters on acutely injured frog limbs.[39,55,56,57] These works concluded that only negative polarity was effective in limiting the amount of edema that formed and that the effects were short lived following the end of the treatment. These studies point out a discrepancy between the clinical practice of administering this modality once a day, three or four times a week and the actual level of treatment required to obtain good results. Multiple daily treatment sessions are recommended for maximal edema reduction.

Wound Healing

A literature review indicates that HVPS has little effect on peripheral blood flow. A controlled study conducted by Walker and associates[58] indicated a slight increase in blood flow when pulsed stimulation was used to elicit isometric contractions of 10 percent and 30 percent of the MVC. This increase was significantly less than the increase in blood flow following voluntary muscle contractions of the same magnitude.

Tracy and associates[59] examined the effect of pulse frequency on changes in blood flow in the human quadriceps femoris muscle group. Their findings demonstrated that pulse frequencies of 10, 20, and 50 pulses per second sig-

Table 4-12 **REDUCTION OF EDEMA USING HIGH-VOLTAGE PULSED STIMULATION (HVPS) (MUSCLE MILKING TECHNIQUE)**

Parameter	Setting
Intensity	Strong, yet comfortable muscle contraction. Avoid joint movement that may be contraindicated.
Pulse Rate	Low
Polarity	Acute—positive
	Subacute—Alternating positive and negative throughout treatment
	Chronic—negative
Mode	Alternating
Electrode Placement	Bipolar—proximal and distal ends of the muscle to be stimulated
	Monopolar—active electrodes following course of venous return system

nificantly increased blood flow, as compared to a frequency of 1 pulse per second. In addition, they concluded that the varying wave forms produced by the various generators used in the study did not influence blood flow.

Kincaid and Lavioe[60] demonstrated that pulsed high-voltage current can inhibit the growth of certain bacteria in infected wounds. The voltage and/or duration of the treatment had to be significantly increased to achieve the same results found with the application of low-voltage direct currents.

Electrode Placement

High-voltage pulsed stimulation may be applied using either a monopolar or bipolar technique. Monopolar application is used when the focus of the treatment is over a wide area, such as in the control and reduction of edema and in sensory-level pain control. Bipolar techniques are most often used when attempting to evoke a contraction from a specific muscle or in motor-level pain control.

Instrumentation

This section generically describes the controls, meters, and leads that are commonly found on a high-voltage pulsed stimulator. These descriptions are provided for introductory purposes only. Consult the user's manual of the device being used for an exact description.

Power: When this switch is in its ON position, the current is allowed to flow to the internal components of the generator.

Reset: This safety feature ensures that the voltage is reduced to zero before each new treatment is started.

Timer: Sets the duration of the treatment and subsequently displays the remaining time. On some units the TIMER serves as the master power switch.

Start/stop: When this button is depressed to start the treatment, the circuit is closed, allowing the current to flow to the athlete's tissues. When it is depressed again, the circuit is opened, interrupting the current flow.

Intensity (voltage): Adjusts the amplitude of the pulse from zero (off) to the maximal value of the unit. The applied output is displayed on the OUTPUT meter.

Pulse rate: This controls the number of pulses (or pulse trains) per second. Low numbers of pulses per second stimulate endorphin release for pain control, moderate levels produce tetanic contractions, while the upper levels are useful in activating the gate mechanism of pain control.

Pulse multiplier: This switch multiplies the number of pulses per second by a selectable value. For example, if the pulse rate is set at 12 pulses per second and the pulse multiplier is set at 10, the resultant output would be 120 pulses per second.

Polarity: This switch determines the polarity (positive or negative) of the ACTIVE electrode(s). Depending on the manufacturer of the product, the polarity may be changed during the course of the treatment without first decreasing the voltage. Other units require that the voltage be reduced before changing polarity.

Mode: When this switch is set to CONTINUOUS, the current is always flowing to each set of active electrodes. Switching to the ALTERNAT-ING modes causes the current to be routed to only one set of active electrodes at a time. Many units also have a PROBE selection that activates the hand-held electrode.

Pad alternating rate: This switch sets the amount of time the current is routed to each active electrode. For example, selecting an electrode alternating rate of 2.5 seconds will route the current to one set of electrodes for 2.5 seconds, then the other set for the same amount of time. On many units, this function is only meaningful when the MODE is set to ALTERNATING and two sets of active electrodes are being used in a monopolar configuration.

Alternating the electrodes is useful for reciprocal stimulation of agonist-antagonist muscle groups. Another use is to stimulate different muscle groups so as to produce a milking action to reduce edema.

Balance: During the course of a treatment, the athlete may experience greater sensation under one set of active electrodes than the other. This situation may be corrected through the BALANCE adjustment dial. When this dial is in its midposition, there is an equal amount of current being routed to both sets of electrodes. If this dial is moved in one direction, towards the "B" electrodes for example, a greater amount of current flows to the "B" electrodes and less to the "A" electrodes.

The imbalance in stimulation under the electrodes can be the result of many factors. These may include improper preparation of the electrodes, the location of the electrodes, and loose connections between the electrodes and the generator, or between the electrodes and the athlete. If adjusting the BALANCE dial does not equalize the sensation, discontinue the treatment, reapply the electrodes, and start again.

Setup and Application

This section describes the basic method of applying high-voltage pulsed stimulation. The use of these devices by inexperienced users should be supervised by qualified personnel. Refer to the section on basic guidelines for the setup and application of electrotherapy at the beginning of this section for details regarding preparation and termination of the treatment.

Initiation of the Treatment

1. Turn on the unit by activating the POWER switch.
2. Fully reduce the INTENSITY control and depress the RESET button.
3. Based on the goal of the treatment, adjust the POLARITY, DURATION (width), FREQUENCY, and electrode ALTERNATING rates.
4. Indicate the duration of the treatment by adjusting the TREATMENT TIME.
5. Press the START button to close the circuit between the generator and the athlete's tissues.
6. *Slowly* increase the INTENSITY control until the appropriate current level is obtained.

7. If necessary, adjust the BALANCE control to maximize the athlete's comfort.

Alternate Methods of Application

Water Immersion

High-voltage pulsed stimulation may be combined with water immersion to treat irregularly shaped areas, such as the hand or foot. The water touching the skin serves as the active electrode. With this in mind, the dispersive electrode should be as large as possible to keep the focus of the electrical stimulation on the part being treated.

The active electrodes are placed in the tub with the insulated (rubber-coated) side facing toward the athlete's skin. Intense stimulation would occur if the athlete were to contact one of the electrodes. The dispersive electrode is placed on the closest large body mass. When treating the foot and/or ankle, the thigh is a logical site. The application of the current is similar to that in all other forms of HVPS. It is important to instruct the athlete not to remove the treated body part from the water (see section on current density).

Treatment of acute injuries with water immersion also raises the same concerns about edema management as ice immersion. Since the limb is placed in a gravity-dependent position, the hydrostatic pressure within the capillaries is increased and the formation of edema is encouraged rather than discouraged. Following treatment, the athlete's limb should be wrapped and elevated to encourage venous return.

Probes

To specifically stimulate trigger points or other localized areas, a probe (tap key) can be employed. The probe serves as a very small active electrode that results in a very high current density being placed on a limited group of tissues. A typical probe consists of a handle with a metal tip that is designed to hold a conductive medium.

The handle contains an intensity control knob and an interrupt button. The probe is activated by setting the electrode alternating switch to PROBE, or by plugging the probe into a separate jack on the generator. In either case, the intensity adjustment on the probe overrides the adjustment on the generator. This allows the operator to remotely adjust the intensity of the treatment. The interrupt button allows the operator to open and close the circuit. When the button is depressed, the circuit is closed and the athlete's tissues are stimulated.

Duration of Treatment

The standard duration of HVPS treatments is 15 to 30 minutes, and the treatments may be repeated as many times a day as needed.

Precautions

- Stimulation of muscles can cause unwanted tension to be placed on the muscle fibers, the tendons, or the bony insertion.
- Improper use can cause electrode burns or irritation.

- Intense or prolonged stimulation may result in muscle spasm and/or muscle soreness.

Indications

- Peripheral nerve injuries
- Delaying denervation and disuse atrophy
- Reduction of posttraumatic edema
- Maintenance of range of motion
  - Reduction of muscle spasm
  - Inhabitation of spasticity
  - Re-education of partially denervated muscle
  - Facilitation of voluntary motor function
- Increasing local blood circulation

Contraindications

- Demand-type pacemakers
- Pregnancy (stimulation of the abdominal and/or pelvic region)
- Areas of particular sensitivity:
  - The carotid sinus
  - The laryngeal and pharyngeal muscles
  - The upper thorax
  - The temporal region
  - Cancerous lesions
  - Sites of infection

TRANSCUTANEOUS ELECTRICAL NERVE STIMULATION

Although all electrical modalities described in this chapter deliver their current transcutaneously, the term transcutaneous electrical nerve stimulation (TENS) has evolved to describe a specific electrotherapeutic approach to pain control. Transcutaneous electrical nerve stimulation describes the process of altering an athlete's perception of pain through the use of an electrical current. Depending on the parameters used during treatment, electrical stimulation may reduce pain through activation of the gate control mechanism or centrally through the release of endogenous opiates.

The use of TENS in the treatment of pain is reported to be a spin-off of work by Melzack and Wall,[61] who described and experimentally investigated the gate control mechanism of pain transmission.[61] Anecdotal claims of permanent relief from chronic pain following a single, brief TENS treatment—although possibly true—are an exaggeration and oversimplification of practical effects and application of TENS. The application of TENS has been found to be effective in the management of acute or chronic musculoskeletal pain but has little effect on reducing *visceral* or psychogenic pain.

The effectiveness of TENS treatment is as varied as its application techniques. The outcome of TENS treatment is dependent on the nature of the pain, the individual's pain threshold, electrode placement, the intensity of the stimulation, and the electrical characteristics of the stimulus[62] (Table 4–13). Traditionally, TENS units incorporate an asymmetrical biphasic pulsed current

---

Viscera: Organs enclosed by the abdominal cavity.

Table 4–13 **ELECTRICAL PARAMETERS USED IN TRANSCUTANEOUS ELECTRICAL NERVE STIMULATORS**

Parameter	Range
Intensity	0–100 mA
Pulse frequency	1–150 pps
Pulse duration	10–500 μsec

(see Fig. 4–6B). However, some manufacturers use variants of this pulsed current including a symmetrical biphasic or monophasic wave form. When this treatment is given for extended periods, the wave form should be designed so that there is no net physiochemical effect on the tissues.

Biophysical Effects

Pain Control

Despite the fact that a TENS unit can provoke muscle contractions, the primary, if not the only, use of TENS is to control pain. The pulse rate and pulse duration, combined with the current intensity, activate responses at different pain modulating levels (Table 4–14).

High-Frequency TENS

Conventional TENS treatment, applied with a high pulse frequency (>50 pps), short pulse duration (30–200 μsec), and sensory-level intensity activates the pain-modulating gate at the spinal cord level. Painful impulses are transmitted along slow-transmitting, small-diameter nerves, while nonpain sensory information travels at a faster rate along neurons of larger diameter. Because of the short pulse duration and high pulse frequency used with conventional TENS, sensory nerve **A-fibers** are selectively stimulated. The increased sensory activity activates **T cells** in the dorsal horn of the spinal cord, closing the gate to pain transmission along the **C-fibers**. This method of TENS application is also referred to as **high TENS**, based on the high pulse rate used.

Accommodation and habituation are concerns when high TENS is used for an extended period of time. If the stimulation parameters are kept constant, the athlete may adapt to the unchanging stimulus. Most TENS generators have current modulation parameters designed to diminish these effects. Even so, the current intensity is normally increased during the course of the treatment.

High TENS is effective in the treatment of acute soft-tissue injury, but care

Table 4–14 **PROTOCOL FOR VARIOUS METHODS OF TRANSCUTANEOUS ELECTRICAL NERVE STIMULATION (TENS) APPLICATION**

Parameter	High TENS	Low TENS	Brief-Intense
Intensity	Sensory	Motor	Noxious
Pulse frequency	50–100 pps	1–5 pps	100–150 pps
Pulse duration	30–200 μsec	200–500 μsec	250–500 μsec
Mode	Modulated rate	Burst	Modulated amplitude
Duration	As needed	30 min	15–30 min
Onset of relief	<10 min	20–40 min	<15 min
Duration of relief	min to hr	hr to days	<30 min

Source: Adapted from: Bechtel, T and Fan, PT,[64] p 41

must be taken to avoid unwanted muscle contractions. Other indications for high TENS include treatment of pain associated with musculoskeletal disorders, postoperative pain, inflammatory conditions, and myofascial pain.

Low-Frequency TENS

Low-frequency TENS (**low TENS**) is applied with a low pulse frequency (1–10 pps), long pulse duration (200–500 µsec), and motor-level intensity, in treatment bouts lasting 15 to 30 minutes. Pain relief obtained through this method is thought to occur by the release of β-endorphin, which results in narcoticlike pain reduction.

Low-frequency, high-intensity stimulation provides pain relief by forming a negative feedback loop within the central nervous system. The intense stimulation activates ascending neural mechanisms that, upon reaching the brain, make the athlete conscious of the pain caused by the stimulation. During the impulse's passage through the midbrain, a "short circuit" occurs, stimulating the release of endogenous opiates in the raphe nuclei. A mechanism is then activated that loops efferent impulses down the spinal cord. Here, the opiates inhibit the release of substance P, a neurotransmitter of noxious impulses, thus blocking the transmission of pain.[63]

Actual relief of pain may not be experienced for some time after the treatment has been completed, but the effects are much longer lasting than with high TENS.[11,64,65] Suggested uses for low TENS include the treatment of chronic pain, pain caused by damage to deep tissues, myofascial pain, and pain caused by muscle spasm. Since this method of TENS application involves muscle contractions, care must be taken to avoid any joint movement that may be contraindicated. Studies have indicated that there is little difference between the degree of pain reduction obtained from high and low TENS treatments.[62,66]

Brief-Intense TENS

This method of TENS application is delivered at a high pulse frequency (>100 pps), long pulse duration (>250 µsec), and motor-level intensity in treatment bouts lasting a few seconds to a few minutes. Pain relief is achieved by activating mechanisms in the brain stem that dampen or amplify pain impulses. This method of TENS application is also referred to as **noxious level TENS**.

A high level of analgesia is achieved through this application protocol, but the effects are more transitory than high and low TENS. Because of the short duration of pain relief, this technique is recommended for pain reduction prior to rehabilitation exercises.[64]

Other Biophysical Effects of TENS

Studies by Denegar and Huff[66] and Denegar and associates[67] examined the effect that TENS has on increasing the range of motion of the elbow joint by decreasing the pain associated with delayed onset muscle soreness (DOMS), with varying conclusions. Both studies showed that TENS was effective in reducing the perception of pain, but one study described no improvement in joint range of motion using a modified high TENS technique.[66] The study by Denegar and associates[67] used low TENS at four sites on the upper arm. This technique did produce a statistically significant improvement in elbow range of motion.

In a study of arthroscopic *menisectomy* patients, the group receiving TENS as an adjunct to a postsurgical physical therapy protocol was described as

---

Meniscectomy: The surgical removal of the knee's meniscal cartilage.

having less pain, requiring less pain medication, and regaining isokinetic torque more rapidly than the group receiving only the postsurgical physical therapy protocol.[31]

Electrode Placement

The placement of TENS electrodes for optimal treatment is not an exact science and many times is derived through trial and error. The determination of electrode placement is made easier if a set of logical constructs is followed. Placement techniques may be described by the electrodes' location relative to the painful area. Methods include direct placement, contiguous placement, placement at stimulation points, dermatome placement, and placement at the spinal nerve root level.

High TENS is most commonly employed with direct, contiguous, dermatome, or nerve root level electrode placement. Low TENS and brief-intense TENS treatments target the stimulation points. This is not an absolute formula, as the parameters can be mixed and matched to obtain the best treatment results.

Most TENS units use four electrodes, two originating from each of two channels used. However, some units may have as few as two electrodes or as many as eight (two electrodes originating from each of four channels). When two or more channels are used, electrode placement is further defined by one channel's electrode placement relative to the other possible placements (Fig. 4–21).

The effects of TENS can be maximized if the nerve(s) involved in the transmission of pain can be identified and stimulated. For example, the reduc-

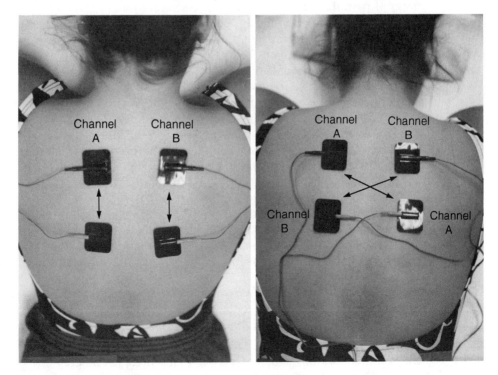

Figure 4–21. Parallel and crossing electrode placements.

tion of pain associated with an injured thumb will be facilitated if the radial nerve, or portions of its path, is stimulated, rather than the median or ulnar nerve.

Direct Placement

The electrodes are placed on the skin directly over or around the painful site. The electrodes are arranged so that each channel runs parallel to the midline of the body part. The electrodes are then connected so that the channels flow parallel to each other and the midline of the body.

Contiguous Placement

In conditions such as postoperative incisions, lacerations, and other situations that contraindicate direct electrode placement on the site of the pain, contiguous electrode placement may be used. In this method, electrodes are placed in the immediate vicinity of the painful site. The currents from each channel may run parallel to each other or they may cross at the center of the painful area.

Stimulation Point Placement

Areas such as motor, trigger, and acupuncture points may be targeted for TENS treatments. These points are very sensitive to stimulation and in many instances are located in close proximity to each other. Because of the close location of these areas, a single TENS electrode may stimulate all three points at once.

Motor points are areas of the skin above the point where a motor nerve enters the muscle mass (Appendix B). **Trigger points** are pathological, localized areas of pain that are hypersensitive to stimulation. Stimulation of these areas "triggers" radiating or referred pain. Unlike motor points, trigger points may be found not only in muscle, but also in other soft tissue such as ligament, tendon, and fascia (Appendix A).

Acupuncture points are specific sites on the skin possessing a decreased electrical skin resistance and increased electrical conductivity. These points are connected by meridians through which blood and energy flow.[64,65,68] Superficial master points, consisting of 12 main channels, 8 secondary channels and a network of subchannels, connect areas of the skin to deeper channels and allow systemic regulation of many body functions. These master points are especially effective in alleviating pain along the entire meridian. Although acupuncture has been successfully used for many centuries, its theoretical basis has never been fully substantiated.

Berlant[68] describes a manual method of determining optimal stimulation sites where one electrode is attached to the athlete and the other to the clinician. The clinician's finger is then used to probe the area and identify those sites that are the most sensitive to stimulation. Some units have a built-in ohmmeter for this purpose.

Dermatome Placement

In cases where the athlete's pain is spread across one or more **dermatomes**, pain reduction can be achieved by placing electrodes along the affected and the contralateral dermatome. One technique involves placing one electrode at the corresponding spinal cord nerve root and the other at the distal end of the dermatome.

Spinal Cord Level Placement

This method stimulates the spinal cord nerve root associated with the pain. The electrode should be placed parallel to the spinal column between the transverse processes.

Both dermatome and spinal cord level placement are unexacting methods of TENS treatment. These forms of application should only be used when the surface area of the afflicted area is inaccessible (e.g., with casts or nonremovable immobilization devices).

Instrumentation

This section generically describes the controls, meters, and leads that are commonly found on a TENS generator. These descriptions are provided for introductory purposes only. Consult the user's manual of the device being used for an exact description.

Intensity: On most units there is one intensity dial for each channel. Although the intensity of each channel is controlled individually, the other current parameters (pulse duration and pulse frequency) regulate the activity in all channels.

Pulse duration: This adjustment is usually labeled "PULSE WIDTH" on the unit. This adjustment should be set according to the treatment method being used.

Pulse frequency: Also labeled "PULSE RATE," this adjustment sets the number of pulses per second used during the treatment.

Mode: Modes are used to alter the current in an attempt to reduce the amount of accommodation that occurs. The various modes that are commonly selectable are:

Constant: Current flow occurs at a constant amplitude, rate, and pulse duration. This mode is best described as unmodulated, in order to avoid confusion with uninterrupted current. This mode is used when the treatment is not required for an extended length of time and accommodation is not a concern.

Burst: In the burst mode, pulse frequencies are interrupted at regular intervals. Bursts allow "OFF" time from stimulation and assist in reducing muscle fatigue in low TENS treatments.

Modulated rate: This setting alters, at a preset percentage, the frequency at which the stimulus is delivered. For example, if the pulse rate was adjusted to 100 pulses per second, the unit would alternate the rate between 90 and 110 pulses per second. Modulating the frequency has been found effective in the treatment of chronic musculoskeletal pain.[64]

Modulated amplitude: The pulse amplitude is increased and decreased by a preset percentage. Modulating the amplitude has been shown to provide short-term analgesia in the area.

Multiple modulation: Intensity, frequency, and pulse duration are alternately modulated in such a way that there is delivery of a steady amount of current to the body, but the body has a varying sensory perception of the treatment. This mode decreases the effects of accommodation during prolonged TENS application.

Setup and Application

This section describes the basic method of applying transcutaneous electrical nerve stimulation. The use of these devices by inexperienced users should be supervised by qualified personnel. Refer to the Basic Guidelines for the Setup and Application of Electrotherapy at the beginning of this section for details regarding preparation for and termination of the treatment.

Initiation of the Treatment

1. Depending on the method of TENS application to be used (see Table 4–14), set the pulse duration (WIDTH) and pulse frequency (RATE) dials to the midrange for the parameter to be used.
2. Select the appropriate MODE for the method and duration of the TENS application.
3. Make sure that the output intensity is reset to zero and turn the unit on. Note that many TENS units have the power switch built into the intensity knob(s). In this case the intensity level of zero (0) is equal to "OFF."
4. Slowly turn up the INTENSITY of channel one. If this treatment involves sensory-level stimulation, continue increasing the intensity until a slight muscle contraction is visible, then reduce the intensity by approximately 10 percent. (The athlete should be monitored for comfort while the intensity is being increased.)
5. If more than one channel is being used, increase the intensity of the remaining channels. The intensity between the channels should be more-or-less balanced to provide approximately equal stimulation.
6. When "fine-tuning" the treatment parameters, most manufacturers recommend first adjusting the intensity, then the pulse duration, and finally the pulse frequency.
7. If the athlete is being sent home or to class wearing this unit, instruction should be provided on how to adjust the intensity. If indicated, instructions should also be provided on how to disconnect the unit before taking a shower or retiring for the night, and during recharging.

Alternate Forms of Application

Point Stimulators

Devices such as the Neuroprobe (Medical Research Lab, Inc., 1 Armour Court, Lake Bluff, IL) are modified TENS devices designed to locate and stimulate trigger and acupuncture points by measuring the amount of resistance provided by the skin.

Auriculotherapy

Researchers have examined the effectiveness of TENS application at acupuncture points on the ear (auriculotherapy).[30,69] These authors state that this method of application is based on the premise that an injured or diseased body will reflect pain or tenderness to specific points on the ear. These points, arranged in the form of an inverted fetus, are said to represent the point where all the acupuncture channels meet. These points respond to stimulation by decreasing the perception of pain in the corresponding area of the body.

A study conducted by Paris and associates[69] examined the time required to regain normal function following second degree inversion ankle sprains. This study examined the recovery time between patients receiving Neuroprobe treatments to acupuncture points on the ear and ankle, and a group receiving standard physical therapy alone. Based on measurable parameters including joint range of motion, pain, and functional gait, the group receiving Neuroprobe™ treatments had decreased recovery time.

Microcurrent Therapy

Microamperage electrical nerve stimulation (MENS or microcurrent) attempts to reduce pain by restoring the biological electrical balance found in normal tissue.[33] The reported pain-controlling effects of this low amperage (10–600 µA) subsensory level of electrotherapy has received much recent attention.

However, as noted by Gersh,[33] "... reports claiming major advantages of microcurrent over conventional forms of TENS and other treatment interventions have remained largely the domain of manufacturer's testimonials, public-interest articles, sports magazine articles, and nonreviewed journals." Although MENS may live up to its manufacturers' claims, the efficacy of this method of pain control has not been experimentally established.

Duration and Frequency of Treatment

Conventional high-frequency TENS may be delivered to the athlete as needed. Caution should be used when the athlete is sleeping. The use of a TENS device during athletic competition has been attempted. However, because of the potential of TENS in masking pain, its use should be discouraged. An alternate approach would be to keep the electrodes affixed to the athlete and apply stimulation while the athlete is on the bench.

Low-frequency TENS may be given as needed in treatment bouts not exceeding 30 minutes. Brief-intense type TENS application should only be performed once a day, in treatment bouts not exceeding 30 minutes.

Precautions

- TENS is a symptomatic treatment that can mask underlying pain and other conditions.
- Improper use can result in electrode burns or skin irritation.
- Intense or prolonged stimulation may result in muscle spasm and/or muscle soreness.

Indications

- Control of chronic pain
- Management of postsurgical pain
- Reduction of posttraumatic acute pain

Contraindications

- Demand-type pacemakers
- Pregnancy (stimulation of the abdominal and/or pelvic region)
- Pain of central origin
- Pain of unknown origin
- Areas of particular sensitivity:
  - The carotid sinus
  - Laryngeal and pharyngeal muscles
  - The upper thorax
  - The temporal region
  - Cancerous lesions
  - Sites of infection

INTERFERENTIAL STIMULATION

Interferential electrical stimulation (IFS) units generate two alternating currents on two separate channels. One channel produces a constant high-frequency sine wave (4000–5000 Hz) and the other channel produces a sine wave with a variable frequency. As theorized, these independent channels combine to produce an interference wave possessing a frequency of 1 to 100 Hz. The high-frequency carrier currents serve to penetrate the tissues with very little resistance, while the resulting interference currents are in a range that allows for effective stimulation of biological tissues (Fig. 4–22).

To realize the combined effects of two separate wave forms, we must first understand the effect that one series of waves has on the other. When two waves are in perfect phase, that is the wavelengths are equal and the phases cross the baseline at the same point, the amplitude of the combined wave is equal to the sum of its two parts. This effect is termed **constructive interference** because the two wave forms build a larger single wave (Fig. 4–23).

The opposite effect occurs in **destructive interference**. In this case two wave forms are perfectly out of phase. The positive peak of the first wave form occurs at the same point on the horizontal baseline as the negative peak of the second wave. When these two waves meet the amplitudes cancel each other out resulting in a wave intensity of zero (Fig. 4–24).

Interferential generators combine constructive and destructive interference patterns to form a **continuous interference** pattern. This occurs when two circuits have slightly different frequencies (±1 Hz). The resultant wave form is one that drifts between constructive and destructive interference patterns (Fig. 4–25). These circuits may be superimposed in the athlete's tissues (quadripolar technique) or within the generator itself (bipolar technique). Superimposing the circuits within the generator itself allows for precise mixing of the waves.[70]

The rate at which the resultant wave form changes is known as the **beat pattern**. The beat pattern frequency is the difference in frequency between the two circuits. One channel has a fixed frequency in the range of 4000 Hz and the frequency of the second channel is variable. By selecting a beat frequency of 1 Hz, the second channel produces a current with a frequency of 4001 Hz. Selecting a beat frequency of 100 Hz increases the frequency of the second channel to 4100 Hz. The beat produced by IFS will elicit responses similar to the wave forms produced by TENS units, but is capable of delivering a greater

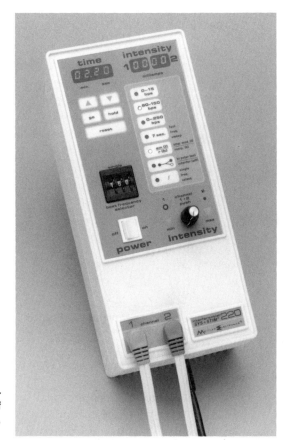

Figure 4–22. An Interferential Stimulator. (The Sys*Stim 220 courtesy of Mettler Electronics Corporation, Inc., Anaheim, CA.)

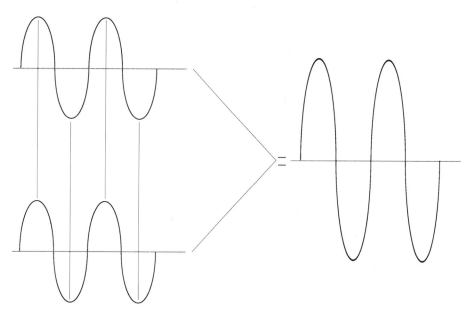

Figure 4–23. Constructive interference. Two waves in perfect phase collide to form one single, larger wave.

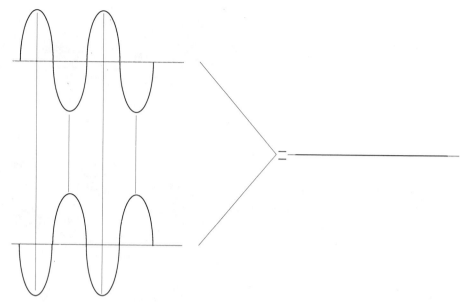

Figure 4–24. Destructive interference. Two waves perfectly out of phase collide, cancel each other out, and produce no wave.

total current to the tissues (70–100 mA).[71] Refer to Table 4–15 for other electrical parameters.

As you will recall, capacitive skin resistance is inversely proportional to the frequency of the current. An alternating current of 50 Hz encounters approximately 3000 ohms of resistance per 100 square centimeters of skin. Increasing the frequency to 4000 Hz reduces capacitive skin resistance to approximately

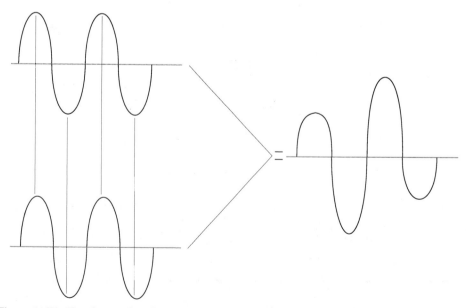

Figure 4–25. Continuous interference. Two waves slightly out of phase collide and form a single wave with progressively increasing and then decreasing amplitude.

Table 4–15 **ELECTRICAL PARAMETERS USED IN INTERFERENTIAL STIMULATORS**

Parameter	Range
Intensity	0–100 mA
Carrier frequency	4000–5000 Hz
Pulse duration	~125 μsec
Beat frequency	0–299 Hz
Sweep frequency	10–500 μsec

40 ohms.[10] Consequently, IFS encounters less skin resistance than other, low-frequency, forms of stimulation. Inside the tissues, the interference between the two waves reduces the frequency to a level that has biological effect on the tissues.

True interferential stimulation involves amplitude modulation as described in the preceding section. Many generators have a "RUSSIAN STIMULATION" setting. This term describes a Soviet neuromuscular stimulation technique where a burst-modulated AC current is used to elicit strong muscle contractions (see Burst-Modulated AC in the following section).

Biophysical Effects

Interferential stimulation has been used to control pain and elicit muscle contractions to increase venous return. A variation of IFS, burst modulation, is used for muscle re-education and to increase muscular strength.

Pain Control

Mechanisms of pain control are similar to those found with TENS. High beat frequencies, in the area of 100 Hz, when accompanied by sensory-level stimulation, activate the spinal gate, inhibiting the transmission of noxious impulses (Table 4–16). Low beat frequencies of 2 to 10 Hz, when combined with motor-level intensities, initiate the release of opiates and result in a narcoticlike pain reduction (Table 4–17).

A study by Taylor and associates[29] examined the effectiveness of high-frequency IFS in reducing pain and increasing range of motion for the jaw in patients experiencing temperomandibular joint dysfunction. The results indicated that the group receiving three 20-minute stimulation bouts did not experience significant pain reduction or increased range of motion when compared to the group receiving placebo treatment.

Table 4–16 **PAIN CONTROL VIA GATE CONTROL USING INTERFERENTIAL THERAPY**

Parameter	Setting
Intensity	Submotor threshold
Mode	Quadripolar is desirable
Beat frequency	High
Sweep	Longer duration, ramped change

Table 4–17 **PAIN CONTROL VIA OPIATE RELEASE USING INTERFERENTIAL THERAPY**

Parameter	Setting
Intensity	Strong, yet comfortable muscle contraction
Mode	Quadripolar is desirable
Beat frequency	Low
Sweep	Longer duration, abrupt shift

Neuromuscular Stimulation

Medium beat frequencies of approximately 15 Hz may be used to reduce edema. Venous and lymphatic return can be increased by way of muscle contractions. A study by Nussbaum and associates[72] indicated that IFS did not significantly increase blood flow to the treated area.

Burst-Modulated Alternating Current

Following the 1972 Summer Olympics, much attention was given to an electrical strength training regime used by Russian athletes. A Soviet physician, Dr. Yakov Kots, reported that athletes training under this technique demonstrated a 30 percent to 40 percent strength improvement over isometric exercise alone. Other reported benefits of this technique included increased muscular endurance and changes in the velocity of muscular contractions. These results, due in part to Dr. Kots' failure to specify the parameters used by these athletes, have never been duplicated in the United States.[3,16,18,19,21,23,24,73] This method of application has gained the name "Russian stimulation" based on its country of origin.

Classical Russian stimulation involves the use of a 2500-Hz carrier sine wave with burst modulation (Table 4–18). The theory behind Russian stimulation, as with IFS, is that the higher frequencies would decrease the amount of capacitive skin resistance and allow more current to reach the motor nerve at lower intensities.[3]

Although sometimes found as dedicated units, IFS units are often capable of modulating bursts, providing for Russian-type stimulation.

Reduction of Edema

Removal of chronic posttraumatic edema through the use of IFS has been documented.[73] This effect is most likely attributable to milking of the venous and lymphatic return systems through electrically evoked muscle contractions. Care must be taken to avoid unwanted joint motion that could produce further injury of the involved structures.

Table 4–18 **ELECTRICAL PARAMETERS USED IN BURST-MODULATED AC STIMULATION**

Parameter	Setting
Intensity	To tolerance
Carrier frequency	2500 Hz
Beat frequency	1–100 Hz
Pulse duration	~125 μsec

Electrode Placement

Quadripolar Technique

The four electrodes are positioned around the painful area so that each channel runs perpendicular to the other and the current will cross at the midpoint (Fig. 4–26). The interference effects branch off at 45-degree angles from the center of the treatment, in the shape of a four-leaf clover. Tissues within in this area receive the maximal treatment effect. When the electrodes are properly positioned, the athlete should feel only the stimulation between the electrodes, not under the electrodes.[10]

Referring to Figure 4–26, you will notice that the interference effect only covers about half of the area between the electrodes. If the athlete has a very discrete area of pain, the interference pattern should be able to encompass the appropriate tissues. However, in those cases where the pain is diffuse, maximal pain reduction may not occur. This problem can be reduced through rotating the interference effect area. By slightly unbalancing the currents, the interference pattern "rotates" or "scans" 45 degrees back and forth between the electrodes, resulting in treatment of a larger area (Fig. 4–27).

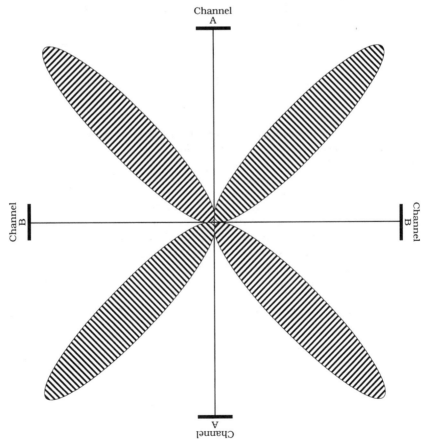

Figure 4–26. Interference Pattern. Maximal benefit from interferential stimulation occurs at 45 degree angles from the intersection of the channels.

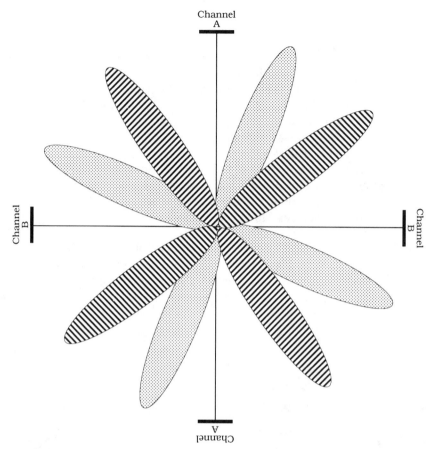

Figure 4-27. Dynamic Interference Vectoring. The normal vector pattern is rotated throughout the treatment to stimulate a broader tissue area.

Bipolar Electrode Placement

When IFS is being applied using a bipolar technique, the mixing of the two channels occurs within the generator rather than in the athlete's tissues. Two channels are used within the generator, with a single output channel applied to the tissues. Although bipolar IFS does not penetrate the tissues as deeply as quadripolar application, a more precise mixing occurs.

When muscle contractions are the goal of the treatment session, either through IFS or Russian stimulation, bipolar electrode placements are used. When the effects are targeted for one specific muscle or muscle group, only one channel is used. Four electrodes are incorporated into a dual channel, agonist-antagonist treatment regime.

Instrumentation

This section generically describes the controls, meters, and leads that are commonly found on an interferential stimulation unit. These descriptions are provided for introductory purposes only. Consult the user's manual of the device being used for an exact description.

Power: When this switch is in its ON position, the current is allowed to flow to the internal components of the generator.

Reset: This ensures that the intensity is reduced to zero (0) before the treatment is initiated.

Treatment time: Sets the duration of the treatment and subsequently displays the remaining time once the treatment has been started.

Start/stop: Used to initiate and terminate the treatment.

Intensity: Adjusts the amplitude of the pulse and is displayed in milliamperes (mA). When quadripolar stimulation is being used, the intensity control regulates both channels simultaneously.

Mode: Allows the user to choose between true interferential therapy and bipolar stimulation. The interferential mode allows the current to stimulate deep tissue. In the bipolar mode only one channel is used and the resultant current flow stimulates relatively subcutaneous nerves.

Russian stimulation: Changes the output from amplitude-modulated to burst-modulated for evoking strong muscle contractions. This technique may use one or both channels. This is an option on many IFS units, while other units provide Russian stimulation.

Beat frequency: The "beat" is the result of the fixed rate of the carrier wave and the variable rate of the second channel.

On/off control: When Russian-type stimulation has been selected from the MODE control, this adjusts the duty cycle by determining the amount of time the current is ON versus OFF.

Balance: This allows the user to control the balance of electrical current under each set of electrodes and equalize the sensory stimulation. This control may only be meaningful during quadripolar stimulation.

Setup and Application

This section describes the basic method of applying IFS. The use of these devices by inexperienced users should be supervised by qualified personnel. Refer to the Basic Guidelines for the Setup and Application of Electrotherapy at the beginning of this section for details regarding preparation for and termination of the treatment.

Initiation of the Treatment

1. If the unit uses electrodes that are secured by means of a vacuum, refer to the operator's manual for instructions on their use.
2. Turn on the unit by activating the POWER switch.
3. Fully reduce the INTENSITY control and depress the RESET button.
4. Determine the MODE of application: quadripolar, bipolar, or Russian stimulation.
5. Based on the goals of the treatment, select the appropriate BEAT frequencies.
6. Indicate the duration of the treatment by adjusting the TREATMENT TIME.
7. Press the START button to close the circuit between the generator and the athlete's tissues.
8. *Slowly* increase the INTENSITY control until the appropriate current level is obtained.

9. If necessary, adjust the BALANCE control to obtain maximal athlete comfort.

Duration of Treatment

Interferential stimulation may be applied once or twice a day in treatment bouts normally ranging from 15 to 30 minutes. Burst-modulated stimulation is normally applied three times a week in 30-minute bouts.

Precautions

- Improper use can result in electrode burns or skin irritation.
- Intense or prolonged stimulation may result in muscle spasm and/or muscle soreness.

Indications

- Acute Pain
- Chronic Pain
- Muscle Spasm

Contraindications

- Demand-type pacemakers
- Pregnancy (stimulation of the abdominal and/or pelvic region)
- Pain of central origin
- Pain of unknown origin
- Areas of particular sensitivity
  - The carotid sinus
  - Laryngeal and pharyngeal muscles
  - The upper thorax
  - The temporal region
  - Cancerous lesions
  - Sites of infection

NEUROMUSCULAR ELECTRICAL STIMULATION

Neuromuscular electrical stimulation (NMES) is used for muscle re-education, reducing spasticity, delaying atrophy, and strengthening muscles (Fig. 4–28). The use of electrical stimulation reverses the order in which muscle fibers are recruited into the contraction. During voluntary muscle contractions, small-diameter type I motor nerves are the first to contract. Because of their construction, type I fibers do not generate much force, but are able to sustain the contraction for a prolonged period of time. Electrical stimulation causes large-diameter type II motor nerves to evoke a contraction before the type I fibers. Since type II fibers are capable of producing more force, the strength of the contraction is increased.

This reversal of the order of motor nerve recruitment is a result of the relative sizes of the nerves and their depths below the surface of the skin. Electrical stimulation will first cause a depolarization of large-diameter nerves

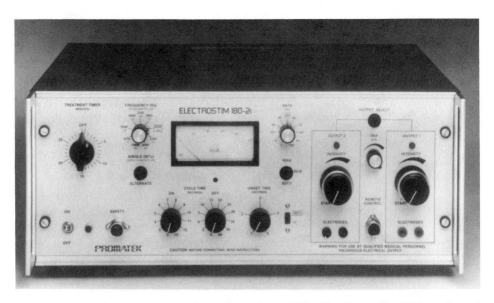

Figure 4–28. A Neuromuscular Electrical Stimulation Unit. (The Electrostim 180-2 courtesy of Promatek Medical Systems, Inc., Joliet, IL.)

because their cross-sectional area provides less resistance to current flow. Additionally, type II motor nerves, being more superficial, will receive greater stimulation than the deeper type I nerves.

The amount of torque produced has been found to be directly related to the amount of current introduced into the muscle.[16] The strength of the contraction can be further altered through manipulation of the electrode placement.

Generators for NMES utilize a wide range of wave forms, but the majority of the units currently on the market use a biphasic wave. A review of the literature indicates that no one wave form is universally comfortable, but that perceived comfort is based on an individual athlete's preference.[17] Symmetric pulses tend to be less painful over a large muscle mass because there is an equal amount of stimulation under both electrodes.[22]

Neuromuscular stimulation is a frequency-dependent modality. The current must be strong enough to overcome the capacitive resistance of the tissues before the motor nerves can be stimulated. The capacitive tissue resistance is inversely proportional to the frequency of the current. Therefore, the relatively low frequencies used by NMES generators must produce a greater current to overcome this resistance. Commonly used electrical parameters in NMES generators are presented in Table 4–19.

Table 4–19 **ELECTRICAL PARAMETERS USED IN NEUROMUSCULAR ELECTRICAL STIMULATION**

Parameter	Setting
Peak amperage	To tolerance
Pulse duration	50–300 μsec
Pulse frequency	1–200 pps
Pulse charge	≤10 mQ

Biophysical Effects

Neuromuscular Stimulation

Because of the large amplitude and long pulse duration, NMES provides stronger stimulation than other forms of electrical stimulation. However, the increased pulse duration and amperage result in a decrease in comfort. Increasing the duration of the pulses results in increased stimulation of pain nerve fibers. When the aim of the treatment session is to increase muscular strength, the output of the treatment should be as high as the athlete will allow; if the aim is muscle re-education, a mild tonic contraction for "cueing" is all that is required.[3]

The efficacy of NMES in improving isometric muscle strength has been substantiated in the literature. The improvement in strength occurs as a result of increasing the functional stress placed on the muscle and as a result of the reversal of motor nerve recruitment, as described by Delitto and Snyder-Mackler.[23] Neuromuscular electrical stimulation has been shown to elicit a contraction which produces torque equal to 90 percent of the maximal voluntary contraction.[17]

Athletes who are re-educating muscle through NMES have the potential of significantly increasing strength compared to athletes who are not exercising. It has been demonstrated that groups using NMES applied with a 60 percent duty cycle displayed a significant increase in strength over an isometrically trained group.[74,75]

Muscular contractions obtained through NMES have been shown to increase peripheral blood flow to the extremity being stimulated. This occurs as a result of the increased metabolic rate associated with the contractions. A study by Currier and Petrilli[76] examined the effects of peripheral blood flow when the ankle plantar flexors were stimulated with burst-modulated alternating currents. Their results indicated that blood flow increased during the first minute and then reached a steady state that was maintained throughout the course of the treatment. The degree of increased blood flow was shown to be unrelated to the stimulation intensity. Another study, using the same parameters, indicated a sympathetic response in blood flow. In this case, stimulation of the ankle plantar flexors resulted in a decreased flow of blood to the fingers of the opposite hand.[77]

Reduction of Edema

In reducing edema, NMES is similar to other forms of electrotherapy. Venous and lymphatic return are enhanced through the milking of these vessels by muscle contractions. Since the aim of this method is to produce individual muscle contractions, a low (1–10 pps) frequency is used. The intensity of the current should produce a visible contraction, but should not cause unwanted movement of the joint. As with other methods of edema reduction, the benefits of this treatment are increased if the limb is placed in a nondependent position.

Electrode Placement

Bipolar electrode placement is commonly employed in NMES treatments. The electrodes are placed over the proximal and distal ends of the muscle or muscle group. Because large electrodes lie over several muscles and/or motor points, a more generalized contraction is obtained. The use of small electrodes may elicit a more specific contraction through direct stimulation of the muscle's motor point. As the electrodes are brought closer together, the effect of the stimulation becomes more superficial, and the relative intensity of the contraction decreases.

Quadripolar application requires the use of two separate channels. This method of application is commonly used when stimulating agonist-antagonist muscle groups.

A monopolar technique may be employed through the use of one small and one large electrode, or through the use of a hand-held applicator. This method of electrode placement is useful when a specific muscle, or a small muscle group, is the target of the treatment.

The size of the electrodes should be only as large as is required to stimulate the desired tissues. Electrodes which are too small will result in a very high current density while electrodes that are larger than needed may stimulate unwanted nerves.

Instrumentation

This section generically describes the controls, meters, and leads that are commonly found on a neuromuscular electrical stimulator. These descriptions are provided for introductory purposes only. Consult the user's manual of the device being used for an exact description.

Power: When this switch is in its ON position, the current is allowed to flow to the internal components of the generator.

Reset: This safety feature ensures that the output is reduced to zero (0) before the treatment is started.

Timer: Sets the duration of the treatment and subsequently displays the remaining time.

Intensity: Adjusts the amplitude of the pulses.

Pulse rate: Determines the type of muscle contraction to be elicited. Depending on the muscle, or muscle group, being stimulated, a pulse rate of less than 15 pulses per second will cause a distinct contraction for each impulse. Between 15 and 25 pulses per second the muscle begins to contract smoothly, eventually leading to a tonic contraction at approximately 35 to 50 pulses per second.

Mode: This allows the user to select the type of wave form used in the treatment.

On/off rate: Allows the user to set the duty cycle for the treatment. Many units have separate dials to independently adjust the number of seconds that the current is flowing and the number of seconds it is not. Other units have preset duty cycles that the user cannot alter. A CONSTANT mode (100% duty cycle) may be provided. This is useful for adjusting the other treatment parameters (intensity, pulse duration, etc.) without waiting for the duty cycle to switch to its ON mode.

External trigger: A hand-held device that allows the user to manually control the ON/OFF time of the stimulation. When the trigger is depressed, current is allowed to flow to the athlete's tissues.

Reciprocal rate: When two channels are being used, this selects the duration of time that the current is flowing to each channel.

Ramp: The RAMP parameter allows the user to determine the amplitude rise time until the peak current is obtained.

Interrupt switch: This device is held by the athlete and is used to terminate the treatment if the intensity becomes too great or too painful.

Setup and Application

This section describes the basic method of applying NMES. The use of these devices by inexperienced users should be supervised by qualified personnel. Refer to the Basic Guidelines for the Setup and Application of Electrotherapy at the beginning of this section for details regarding preparation for and termination of the treatment.

Initiation of the Treatment

1. Set the pulse duration (WIDTH) and pulse frequency (RATE) to the midrange of the parameters to be used.
2. Reduce the output intensity to zero and turn the unit on. If applicable, press the RESET button.
3. Connect the leads to the unit and to the electrodes.
4. Secure the electrodes with elastic straps.
5. Give the athlete the INTERRUPT SWITCH and provide instruction on its purpose and use.
6. If the RAMP and ON/OFF parameters are manually adjustable on the unit, increase the RAMP to a rapid rise and adjust the ON/OFF controls to a 100 percent duty cycle. This configuration allows the INTENSITY to be increased without waiting for the generator to run through its duty cycle. If these parameters cannot be changed during the course of the treatment adjust them to the desired settings now.
7. Set the TREATMENT TIME for this session.
8. Begin the treatment by *slowly* increasing the INTENSITY until the desired tension is developed in the muscle.
9. If applicable, reset the RAMP and ON/OFF time to match the treatment goals.

Duration and Frequency of Treatment

Treatments used for muscular re-education may be given daily, but as with any muscle-building program, the athlete should be monitored for undue pain. Treatments for the delay of atrophy are given constantly through the use of a portable stimulator.

Precautions

- Improper use may result in electrode burns or skin irritation.
- Intense or prolonged stimulation may result in muscle spasm and/or muscle soreness.

Indications

- Maintaining range of motion
- Re-education of muscles
- Prevention of joint contractures
- Prevention of disuse atrophy
- Increasing local blood flow
- Decreasing muscle spasm

Contraindications

- Musculotendinous lesions where the tension produced by the contraction will further damage the muscle or tendon fibers
- There is not a secure bony attachment of the muscle.
- Demand-type pacemakers
- Pregnancy (stimulation of the abdominal and/or pelvic region)
- Areas of particular sensitivity
  - The carotid sinus
  - Laryngeal and pharyngeal muscles
  - The upper thorax
  - The temporal region
  - Cancerous lesions
  - Sites of infection

CHAPTER QUIZ

• •

1. Electrons travel from the ____, which has a ____ of electrons to the ____ which has a ____ of electrons.
   A. Anode • high concentration • cathode • low concentration
   B. Anode • low concentration • cathode • high concentration
   C. Cathode • high concentration • anode • low concentration
   D. Cathode • low concentration • anode • high concentration

2. The ability of a material to store energy by means of an electrostatic field is called:
   A. Capacitance
   B. Inductance
   C. Impedance
   D. Work.

3. What is the current flow in a 40-volt circuit possessing 10 ohms of resistance?
   A. 0.25 amps
   B. 50 amps
   C. 4 amps
   D. 30 amps

4. What is the resistance found in a 40-volt circuit possessing a current flow of 10 amperes?
   A. 4 ohms
   B. 400 ohms
   C. 0.25 ohms
   D. 30 ohms

5. What is the voltage of a circuit providing 4 ohms of resistance when 10 amperes are flowing?
   A. 0.4 volts
   B. 2.5 volts
   C. 6 volts
   D. 40 volts

6. What is the amount of power used by a device drawing 2 amperes from a 120-volt source?
   A. 0.02 watts
   B. 60 watts
   C. 240 watts
   D. Unable to calculate because the resistance is not provided

7. What is the total amount of resistance to current flow in a **series circuit** possessing two resistors, one of 10 ohms and another of 30 ohms?
   A. 4 ohms
   B. 7.5 ohms
   C. 20 ohms
   D. 40 ohms

8. What is the total amount of resistance to current flow in a **parallel circuit** possessing two resistors, one of 10 ohms and another of 30 ohms?
   A. 4 ohms
   B. 7.5 ohms
   C. 20 ohms
   D. 40 ohms

9. Monopolar stimulation involves the use of active and dispersive electrodes. The parameter that determines which pad(s) will be active is:
   A. The POLARITY adjustment
   B. The average current
   C. The pulse duration
   D. The current density.

10. What is the percent duty cycle for an electrical current that flows for 30 seconds and has no flow for 10 seconds?
    A. 300%
    B. 25%
    C. 75%
    D. 3:1

11. All of the following are excitable tissues **except**:
    A. Muscle fiber
    B. Meniscal cartilage
    C. Sensory nerves
    D. Secretory cells.

12. Which of the following would be the modality of choice to cause physiochemical changes within the tissues?
    A. High-voltage pulsed stimulation
    B. Interferential stimulation
    C. Low-voltage alternating current
    D. Low-voltage direct current

13. Under normal circumstances, which of the following nerves would be the first to be stimulated by an electrical current?
    A. A superficial large-diameter nerve
    B. A deep large-diameter nerve
    C. A superficial small-diameter nerve
    D. A deep small-diameter nerve

14. Most tissues provide capacitive resistance to electrical current flow. Which of the following currents would meet the least amount of capacitive resistance?
    A. 1 Hz
    B. 10 Hz
    C. 50 Hz
    D. 100 Hz

15. High-frequency stimulation possessing pulses of a short duration and applied at the sensory level is thought to activate which pain control mechanism?
    A. Gate mechanism
    B. Endogenous opiate
    C. Central biasing
    D. Specificity

16. The electrodes from lead (A) have an area of 10 square inches and 5 square inches while the electrodes originating from lead (B) have an area of 7.5 square inches and 7.5 square inches. This type of stimulation would be classified as:
    A. Monopolar
    B. Bipolar
    C. Quadripolar
    D. Polypolar.

REFERENCES

1. Kloth, LC and Cummings, JP: Electrotherapeutic Terminology in Physical Therapy. Section on Clinical Electrophysiology and the American Physical Therapy Association, Alexandria, VA, 1990.

2. Urbscheit, NL: Review of Physiology. In Nelson, RM and Currier, DP (eds): Clinical Electrotherapy. Appleton and Lange, Norwalk, CT, 1987, pp 1–9.

3. Lake, DA: Neuromuscular electrical stimulation: An overview and its application in the treatment of sports injuries. Sports Med 13:320, 1992.

4. Robinson, AJ: Basic concepts and terminology in electricity. In Snyder-Mackler, L and Robinson, AJ (eds): Clinical Electrophysiology: Electrotherapy and Electrophysiologic Testing. Williams & Wilkins, Baltimore, 1989, pp 1–19.

5. Alon, G: Principles of electrical stimulation. In Nelson, RM and Currier, DP (eds): Clinical Electrotherapy. Appleton and Lange, Norwalk, CT, 1987, pp 29–80.

6. Cook, TM: Instrumentation. In Nelson, RM and Currier, DP (eds): Clinical Electrotherapy. Appleton and Lange, Norwalk, CT, 1987, pp 11–28.

7. Baker, LL: Neuromuscular electrical stimulation in the restoration of purposeful limb movements. In Wolf, SL (ed): Electrotherapy. Churchill Livingstone, New York, 1981, pp 25–48.

8. Binder, SA: Application of low- and high-voltage electrotherapeutic currents. In Wolf, SL (ed): Electrotherapy. Churchill Livingstone, New York, 1981, pp 1–24.

9. DeVahl, J: Neuromuscular electrical stimulation (NMES) in rehabilitation. In Gersh, MR (ed): Electrotherapy in Rehabilitation. FA Davis, Philadelphia, 1992, pp 218–268.

10. Gieck, JH and Salbina, EN: The athletic trainer and rehabilitation. In Kuland, DN: The Injured Athlete, ed 2. JB Lippincott, Philadelphia, 1988, pp 165–240.

11. De Domenico, G: Interferential Stimulation (monograph). Chattanooga Group, Inc., Chattanooga, TN, 1988.

12. Nolan, MF: Conductive differences in electrodes used with transcutaneous electrical nerve stimulation devices. Phys Ther 71:746, 1991.

13. Lieber, RL and Kelly, MJ: Factors influencing quadriceps femoris muscle torque using transcutaneous neuromuscular stimulation. Phys Ther 71:715, 1991.

14. Baker, LL, Bowman, BR, and McNeal, DR: Effects of wave form on comfort during neuromuscular electrical stimulation. Clin Orthop 223:75, 1988.

15. Killian, CB: Electrical Stimulation Overview: Introduction to High Frequency Stimulation. Presented to the Physical Therapy Combined Section Meeting, Orlando, FL, 1985.

16. Ferguson, JP, et al: Effects of varying electrode site placements on the torque output of an electrically stimulated involuntary quadriceps femoris muscle contraction. JOSPT, 11:24, 1989.

17. Delitto, A and Rose, SJ: Comparative comfort of three wave forms used in electrically eliciting quadriceps femoris muscle contractions. Phys Ther 66:1704, 1986

18. Miller, CR and Webers, RL: The effects of ice massage on an individual's pain tolerance level to electrical stimulation. JOSPT 12:105, 1990.

19. Durst, JW, et al: Effects of ice and recovery time on maximal involuntary isometric torque production using electrical stimulation. JOSPT 13:240, 1991.

20. Singer, K, et al: Electrical modalities. In Drez, D (ed): Therapeutic Modalities for Sports Injuries. Year Book Medical Publishers, Chicago, 1989, p 42.

21. Parker, MG, et al: Fatigue response in human quadriceps femoris muscle during high frequency electrical stimulation. JOSPT 7:145, 1986.

22. Bowman, BR and Baker, LL: Effects of wave form parameters on comfort during transcutaneous neuromuscular electrical stimulation. Ann Biom Eng 13:59, 1985.

23. Delitto, A and Snyder-Mackler, L: Two theories of muscle strength augmentation using percutaneous electrical stimulation. Phys Ther 70:158, 1990.

24. Kramer, JF: Effect of electrical stimulation frequencies on isometric knee extension torque. Phys Ther 67:31, 1987.

25. Trimble, MH and Enoka, RM: Mechanisms underlying the training effects associated with neuromuscular electrical stimulation. Phys Ther 71:273, 1991.

26. Sinacore, DR, et al: Type II fiber activation with electrical stimulation: A preliminary report. Phys Ther 70:416, 1990.

27. Draper, U and Ballard, L: Electrical stimulation versus electromyographic biofeedback in the recovery of quadriceps femoris muscle function following anterior cruciate ligament surgery. Phys Ther 71:455, 1991.

28. Currier, DP and Mann, R: Muscular strength development by electrical stimulation in healthy individuals. Phys Ther 63:915, 1983.

29. Taylor, K, et al: Effects of interferential current stimulation for treatment of subjects with recurrent jaw pain. Phys Ther 67:346, 1987.

30. Longobardi, AG, et al: Effects of auricular transcutaneous electrical nerve stimulation on distal extremity pain. Phys Ther 69:10, 1989.

31. Jensen, JE, et al: The use of transcutaneous neural stimulation and isokinetic testing in arthroscopic knee surgery. Am J Sports Med 13:27, 1985.

32. Lewers, D, et al: Transcutaneous electrical nerve stimulation in the relief of primary dysmenorrhea. Phys Ther 69:3, 1989.

33. Gersh, MR: Transcutaneous electrical nerve stimulation (TENS) for management of pain and sensory pathology. In Gersh, MR (ed): Electrotherapy in Rehabilitation. FA Davis, Philadelphia, 1992, pp 149–196.

34. French, S: Pain: Some psychological and sociological aspects. Physiotherapy 75:255, 1989.

35. Feedar, JA, Kloth, LC, and Gentzkow, GD: Chronic dermal ulcer healing enhanced with monophasic pulsed electrical stimulation. Phys Ther 71:639, 1991.

36. Snyder-Mackler, L: Electrical stimulation for tissue repair. In: Snyder-Mackler, L and Robinson, AJ (eds): Clinical Electrophysiology: Electrotherapy and Electrophysiologic Testing. Williams & Wilkins, Baltimore, 1989, pp 229–244.

37. Kloth, LC and Feedar, JA: Electrical stimulation in tissue repair. In Kloth, LC, McCulloch, JM, and Feedar, JA (eds): Wound Healing: Alternatives in Management. FA Davis, Philadelphia, 1990, pp 221–258.

38. Newton, R: High-voltage pulsed galvanic stimulation: Theoretical bases and clinical application. In Nelson, RM and Currier, DP (eds): Clinical Electrotherapy. Appleton and Lange, Norwalk, CT, 1987, pp 165–182.

39. Bettany, JA, Fish, DR, and Mendel, FC: Influence of high voltage pulsed direct current on edema formation following impact injury. Phys Ther 70:219, 1990.

40. Cummings, JP: Additional uses of electricity. In Gersh, MR (ed): Electrotherapy in Rehabilitation. FA Davis, Philadelphia, 1992, p 337.

41. Michlovitz, S, Smith, W, and Watkins, M: Ice and high voltage pulsed stimulation in treatment of lateral ankle sprains. JOSPT 9:301, 1988.

42. Griffin, JW, et al: Reduction of chronic posttraumatic hand edema: A comparison of high voltage pulsed current, intermittent pneumatic compression, and placebo treatments. Phys Ther 70:279, 1990.

43. Lilly-Masuda, D and Towne, S: Bioelectricity and bone healing. JOSPT 7:54, 1985.

44. Nash, HL and Rogers, CC: Does electricity speed the healing of non-union fractures. Physician and Sportsmedicine 16:156, 1988.

45. Stanish, WD, et al: The use of electricity in ligament and tendon repair. The Physician and Sportsmedicine 13:110, 1985.

46. Hasson, SH, et al: Exercise training and dexamethasone iontophoresis in rheumatoid arthritis: A case study. Physiotherapy Canada 43:11, 1991.

47. Henley, EJ: Transcutaneous drug delivery: Iontophoresis, phonophoresis. Physical and Rehabilitation Medicine 2:139, 1991.

48. Harris, PR: Iontophoresis: Clinical research in musculoskeletal inflammatory conditions. JOSPT 4:109, 1982.

49. Newton, RA and Karselis, TC: Skin pH following high voltage pulsed galvanic stimulation. Phys Ther 63:1593, 1983.

50. Mohr, T, et al: The effect of high volt galvanic stimulation on quadriceps femoris muscle torque. JOSPT 7:314, 1986.

51. Mohr, T, et al: Comparison of isometric exercise and high volt galvanic stimulation

on quadriceps femoris muscle strength 65:606, 1985.

52. Ralston, DJ: High voltage galvanic stimulation: Can there be a "state of the art?" Athletic Training 20:291, 1985.

53. Voight, ML: Reduction of post traumatic ankle edema with high voltage pulsed galvanic stimulation. Athletic Training 19:278, 1984.

54. Mohr, TM, Akers, TK, and Landry, RG: Effect of high voltage stimulation on edema reduction in the rat hind limb. Phys Ther 67:1703, 1987.

55. Taylor, K, et al: Effect of electrically induced muscle contractions on post traumatic edema formation in frog hind limbs. Phys Ther 72:127, 1992.

56. Taylor, K, et al: Effect of a single 30-minute treatment of high voltage pulsed current on edema formation in frog hind limbs. Phys Ther 72:63, 1992.

57. Fish, DR, et al: Effect of anodal high voltage pulsed current on edema formation in frog hind limbs. Phys Ther 71:724, 1991.

58. Walker, DC, Currier, DP, and Threlkeld, AJ: Effects of high voltage pulsed electrical stimulation on blood flow. Phys Ther 68:481, 1988.

59. Tracy, JE, Currier, DP, and Threlkeld, AJ: Comparison of selected pulse frequencies from different electrical stimulators on blood flow in healthy subjects. Phys Ther 68:1526, 1988.

60. Kincaid, CB and Lavoie, KH: Inhibition of bacterial growth in vitro following stimulation with high voltage, monophasic, pulsed current. Phys Ther 69:651, 1989.

61. Roeser, WM, et al: The use of transcutaneous nerve stimulation for pain control in athletic medicine. A preliminary report. Am J Sports Med 4:210, 1976.

62. Jette, DU: Effect of different forms of transcutaneous electrical nerve stimulation on experimental pain. Phys Ther 66:187, 1986.

63. Gersh, MR and Wolf, SL: Applications of transcutaneous electrical nerve stimulation in the management of patients with pain. Phys Ther 65:314, 1985.

64. Bechtel, TB and Fan, PT: When is TENS effective and practical for pain relief? J Musculoskel Medicine 2:37, 1985.

65. Ottoson, D and Lundeberg, T: Pain Treatment by Transcutaneous Electrical Nerve Stimulation: A Practical Manual. Springer-Verlag, New York, 1988.

66. Denegar, CR and Huff, CB: High and low frequency TENS in the treatment of induced musculoskeletal pain: A comparison study. Athletic Training 23:235, 1988.

67. Denegar, CR, et al: Influence of transcutaneous electrical nerve stimulation on pain, range of motion, and serum cortisol concentration in females experiencing delayed onset muscle soreness. JOSPT 11:100, 1989.

68. Berlant, SR: Method of determining optimal stimulation sites for transcutaneous electrical nerve stimulation. Phys Ther 64:924, 1984.

69. Paris, DL, Baynes, F, and Gucker, B: Effects of the neuroprobe in the treatment of second-degree ankle sprains. Phys Ther 63:35, 1983.

70. Snyder-Mackler, L: Electrical stimulation for pain modulation. In Snyder-Mackler, L and Robinson, AJ: Clinical Electrophysiology: Electrotherapy and Electrophysiologic Testing. Williams & Wilkins, Baltimore, pp 205–227.

71. Kloth, LC: Electrotherapeutic alternatives for the treatment of pain. In Gersh, MR (ed): Electrotherapy in Rehabilitation. FA Davis, Philadelphia, 1992, pp 197–217.

72. Nussbaum, E, Rush, P, and Disenhaus, L: The effects of interferential therapy on peripheral blood flow. Physiotherapy 76:803, 1990.

73. Hobler, CK: Case study: Reduction of chronic posttraumatic knee edema using interferential stimulation. Athletic Training 26:364, 1991.

74. Selkowitz, DM: Improvement in isometric strength of the quadriceps femoris muscle after training with electrical stimulation. Phys Ther 65:186, 1988.

75. Laughman, RK, et al: Strength changes in the normal quadriceps femoris muscle group as a result of electrical stimulation. Phys Ther 63:494, 1983.

76. Currier, DP, Petrilli, CR, and Therlkeld, JA: Effect of graded electrical stimulation on blood flow to healthy muscle. Phys Ther 66:937, 1986.

77. Liu, H, Currier, DP, and Threlkeld, AJ: Circulatory response of digital arteries associated with electrical stimulation of calf muscle in healthy subjects. Phys Ther 67:340, 1987.

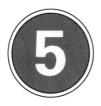

Mechanical Agents

. . . .

This section presents those therapeutic modalities utilizing mechanical energy to elicit involuntary responses in the human body. Ultrasound is presented in this section because of its presence on the acoustical spectrum rather than the electromagnetic spectrum.

Ultrasound

Ultrasound is a deep penetrating modality capable of producing changes in tissue through both thermal and nonthermal (mechanical) mechanisms (Fig. 5–1). Unlike most other electrically driven modalities in this book, ultrasonic energy is not a part of the electromagnetic spectrum. Rather, it is located on the **acoustical spectrum** (see Chapter 2, Box 2–1). Depending on the frequency of the waves, ultrasound is used for diagnostic imaging, therapeutic tissue healing, or tissue destruction. This chapter will focus on the therapeutic effects of ultrasound. Many textbooks place the discussion of ultrasound in the section on thermal agents, but it is classified here as a mechanical agent to reinforce the fact that its application results in both thermal and nonthermal effects.

Traditionally, ultrasound has been used in the athletic training room for its deep-heating effects. Although ultrasound does increase the temperature of deeply located structures, it is not necessarily interchangeable with other forms of thermotherapy. Other benefits of ultrasound application include increased rate of tissue repair and the reduction of pain and spasticity through alteration of nerve conduction velocities.

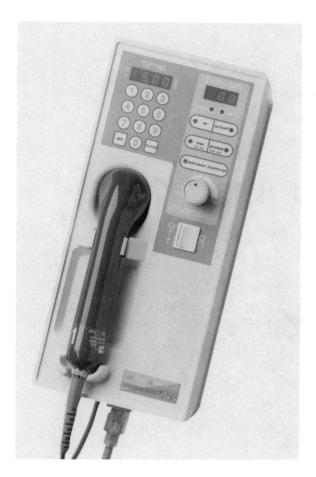

Figure 5–1. An ultrasound unit with a 1-MHz sound head. (The Sonicator 720 courtesy of Mettler Electronics Corporation, Inc., Anaheim, CA.)

PRODUCTION OF ULTRASOUND

Ultrasound is produced by an alternating current flowing through a **piezoelectric crystal** such as quartz, barium titanate, lead zirconate or titanate housed in a *transducer*. Piezoelectric crystals produce positive and negative electrical charges when they contract or expand (Fig. 5–2). A reverse (indirect) piezoelectric effect occurs when an alternating current is passed through a piezoelectric crystal, resulting in the contraction and expansion of the crystals. It is through the reverse piezoelectric effect that ultrasound is produced. This vibration of the crystals results in the mechanical production of sound waves.

The human ear is capable of hearing sound waves ranging between 16 and 20,000 Hz. Any sound wave above this range is considered to be ultrasound. Therapeutic ultrasound ranges between 750,000 and 3,000,000 Hz (0.8 to 3 MHz). In the United States, the most frequently used ultrasound frequency is 1 MHz (Box 5–1).

Transducer: A device that converts one form of energy to another.

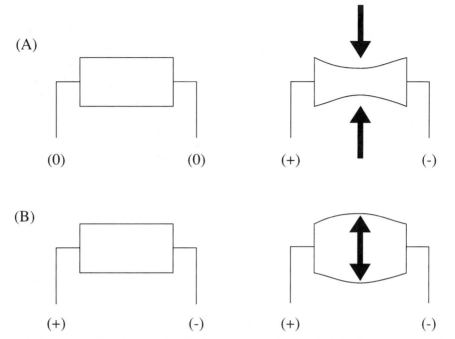

Figure 5–2. Piezoelectric crystals. (A) The direct piezoelectric effect. Crystals possessing piezo-electric properties produce positive and negative electrical charges when they are compressed or expanded. (B) The reverse (indirect) piezoelectric effect. These same crystals will expand and contract when an electrical current is passed through them.

Box 5–1 CONTRAST AND COMPARISON OF ULTRASOUND AND AUDIBLE SOUND

The way that piezoelectric crystals produce ultrasound bears some striking resemblances to the way in which a stereo produces audible sound. When a stereo plays music, it detects the patterns of recorded sound impulses. These patterns are converted to electrical energy that is transferred to a speaker. Once the energy reaches the speaker, it activates a magnet causing a cone to expand and contract. The vibration of the cone produces mechanical waves that are transmitted through the air and subsequently strike our eardrums.

Ultrasound generators operate on basically the same principle. An alternating current is passed through a crystal, causing it to expand and contract. The vibration of this crystal produces mechanical waves that are passed along to the body.

The difference between the production of these two sound waves lies in the frequency that the "speaker" vibrates. Stereos use a much lower frequency than ultrasound, so the waves can be transmitted through the air and be detected by the human ear. Ultrasound units use such a high frequency that the waves cannot be transmitted without the use of a dense medium and cannot be detected by the human ear.

TRANSMISSION OF ULTRASOUND WAVES

Because of the high frequencies involved, ultrasound requires a dense medium through which to travel. Ultrasound waves are therefore unable to pass through the air. Electromagnetic energy (such as a radio wave) prefers to travel through a vacuum and does so at a speed at, or near, the speed of light. Acoustical energy prefers a dense medium and travels through it at a much slower speed. Ultrasound has a sinusoidal wave form and displays the properties of wavelength, frequency, amplitude, and velocity.

Wave energy is transferred by one molecule jostling against its neighbor, without actual displacement of the molecules. Consider a leaf floating in a pond. If a pebble is dropped near it, the leaf will bob up and down as the ripples pass beneath it, but it does not change its position.

Longitudinal Waves

Particle displacement in longitudinal waves occurs parallel to the direction of the sound. An example of longitudinal waves may be seen at the end of a bungee jump. As the jumper bobs up and down, the elastic band is elongating and contracting. In this case the energy, as represented by the jumper, is transmitted parallel to the direction of the wave.

The alternation of high and low pressure exerted by the ultrasound beam results in regions of high particle density (compression) and low particle density (rarefaction) along the path of the wave (Fig. 5–3). These pressure fluctuations serve to transmit the energy within the tissues and, as discussed in subsequent sections, produces physiological effects. Longitudinal waves are

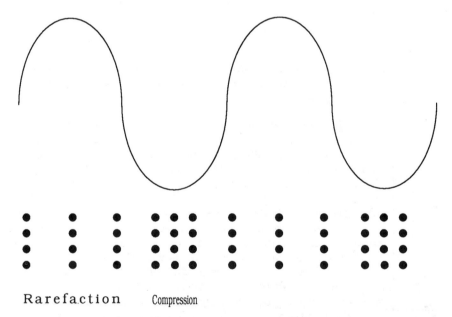

Rarefaction   Compression

Figure 5–3. Rarefaction and compression of molecules. An ultrasound wave passing through the tissues will create alternating periods of low and high pressure. Molecules in the low pressure areas will expand (rarefaction) and molecules in high pressure areas will compress.

capable of traveling through both solid and liquid media, and ultrasound passes through soft tissue in this form.

Transverse (Shear) Waves

Particle displacement in transverse waves occurs perpendicular to the direction of the sound wave. A vibrating guitar string is an example of this type of wave. Plucking a guitar string causes it to vibrate parallel to its length. Transverse waves cannot pass through fluids and are only found in the body when ultrasound strikes bone.

THE ULTRASOUND WAVE

Low-frequency sound waves, such as those produced by the human voice, diverge in all directions, making it possible to hear the voice of a person behind you. As the frequency of the sound wave increases, the less the sound beam diverges.[1] The frequencies used in therapeutic ultrasound produce cylindrical beams that have a width somewhat smaller than the diameter of the sound head (see below). The **effective radiating area** (ERA) represents the portion of the transducer's surface area that actually produces ultrasound waves.

As ultrasound waves travel there is some degree of divergence, but it is not as pronounced as with waves of lower frequency (within the range of human hearing). Consider the difference between a beam of light produced by a spotlight and an ordinary light bulb. If the spotlight and lamp were held 1 foot from a wall, the spotlight would concentrate the light within an area approximately the same diameter as the lens. The light produced from the bare bulb would illuminate an area significantly larger than the bulb itself. As the distance between each source of light and the wall is increased, the diameter of each beam would increase, but much more so with the bare bulb than with the spotlight. Likewise, the treatment area effectively exposed to the ultrasonic energy is limited to the diameter of the sound head.

Ultrasound heads are available in different sizes and with different crystal frequencies (Fig. 5–4). Each transducer head must be labeled with its frequency, effective radiating area, and the beam nonuniformity ratio (covered later). Large-diameter heads produce a beam that is more *collimated* while smaller heads yield a diverging beam.

Close to the transducer head, the pressure of the sound field is very nonuniform, forming peaks of high intensity and valleys of low intensity (Fig. 5–5). This area, the **near field**, is the portion of the ultrasound beam used for therapeutic purposes. The variation in pressure occurs because the transducer head acts as if it were made up of many smaller heads, each producing its own sound wave. Close to the transducer, these areas are individually distinguishable. As the distance from the head is increased, the waves begin to interact to produce a more unified beam. An example of this can be found in a television set. If you look very closely at the screen, individual colored elements are seen. As the distance between your eye and the screen is increased, the dots lose their individuality and a complete picture is formed.

Collimated: Possessing a beam of parallel rays or waves which form a column of energy.

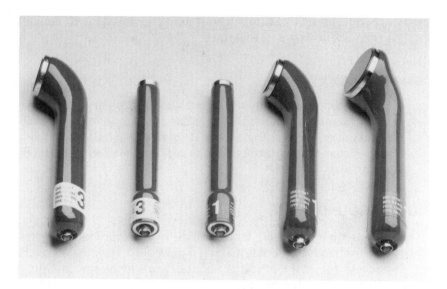

Figure 5–4. Range of Ultrasound Heads. Ultrasound transducers are available in a range of sizes and frequencies. Note the labels indicating the effective radiating area (ERA), beam nonuniformity ratio (BNR), and frequency (1 or 3 MHz). (Courtesy of Mettler Electronics Corporation, Inc., Anaheim, CA.)

Frequency

The frequency of an ultrasound wave is measured in megahertz (MHz) and represents the number of waves occurring in 1 second. Low-frequency (0.75 MHz) ultrasound produces a more diverging beam than high-frequency (3.0 MHz) ultrasound, which produces a collimated beam.

It is the frequency of the ultrasound that determines the depth of penetration of the energy. A linear correlation exists between the frequency of the

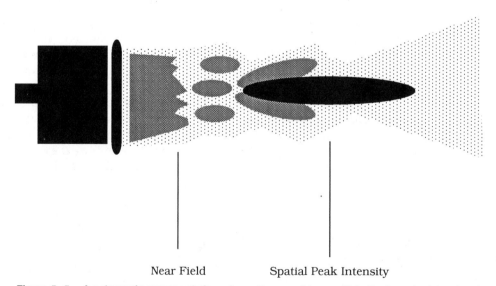

Near Field   Spatial Peak Intensity

Figure 5–5. A schematic representation of an ultrasound beam. Note the irregular intensity of the near field and the spatial peak intensity.

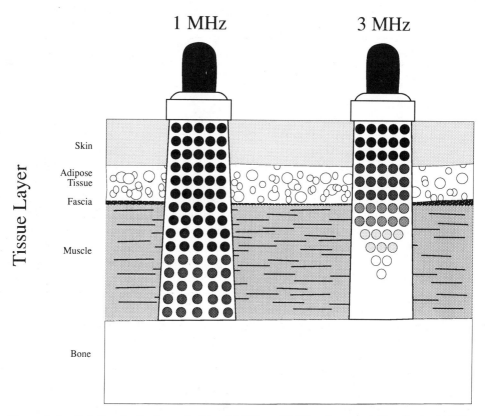

Figure 5–6. **Relative depth of penetration of 1 MHz and 3 MHz ultrasound**. The effects of 1 MHz ultrasound occur deeper within the tissues than 3 MHz ultrasound, which attenuates in the superficial tissues. Note that the 1 MHz beam has a greater degree of divergence than the 3 MHz beam.

ultrasound and the depth at which energy is absorped.[2] High-frequency ultrasound generators of 3.0 MHz provide treatment to superficial tissues because the energy is rapidly absorbed (Fig. 5–6). The commonly used 1.0-MHz generator offers a compromise between deep penetration and adequate heating due to the relatively low frequency used.[1]

The frequency of the ultrasound is dependent on the crystal used in the sound head. Changing the frequency of the ultrasound involves changing to the appropriate sound head (see Fig. 5–4). Do not attempt to change the sound head of units not specifically designed to do so.

Power and Intensity

The **power** produced by an ultrasonic generator is described in watts and represents the amount of energy being produced by the transducer. **Intensity** describes the strength of the sound waves at a given location within the tissues being treated. There are two primary measures of intensity: the spatial average intensity and the temporal (time) average intensity.

Spatial Average Intensity

Spatial average intensity describes the amount of energy passing through a specified area, in this case, the transducer head. This gives a description of

Table 5-1. **EFFECT OF ULTRASOUND RADIATING AREA ON THE TOTAL AMOUNT OF ENERGY PRODUCED**

Intensity (W/cm²)	Effective Radiating Area of the Sound Head (cm²)	Total Power Produced (W)
1.5	5	7.5
1.5	6	9.0
1.5	10	15.0

the power per unit area and is expressed in watts per square centimeter (W/cm²). This measure can be calculated by dividing the power of the output (watts) by the ERA of the transducer head (square centimeters). For example, if 10 watts are being delivered through a transducer head with an effective radiating area of 5 square centimeters, the spatial average intensity would be 2 watts per square centimeter.

Ultrasonic generators can express their output as either **total watts** or **watts per square centimeter**. Standard treatment doses range from 0.5 to 5.0 watts per square centimeter. If the radiating area of the sound head is smaller than specified, or if a portion of the sound head is obstructed from transmitting sound, a higher spatial average intensity is produced than that indicated on the meter.

As seen with electrical current density, altering the size of the sound head affects the power density. Passing 10 watts of energy through a transducer of 10 square centimeters results in a lower density than if a head of 5 square centimeters is used (Table 5-1).

Temporal Average Intensity

Temporal average intensity measures the power of ultrasonic energy over a given period of time and is only meaningful for the application of pulsed ultrasound. The energy delivered to the tissues per unit time with ultrasound operating at a 50 percent duty cycle will be half of that delivered in a continuous mode. If we take a spatial average intensity of 2 watts per square centimeter and pulse with a 50 percent duty cycle, the temporal average intensity of the treatment would be 1.0 watts per square centimeter (2.0 W/cm² × 0.5 = 1.0 W/cm²). It is important to distinguish between the temporal average intensity, the average amount of power delivered during a single cycle, and the temporal peak intensity, the maximum amount of energy delivered by a single pulse (Fig. 5-7).

Ultrasound Beam Nonuniformity

The degree to which the intensity within the ultrasound beam varies is measured by the **beam nonuniformity ratio** (BNR). This is the ratio of the highest intensity within the beam, the spatial peak intensity (see Figure 5-5), to the average intensity reported on the output meter. The BNR must be indicated on the ultrasound unit.[3]

If the BNR is indicated as 3:1 and the meter indicates an output of 2.0 watts per square centimeter, then at some point in the beam the actual intensity is 6.0 watts per centimeter squared. The existence of high-intensity areas in

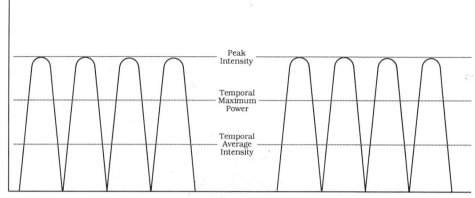

Figure 5–7. Peak intensity, temporal maximum power, and temporal average intensity of a pulsed ultrasound beam. The peak intensity represents the amplitude of a single wave. The temporal maximum power is the average amount of power delivered by a single pulse. The temporal average intensity is the average amount of energy delivered to the tissues during the application of pulsed ultrasound.

the beam is a primary reason for keeping the sound head moving during the treatment. The optimal, although clinically unobtainable, BNR is 1:1, and a BNR greater than 8:1 may be considered unacceptable.

TRANSFER OF ULTRASOUND THROUGH THE TISSUES

Like all sound waves, ultrasonic waves are capable of reflection, refraction, penetration, and absorption. Ultrasound passes through soft tissue in the form of longitudinal waves until it strikes bone, at which time some of the energy is reflected and the rest is converted into transverse waves. The *propagation* of ultrasonic energy is dependent on the frequency of the sound waves and the density of the tissues. Passage of ultrasound through the body causes the tissues to acquire kinetic energy, resulting in cellular vibration.

When the ultrasound beam strikes an *acoustical interface*, some of the energy is reflected or refracted. The amount of reflection is dependent on the degree of change in density at the junction (Table 5–2). Ultrasound meeting with air produces almost total reflection of the energy. The interface between

Table 5–2 **PERCENT REFLECTION OF ULTRASONIC ENERGY AT VARIOUS INTERFACES**

Interface	Energy Reflected (%)
Water–Soft tissue	0.2
Soft tissue–Fat	1
Soft tissue–Bone	15–40
Soft tissue–Air	99.9

Source: Adapted from Williams, R: Production and transmission of ultrasound. Physiotherapy 73:113, 1987.

Propagation: Transmission through a medium.
Acoustical Interface: A surface where two materials of different densities meet.

soft tissue and bone is also highly reflective. Other highly reflective interfaces include the musculotendinous junction and intermuscular interfaces. Unlike infrared energy, ultrasound is not greatly affected by, and therefore passes through, adipose tissue.

If the reflected wave meets the incoming incident wave, a *standing wave* is formed. The standing wave increases the intensity of the energy by creating areas of high and low pressure. Free-floating gas bubbles move toward the low-pressure areas while freely moving cells collect at the high-pressure centers.[4] Because of this, a high level of energy is formed in a limited amount of space, increasing the risk of tissue damage. Standing waves can be avoided by keeping the sound head moving.

Reflection of intense ultrasonic energy from bone produces **periosteal pain**, a deep-seated burning or aching. This effect is to be avoided during the treatment. Caution must be used when applying ultrasound to areas having bony protuberances, such as the elbow's olecranon process. The intensity used to treat the muscle or tendon can produce periosteal pain if applied over these protuberances.

Any energy not reflected or absorbed is passed on to the underlying tissues.

The intensity of ultrasonic energy decreases as the distance it travels through the tissues increases. This process, **attenuation**, occurs through the **scattering** and **absorption** of the waves within the tissues. Absorption of the sound waves transfers energy from the beam into the surrounding tissues through conversion of mechanical energy into thermal energy. The amount of absorption that occurs is related to the protein (especially collagen) content of the tissues. Tissues such as bone, cartilage, and tendon absorb much more ultrasonic energy than muscle, fat, or blood.[1] Scattering occurs when the sound waves strike an acoustical interface where there is reflection or refraction of the wave.

The rate of absorption, and therefore attenuation, increases as the frequency of the ultrasound is increased.[5] The increased absorption occurs because of the molecular friction that the sound waves must overcome in order to pass through the tissues. Because of this, less energy is available to pass deeper into the tissues.[1]

TYPES OF ULTRASOUND APPLICATION

Continuous

Continuous ultrasound application can effectively heat tissues located 5 centimeters deep, or deeper. Since the output is flowing 100 percent of the time, the ultrasonic energy is measured in terms of the spatial average intensity (watts per square centimeter). The spatial peak intensity, as determined by the BNR, should not be allowed to exceed 8 watts per square centimeter (metered output × BNR).

Standing Wave: A single-frequency wave formed by the collision of two waves of equal frequency and speed traveling in opposite directions. The energy with a standing wave cannot be transmitted from one area to another and is focused in a confined area.

Pulsed

Pulsing the ultrasound beam decreases the temporal average intensity of the output, reducing the thermal effects while still allowing for nonthermal effects. The ratio between the pulse length and the pulse interval is expressed as a percentage **duty cycle**:

$$\text{Duty cycle} = \frac{\text{Pulse length}}{(\text{Pulse length} + \text{Pulse interval})} \times 100$$

The closer the duty cycle is to 100 percent, the greater the net thermal effects of the treatment. The output of pulsed ultrasound is measured by the temporal maximal intensity, but the actual amount of energy delivered to the tissue is dependent on the duty cycle. The average treatment doses are presented in Figure 5–8. Note that this chart indicates the output in terms of total watts.

COUPLING AGENTS

Since ultrasonic waves cannot pass through the air, a coupling agent must be used to allow the waves to pass out of the transducer head into the tissue. A good medium is characterized by the ability to transmit a significant percentage of the ultrasound. Therefore it should be nonreflective. The optimal medium for transmission is distilled water, which reflects only 0.2 percent of the energy.[6]

Attempting to pass ultrasound through a nonconductive medium can damage the crystal. For this reason, only approved conducting agents should be used, and the intensity of the unit should not be increased without the sound head in proper contact with the body. Most modern ultrasound generators will automatically shut down if application is attempted without a medium or if an unacceptable medium is used.

COUPLING METHODS

Direct Coupling

In this method of ultrasound application, the transducer is applied directly to the skin, with a gel serving to exclude air between the skin and the sound head. Coupling gels consist of distilled water and an inert, nonreflective material that increases the viscosity of the mixture. This gel should be applied liberally to the area to ensure that a consistent coat is available throughout the treatment.

The effectiveness of gels is decreased if the body part is hairy or irregularly shaped. Each of these conditions can increase the spatial average intensity by decreasing the contact area between the transducer and the tissues. The application of gels causes air bubbles to cling to hair. The greater amount of hair on the body part, the greater the reduction of ultrasound delivered to the tissues. Every effort should be made to eliminate these bubbles while spreading on the coupling agent. Irregularly shaped areas decrease the contact area between the transducer and the skin, resulting in uneven amounts of sound energy being delivered to the tissues.

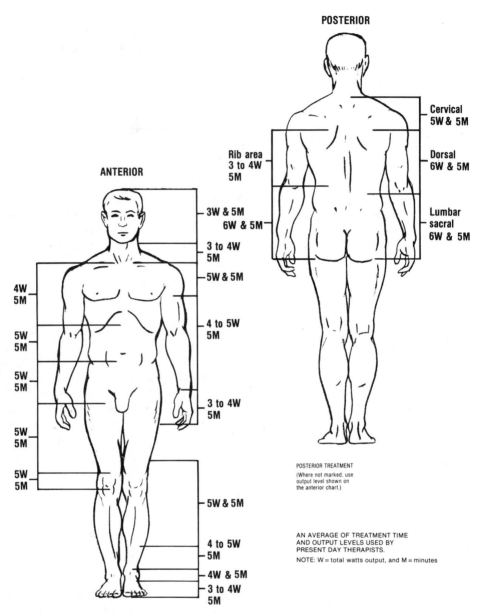

Figure 5–8. Suggested ultrasound intensities and durations for various body areas. The duration of the treatment is 1 to 2 minutes for each area 1½ times the size of the transducer face. The actual intensity and mode of the treatment should be adjusted according to the desired outcomes of the treatment. (Courtesy of Mettler Electronics Corporation, Inc., Anaheim, CA.)

Water Immersion

When treating irregularly shaped areas such as the foot, ankle, or toes, a more uniform dose of ultrasound can be given through water. The body part is immersed in a tub of water (distilled water is the ideal medium, but is seldom used). The transducer is then placed in the water with the sound head facing the body part (Fig. 5–9). The operator's hand should not be immersed in the water.

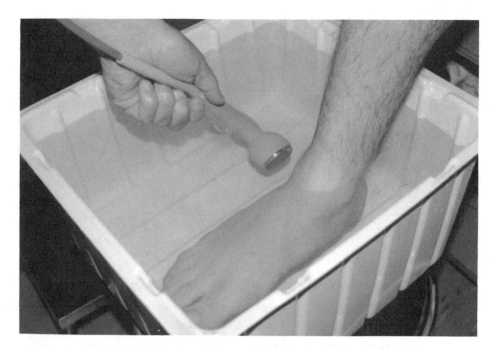

Figure 5–9. Underwater application of ultrasound. Water is used as a coupling medium to evenly distribute ultrasound over irregularly shaped areas. The sound head does not come in contact with the body part.

Although not necessarily dangerous in a single treatment, immersion could unnecessarily expose the hand to ultrasonic energy over repeated exposures.

The use of a ceramic tube for underwater ultrasound application has been recommended.[6] The ceramic sides make an excellent reflective surface, creating an "echo chamber" allowing the sound waves to strike the body part from all angles. If nondistilled water is being used, the intensity of the ultrasound can be increased by approximately 0.5 watts per square centimeter to account for attenuation caused by air and minerals in the water.

Bladder Method

This technique typically employs a water-filled balloon or plastic bag that is coated with a coupling gel. The bladder can conform to irregularly shaped areas such as the acromioclavicular or talocrural joints (Fig. 5–10). The bladder is held against the body part and the sound applicator is moved over the bladder. Because balloons are relatively fragile, condoms are often substituted.

Regardless of the type of bladder used, all air pockets must be removed before sealing. If the ultrasound wave comes into contact with a large air pocket, the energy will not be transmitted.

BIOPHYSICAL EFFECTS OF ULTRASOUND APPLICATION

The physiological changes within the tissues associated with ultrasound application can be grouped into two classes:[1]

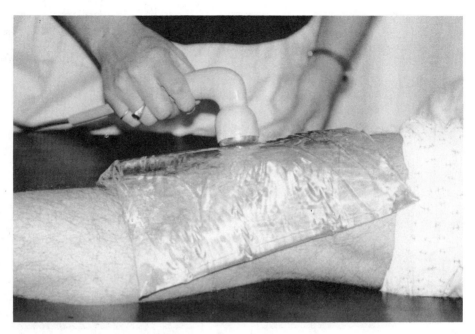

Figure 5–10. Ultrasound application using the bladder coupling method. This method can be used to deliver ultrasound to irregularly shaped areas when the underwater method is not practical.

Nonthermal effects—changes within the tissues resulting from the mechanical effect of ultrasonic energy.

Thermal effects—changes within the tissues as a direct result of ultrasound's elevation of the tissue temperature.

The relationship between the mechanisms responsible for these effects has not been fully determined.

Nonthermal Effects

Passage of ultrasonic energy through liquids leads to the formation of microscopic bubbles that flow along the path of the beam. The process of bubble formation, **cavitation**, is classified into one of two types:[2] (1) **stable cavitation** producing small expansions and contractions of the bubbles or (2) **unstable cavitation** where the bubbles oscillate in a violent manner and then completely collapse. Stable cavitation can produce therapeutic effects while unstable cavitation leads to tissue damage.[4] Unstable cavitation occurs when the intensity or duration of the treatment is too great.

Either type of cavitation leads to localized flow in the fluids surrounding the vibrating bubble; this is known as **microstreaming** or acoustical streaming. The circular flow of bubbles in the microstreams causes a change in cell membrane structure and function, facilitating the passage of calcium and other ions and metabolites into and out of the cell. So long as the cell membrane is not damaged by this process, the response to cavitation and microstreaming can be synthesis of collagen, secretion of chemotactics, and increased cell permeability, all of which assist the healing process[4] (Table 5–3). If microstreaming

Table 5–3 **PHYSIOLOGICAL EFFECTS OF ULTRASOUND APPLICATION**

Nonthermal Effects	Thermal Effects
Increased cell membrane permeability	Increased sensory and motor nerve conduction velocity
Increased vascular permeability	
Increased blood flow	Increased extensibility in collagen-rich structures
Synthesis of protein	Reduction of muscle spasm
Reduction of edema	Increased blood flow
Tissue regeneration	Reduction of pain

occurs in the presence of a standing wave, damage can result to immobile tissue or free-floating blood cells.

Thermal Effects

The degree of temperature increase from ultrasound application is dependent on the mode of application (continuous or pulsed), the intensity and frequency of the output, the vascularity and type of tissues, and the speed with which the sound head is moved over the tissues. Thermal effects are greatest when the ultrasound is delivered in the continuous mode.

Heat production is dependent on the amount of attenuation of the sound waves in the tissues.[7] The process involved in attenuation, absorption, and scattering create friction between the molecules and result in a temperature increase. Tissues that are collagen-rich, such as tendon, joint menisci, superficial bone, large nerve roots, and intermuscular fascia are preferentially heated.[4] Tissues that are largely fluid-filled, such as the fat layer, are relatively transparent to ultrasonic energy.

Temperatures in poorly vascularized tissues increase by 0.8°C per minute during the application of continuous ultrasound with a frequency of 1 MHz.[2] In highly vascularized areas like muscle, the temperature rise is not as great. Blood flow tends to minimize the degree of temperature increase through the continuous replacement of warmed blood with fresh, cool blood.

Tissue temperatures increase at higher frequencies, especially in the superficial tissues, as seen with ultrasound generators operating at 3.0 MHz. Reflected waves also increase the amount of heating. When ultrasound waves are reflected, the energy passes through the tissues more than once, increasing the thermal effects. Standing waves greatly exaggerate the rise in temperature.

To achieve a therapeutic effect through ultrasound heating, the tissue temperatures must be maintained between 40°C and 45°C for at least 5 minutes.[4] The thermal effects associated with ultrasound application are presented in Table 5–3.

EFFECT ON THE INJURY RESPONSE CYCLE

The effects of ultrasound application are dependent on the mode of application (continuous or pulsed), the frequency of the sound, the size of the area treated, the tissues being treated (vascularity and density), and the size of the area being treated. The deep thermal effects are similar to those described in the thermotherapy section. Mechanical changes resulting from the nonthermal effects are discussed, where relevant, in each of the following sections.

Because of similarities in the biophysical effects, the use of laser energy has been suggested as an alternative to ultrasound. Presently, this modality is only available for experimental use in the United States although its use in other countries is widespread (Box 5–2).

Blood Flow

Ultrasound applied at 5 watts per square centimeter has been shown to increase local blood flow for up to 45 minutes after treatment.[8] This study also produced

---

Box 5–2	LASER THERAPY

Laser, an acronym for light amplification by stimulated emission of radiation, employs highly organized light to elicit physiological changes in the tissues. Therapeutic "cold" lasers, which do not normally result in tissue destruction, have been introduced in European countries as an alternative to ultrasound.[60] Material such as helium-neon (HeNe) gas is electrically energized to produce an output of photon radiation to stimulate areas such as acupuncture and trigger points and to assist in superficial wound healing.

The energy produced by therapeutic lasers has a wavelength ranging from 1 *nanometer* (nm) to 1 millimeter (mm). This range includes ultraviolet, visible, and infrared light, and lasers are considered to be an electromagnetic modality. Lasers in the ultraviolet range produce photochemical effects within the tissues, while lasers in the infrared range produce deeper thermal effects. Visible lasers, like the HeNe laser, produce wavelengths that fall in between ultraviolet and infrared lasers, and possess characteristics of both.[61]

The effects of laser energy in the tissues are similar to the effects of ultrasound. Laser energy can effectively stimulate tissues at depths up to 15 millimeters below the surface of the skin.[62,63] When the energy is absorbed by the tissues, it is converted into thermal vibration or it may produce a photobiological effect similar to the way that plants utilize light.

Application of laser energy is thought to activate many events at the molecular level, including short-term stimulation of the electron transport chain, increased synthesis of adenosine triphosphate (ATP), and a reduction in intracellular pH. These actions are theorized to affect pain-producing tissue, such as areas of muscle spasm, by restoring the normal properties of muscle tissue via the increased formation of ATP and increased enzyme activity.[63] Extreme exposure to cold lasers can result in tissue destruction through *thermolysis.*

Pain reduction is thought to occur as a result of decreasing muscle spasm or altering nerve conduction velocity. Tissue healing is proposed to occur through increased collagen production.

Laser therapy is tightly controlled in the United States. An investigational device exemption from the Food and Drug Administration is required for its use. For this reason, therapeutic laser devices are not available for general use. For more information regarding laser therapy, readers are encouraged to refer to "Therapeutic Uses of Light in Rehabilitation" by Snyder-Mackler and Seitz in Michlovitz's, *Thermal Agents in Rehabilitation* (FA Davis).

Nanometer: One billionth (10^{-9}) of a meter.
Thermolysis: Chemical decomposition due to heating.

some interesting results regarding the effect on blood flow of heat and ice massage application prior to the administration of ultrasound. Heat application prior to ultrasound greatly reduced the increase in blood flow. The application of ice massage prior to ultrasound maintained the increased blood flow at the level found with ultrasound application alone.

Tissue Healing

Ultrasound application accelerates the inflammatory phase of tissue healing.[9] The application of continuous ultrasound has been shown to positively influence macrophage activity.[10] Low-frequency (0.75 MHz) ultrasound displayed the ability to cause the release of preformed fibroblasts, while high-frequency (3.0 MHz) ultrasound increased the cell's ability to synthesize and secrete the building blocks of fibroblasts.

This response appears to be localized to those areas with a high collagen content, especially tendons. Studies on animals have shown that the application of ultrasound increased the rate of tendon healing[11] and increased the tensile strength of tendons.[12]

The thermal effect of increased extensibility in collagen-rich tissues may be used advantageously by incorporating range-of-motion exercises following the application of continuous ultrasound. Gentle passive or active stretching is needed to elongate these tissues. As scar tissue possesses a high concentration of collagen, these areas are preferentially heated with ultrasound.

Pain Control

Ultrasound may control pain through the direct effect that the energy has on the peripheral nervous system or pain control may be the result of the other benefits of ultrasound application. Ultrasound directly influences the transmission of painful impulses by eliciting changes within the nerve fibers themselves. Cell membrane permeability to sodium ions is changed, altering the electrical activity of the nerve fiber[4] and elevating the pain threshold.[13] Nerve conduction velocity is increased as a result of the thermal effects of ultrasound application[9] and may produce a counterirritant effect.[1]

Indirect pain reduction results from the other effects of ultrasound application. Increased blood flow and increased capillary permeability augment the delivery of oxygen to hypoxic areas, reducing the activity of chemosensitive pain receptors. Input from mechanical pain receptors is reduced due to a reduction in the amount of muscle spasm and to increased muscular relaxation.[13]

PHONOPHORESIS

Ultrasonic fields can be used to deliver medication into tissues through the process of **phonophoresis**. This technique utilizes the mechanical pressure of ultrasonic waves to drive medication such as anti-inflammatories, *salicylates*, and analgesics deep into the tissues. The advantage of introducing these substances into the body through phonophoresis rather than by injection is that

---

Salicylates: A family of compounds that includes aspirin.

the medication is spread over a larger area and is noninvasive.[14] The philosophy behind phonophoresis is similar to iontophoresis (see Chapter 4), but this technique does not require that the medication be electrically charged.[15]

In order for these medications to be absorbed by the viable subcutaneous tissues, they must first be driven past the *stratum corneum*. Some substances can be moved past this barrier by simply massaging them into the skin. However, some medications have been shown to be driven to a depth of 6 centimeters into the tissues with the assistance of ultrasound.[16,17]

The thermal and nonthermal effects associated with standard ultrasound application may increase the rate and amount of medication absorbed. Increased capillary permeability due to the thermal effect of ultrasound and the increased cell membrane permeability associated with the nonthermal effect may increase medication absorption by the tissues.[18] However, these same effects may remove the medication from the treated area to such an extent that no therapeutic benefits are seen.

In the application of phonophoresis, the standard coupling gel is replaced by a gel or cream containing medication. The type of medication used during phonophoresis is quite varied. Many commercially available creams containing a counterirritant, or an over-the-counter dosage of *hydrocortisone*, are used. Another technique involves mixing 10 to 15 percent hydrocortisone in an inert base, such as skin cream or ultrasound gel. Many of the medications used during phonophoresis require a physician's prescription.

The use of medication mixtures not specifically designed for phonophoresis use should be avoided. Research has shown that the majority of commonly used phonophoresis coupling agents reflect most of the ultrasonic energy; some even resulted in 100 percent reflection.[15,18] The majority of thick, white, corticosteroid creams are poor conductors of ultrasound, while topical gel-mixed media, such as commercially available transmission gels, are good conductors.[19]

The efficacy of phonophoresis has not been fully substantiated and confusion still exists.[14,17,18,20] Many of the contradictions in the results of these studies can be related to the type of coupling agent used and the concentration of the medication. For example, one study examined the subcutaneous absorption of a commercially available salicylate, Myoflex (Rorer Consumer Pharmaceuticals, Fort Washington, PA), and found no difference in the level of salicylates in the bloodstream with or without the use of ultrasound.[18] A later study revealed that Myoflex transmitted no ultrasonic energy compared to water.[19]

CLINICAL APPLICATION OF ULTRASOUND

Instrumentation

> **Power:** Allows the source current to flow into the internal components of the generator. On many units a POWER light will go on, or the WATT METER will illuminate.
>
> **Timer:** Sets the duration of the treatment. The time remaining will be

---

Stratum Corneum: The outermost, nonliving portion of the epidermis.
Hydrocortisone: An anti-inflammatory drug that closely resembles cortisol.

displayed on the console, or the timer rotates to display the time remaining.

Start/Stop: Initiates or terminates the production of ultrasound from the transducer.

Pause: Interrupts the treatment, but retains the remaining amount of treatment time when the treatment is reinstated.

Intensity: Adjusts the intensity of the ultrasound beam. The WATT METER displays the output in total watts and watts per square centimeter.

Duty cycle: Adjusts between continuous and pulsed ultrasound application. Most units display the duty cycle as a percentage, with 100 percent representing continuous ultrasound.

Watt meter: Displays the output of ultrasound in total watts or watts per square centimeter. Digital meters may require that the user manually switch between the two displays. Most *analog* meters will display the total watts on an upper scale while simultaneously displaying output in watts per square centimeter on the lower scale.

Setup and Application

Preparation of the Athlete

1. Determine the method and mode of ultrasound application to be used during this treatment.
2. Clean the area to be treated to remove any body oils, dirt, or grime.
3. Determine the type of cooling method to be used. The efficacy of phonophoresis for the bladder and immersion methods has not been established.
4. If the direct coupling method is being used, spread the gel over the area to be treated. Use the sound head to evenly distribute the gel.
5. Explain to the athlete the sensations to be expected during the treatment. During the application of continuous ultrasound, the only expected sensation is that of mild warmth. The athlete should not experience any subcutaneous sensations during the application of pulsed ultrasound. Advise the athlete to inform you of any unexpected sensations.
6. If phonophoresis is being employed, preheating of the area to be treated is recommended to decrease skin resistance and increase the absorption of the medication.[16]

Initiation of the Treatment

1. Reduce the INTENSITY to zero before turning on the POWER.
2. Select the appropriate mode for the output. Use CONTINUOUS to increase the thermal effects of ultrasound application, or PULSED output for nonthermal effects. The more acute the injury, the lower the duty cycle that is used.
3. Ensure that the WATT METER is displaying the appropriate output for the type of treatment you are giving.

Analog: A readout on continuously variable scale. A clock with hands is a type of analog display.

4. Set the TIMER to the appropriate treatment length. Use the guideline of 1 to 2 minutes for each area 1.5 times the size of the transducer face.[21] If your unit has a face of 10 square centimeters, and you are treating an area of 30 square centimeters, the treatment time should be approximately 2 to 4 minutes.
5. Begin slowly moving the sound head over the medium and depress the START button to begin the treatment session. Units having low BNR may be moved at a slower rate than those with a higher BNR.
6. Slowly increase the INTENSITY to the appropriate level while keeping the sound head moving. A general guideline for determining the intensity of the treatment is that the lowest intensity that produces the desired effects should be used.[21]
7. The sound head is moved at a moderate pace with overlapping strokes.
8. If periosteal pain is experienced, move the sound head at a faster rate, use a reduced duty cycle, and/or lower the intensity. If the pain continues, discontinue the treatment.
9. If the gel begins to wear away, or if the sound head begins sticking on the skin, depress the PAUSE button and apply more gel.

Termination of the Treatment

1. Most units will automatically terminate the production of ultrasound when the time expires. If this is not the case, or if the treatment is being terminated prematurely, the intensity must be reduced prior to removing the transducer from the medium.
2. Remove the remaining gel or water from the athlete's skin.
3. To ensure continuity between treatment, record the parameters used for this treatment in the athlete's file.

Duration and Frequency of the Treatment

The treatment time is from 3 to 10 minutes, depending on the size of the area being treated, the intensity of the treatment, and the goal of the treatment. Ultrasound is normally given once a day for 10 to 14 days.

Precautions

- Symptoms may increase following the first two treatments because of an increase in inflammation in the area. If the symptoms do not improve after the third or fourth treatment, the use of the modality should be discontinued.[21]
- EXTREME caution should be used when applying ultrasound around the spinal cord especially after *laminectomy*. Many manufacturers list this as a contraindication to ultrasound application.
- The use of ultrasound over metal implants is not contraindicated so long as the sound head is kept moving and the athlete has normal sensory function.

Laminectomy: Surgical removal of the lamina from a vertebra.

- The use of ultrasound over the epiphyseal plates of growing bone should be performed with caution. Many authors cite this as a contraindication to ultrasound use.

Indications

- Joint contractures
- Muscle spasm
- Neuroma
- Scar tissue
- Sympathetic nervous system disorders
- Trigger areas
- Warts
- Spasticity
- Postacute reduction of myositis ossificans
- Acute inflammatory conditions (pulsed output)
- Chronic inflammatory conditions (pulsed or continuous output)

Contraindications

- Acute conditions (continuous output)
- Ischemic areas
- Tendency to hemorrhage
- Around the eyes, heart, skull, or genitals
- Pregnancy when used over the pelvic or lumbar areas
- Cancer
- Over the spinal cord or large nerve plexus in high doses
- Anesthetic areas
- Over a fracture site before healing is complete
- Stress fracture sites
- Active infection
- Over the pelvic or lumbar area in menstruating females
- Areas of impaired circulation

Continuous Passive Motion

The concept of applying continuous passive motion to an injured or repaired joint is the antithesis of immobilization, a common postsurgical management technique. To thwart the deleterious effects of immobilization, continuous passive motion (CPM) devices are used to deliver gentle stresses to the healing tissues. Still predominantly used for knee injuries, CPM units have been designed for the hand, wrist, hip, shoulder, elbow, and ankle (Fig. 5–11). Although passive motion can be applied through a dedicated CPM unit, it can be delivered manually or through a number of other methods. Many isokinetic units incorporate "robotics" to deliver short-term passive motion.

Dr. Robert Salter, a Canadian physician, originally proposed the use of CPM to assist in the healing of synovial joints. Based on his clinical observations, Dr. Salter hypothesized that the application of CPM would be beneficial for three reasons:[22]

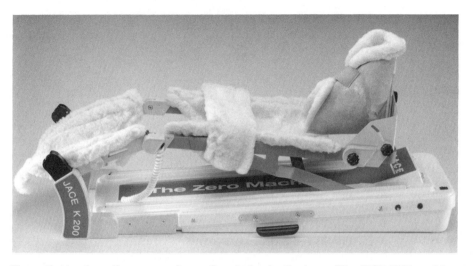

Figure 5–11. A continuous passive motion device for the knee. (The JACE K200 model manufactured by JACE Systems, Inc. Courtesy of Thera Kinetics, Inc., Mount Laurel, NJ.)

1. Nutrition and metabolic activity of articular cartilage would be enhanced.
2. Articular cartilage regrowth would be achieved by stimulating tissue remodeling.
3. Healing of articular cartilage, tendons, and ligaments would be accelerated.

Continuous passive motion devices have been categorized into two types:[23] (1) The *anatomical design* that moves the joint in a manner similar to the natural motion of the joint and (2) the *free linkage design* that allows motion in the structures adjacent to the joint, thus allowing the limb to seek its own anatomical motion.

EFFECT ON THE INJURY RESPONSE CYCLE

By providing a constant gentle stress to the injured structure, remodeling of collagen along the lines of force is enhanced and the negative effects of joint immobilization are reduced.[24] By keeping the injured joint in motion, the unwanted effects of immobilization on muscle, tendons, ligaments, articular and hyaline cartilage, blood supply, and nerve supply are reduced. The philosophy regarding the effects of CPM may be summarized by: "Motion that is never lost need never be regained. It is the regaining of movement that is painful . . ."[25]

Under the stress of motion, collagen that would normally be deposited in a random order aligns along the line of stress. This realignment reduces functional shortening and capsular adhesions, and therefore maintains the range of motion[23,26] and enhances the tensile strength of tendons and *allografts*.[22]

Both meniscal and articular cartilage are relatively avascular and derive the majority of their nutrients from synovial fluid. Similarly to a sponge absorbing water, meniscal cartilage is like a sponge and is nourished by being expanded

---

Allograft: A replacement or augmentation of a biological structure with a synthetic one.

and compressed so that by the natural movement of the joint the synovial fluid is alternately absorbed by and squeezed out of the cartilage. During immobilization, synovial fluid is not distributed throughout the joint. The application of CPM stimulates the circulation of synovial fluids and causes the meniscal cartilage to increase its uptake of nutrients. The delivery and the subsequent absorption of nutrients assists both types of cartilage in the healing process.[27,28] This effect has not been seen to improve the nonvascular nutrition of the anterior cruciate ligament.[29]

Literature reports on the effectiveness of CPM in the reduction of edema are not conclusive. The passive movements of the limb and the elevation of the body part should assist in venous and lymphatic return. A review of the literature indicates that some studies concluded that CPM was effective in reducing edema[30,31] while a single study[26] concluded that there was no effect.

The movement of the joint activates afferent nerves located in the muscle, joint, and skin, and possibly provides pain control through the gate mechanism. Any associated reduction in edema or muscle spasm, as well as deterring functional shortening, aids in limiting pain.

Some units with a proximal posterior tibial bar have been shown to induce an excessive amount of *translation* of one bone on the other. In cases such as anterior cruciate ligament repair, this movement could produce stress sufficient to damage the healing tissue.[32]

CLINICAL APPLICATION OF CONTINUOUS PASSIVE MOTION

Instrumentation

Power: Activates the internal circuits of the CPM unit.

Reset: Clears all previous settings from the CPM unit's memory.

Timer: Sets the duration of the treatment. A CONTINUOUS setting is provided for long-term treatments.

ROM: Adjusts the range of motion (ROM) from slight hyperextension to full flexion. Some units have separate controls to adjust the amount of flexion and extension.

Speed: Adjusts the rate of motion between 10 and 120 degrees per second. Increased speed (cycles per second) has been theorized to produce better tensile properties of healing tendons than lower frequencies.[33]

Pause: Stops the motion at the extreme range of motion (flexion and/or extension) to allow a passive stretching of the fibers to occur.

Interrupt: This control allows the athlete to discontinue the CPM.

Trigger jack: Some units allow for synchronization of CPM and electrical stimulation. The TRIGGER JACK allows for neuromuscular electrical stimulation unit to be activated during the PAUSE function.

Setup and Application

In many instances, the CPM unit is applied in the recovery room following surgery. The following protocol is provided for those athletes who have CPM

Translation: Sliding or gliding of opposing articular surfaces.

prescribed for short-term treatments (i.e., less than 24 hours), and a post-anterior cruciate ligament reconstructive surgery is used as an example.

1. Most CPM devices can be adjusted to fit athletes whether or not they are wearing a brace or surgical bandages.
2. Measure the length of the athlete's thigh from the ischial tuberosity to the joint line. Adjust the proximal carriage so that the proximal end meets the bottom of the buttocks.
3. Determine the length of the athlete's lower leg by measuring from the joint line of the knee to approximately 0.25 inch below the heel. Adjust the distal portion of the carriage accordingly.
4. Place the athlete's lower extremity in the unit. The joint line of the knee should match the articular hinge of the CPM unit.
5. Adjust the foot in the foot plate so that the tibia is placed in the neutral position. Internally or externally rotating the tibia can result in increased stress being placed on the anterior cruciate ligament.
6. Set the range of motion as prescribed by the physician. Generally the athlete is started with a low ROM and progresses to the full range of motion as healing occurs.
7. Set the SPEED of the treatment. Most acute users begin their therapy at 1 or 2 cycles per minute. The speed of movement is then increased to the athlete's tolerance.
8. Give the athlete the INTERRUPT control and provide instruction on how and when to use it.

Termination of the Treatment

1. Clean the mechanical housings with soap. The use of a 10 percent solution of household bleach and water is required if the unit becomes soiled with blood, synovial fluid, and so on.
2. Dispose of the carriage cover or wash it according to the manufacturer's instructions.

Duration and Frequency of Treatment

Continuous passive motion may be applied in long-term bouts where the athlete is continuously attached to the unit, or the device may be applied in 1-hour treatment bouts three times a day. After surgery, use is for 6 to 8 hours a day.

Precautions

- The use of continuous passive motion in conjunction with anticoagulation therapy may produce an intracompartmental hematoma.[34]

Indications

- Following surgical repair of stable intra-articular or extra-articular joint fractures
- After joint surgery, including surgery on the anterior cruciate ligament

- Following knee *arthroplasty*
- After surgery on, or chronic injuries to, the knee extensor mechanisms
- Joint contractures
- After meniscectomy
- Following knee manipulations
- Following joint debridement
- Tendon lacerations
- Following osteochondral repair

Contraindications

- Cases where the device causes an unwanted translation of opposing bones, overstressing the healing tissues

Cervical Traction

Cervical traction is a manipulative technique that elongates the cervical spine and associated structures. This force can be applied with continuous or intermittent tension. Continuous traction is used to maintain the cervical region in an elongated position and is applied with a small weight for a long time. This method of application replaces the supporting and stabilizing functions of the cervical structures and by assisting in support of the head allows the cervical musculature to "rest."

Intermittent cervical traction alternates periods of traction force with intervals of relaxation in the tension. During the traction, the cervical structures are elongated and the posterior articulating surfaces widen. The relaxation phase allows for a decrease in the amount of cervical neuromuscular activity.

Continuous cervical traction may be applied through a weight-and-pulley system, pneumatic systems, or a motorized device. Intermittent cervical traction is most commonly applied through the use of a motorized system (Fig. 5–12). Another type of spinal traction, lumbar (or pelvic) traction, is used for the treatment of lumbar spine dysfunction (Box 5–3).

BIOPHYSICAL EFFECTS

The effectiveness of cervical traction has been linked to five mechanical factors: (1) the position of the neck, (2) the force of the applied traction, (3) the duration of the traction, (4) the angle of pull, and (5) the position of the athlete.[36]

During the application of cervical traction, the neck is placed in approximately 25 degrees of flexion. This position straightens the normal *lordosis* of the cervical spine and allows the posterior articulations to open, widening the intervertebral *foramen* and stretching the posterior soft tissue. The anterior portion of an intervertebral disc is compressed and the posterior portion elon-

---

Arthroplasty: Surgical reconstruction or replacement of an articular joint.
Lordosis: The forward curvature of the cervical and lumbar spine.
Foramen: An opening (e.g., in a bone) to allow the passage of blood vessels or nerves.

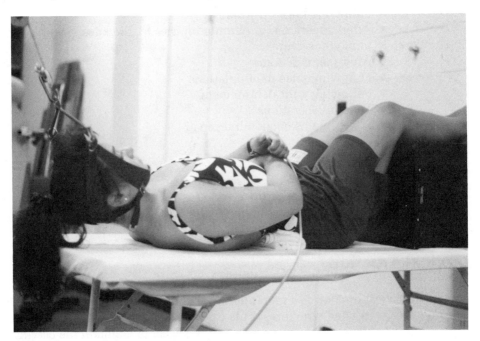

Figure 5–12. Mechanical cervical intermittent traction. Note the lumbar support and flexion of the knees.

gates when the neck is placed in flexion. When the cervical spine is placed in extension, the opposite effect occurs.

Vertebral discs consist of two distinct portions. The outer portion of the disc, the **annulus fibrosis**, is a relatively inflexible, dense substance that is rich in collagen. The middle section, the **nucleus pulposus**, is a shock-absorbing substance having a gelatinous consistency. A herniated disk refers to a condition where the nucleus pulposus protrudes through the annulus fibrosis and places pressure on the nerve root.

The amount of tension applied to the body can be expressed in terms of pounds or as a percentage of the athlete's body weight. In most pathologies, when the athlete is reclining, spinal separation begins to occur with an applied

---

| Box 5–3 | LUMBAR TRACTION |

Traction applied to the lumbar area is useful in treating many of the same conditions as cervical traction, and is especially useful in the treatment of *spondylolisthesis*. Impingement of the lumbar nerve roots can be reduced by increasing the amount of separation between the vertebra. Likewise, nerve entrapment as a result of a herniated disc is reduced by allowing the disc to return to its original shape.

This method of traction can be applied manually or through the use of a pelvic halter in a manner similar to cervical traction. An adjunct method of delivering lumbar traction uses a split table that reduces the amount of frictional forces placed on the lumbar spine.

Spondylolisthesis: Forward slippage of the lower lumbar vertebrae on the sacrum.

force equal to about 20 percent of the body weight. Specific styles of halters have been designed that allow for specificity of spinal separation. Because of this specificity, spinal separation occurs at a lower percentage of the athlete's body weight.[35]

The force applied to the cervical spine during traction has been suspected of being transmitted to the lumbar area through the dural covering of the spinal cord.[36] This can lead to residual lumbar nerve root impingement and subsequent pain.

Although cervical traction can last for treatment bouts measured in hours, the mechanical benefits appear to occur in the first few minutes of treatment.[37] Cervical traction may be applied with the athlete in one of several positions, but the two most common are the seated and supine positions. When the athlete is in a seated position, the traction must first overcome the force of gravity before therapeutic forces are placed on the cervical region. The supine position has several advantages. With the athlete lying down, the cervical musculature is allowed to relax because it is not supporting the weight of the head. Therefore, a lower amount of tension is required to obtain therapeutic effects.

EFFECT ON THE INJURY RESPONSE CYCLE

Intermittent cervical traction is incorporated into the athlete's treatment to reduce the pain and paresthesia associated with cervical nerve root impingement, muscle spasm, or articular dysfunction. This passive treatment can be combined with active exercise to enhance the benefits of the treatment.

Application of cervical traction acts to reduce the amount of pressure on nerve roots as a result of mechanical pressure from bony protuberances or intervertebral discs. Elongating the cervical spine will allow for separation of the vertebrae and result in decompression of the disc.

Muscle Spasm

Traction is often applied in an effort to interrupt the pain-spasm pain cycle through lengthening of the affected musculature. However, following treatment bouts of intermittent cervical traction, an analysis of *electromyograms* showed no decrease in the amount of spasm in the treated tissues when compared with pretreatment activity.[38,39]

The reduction of cervical muscle spasm is contingent on finding the optimal amount of traction force. Too little force will not sufficiently elongate the musculature or open the intervertebral foramen and little or no benefit will be gained. If too much force is applied, an unwanted muscle contraction will ensue as the body attempts to protect itself, resulting in the opposite effect of that desired.

Reduction of Pain

In addition to breaking the pain-spasm pain cycle as described in the previous section, several other factors have been linked to the reduction of pain. Mechanically, traction can reduce pain by decreasing the amount of mechanical pres-

---

Electromyogram: A recording of the electrical charges associated with the contraction of a muscle.

sure placed in the cervical nerve roots. The rhythmical pressure is thought to improve blood flow and to decrease myofascial adhesions. This same rhythm may also stimulate joint and muscular sensory nerves and inhibit the transmission of pain through the gate mechanism.[40]

If the pain results from a disc lesion, the bulging nucleus pulposus returns to normal position. Although a disc lesion is not normally responsive to intermittent traction, continuous traction can provide the time necessary for healing to occur.

CLINICAL APPLICATION OF CERVICAL TRACTION

Instrumentation

Mode: Allows the traction to be applied intermittently or continuously.

Hold time: Adjusts the duration of the traction phase (in seconds).

Rest time: Adjusts the duration of the relaxation phase (in seconds).

Tension: Controls the amount of tension, in pounds, applied to the halter.

Duration: Selects the total duration of the treatment.

Halter (harness): The "standard" halter applies force to the mandible and *occiput*. Modified halters have been designed that reduce the amount of force applied to the chin, allow specificity regarding the cervical level where the separation occurs, and decrease the forces placed on the temporomandibular joint (TMJ).

Spreader bar: Connects the halter to the traction device through a pulley cable.

Safety switch: Allows the athlete to interrupt the treatment and decrease tension.

Setup and Application

Preparation of the Treatment

1. Determine the athlete's weight.
2. Instruct the athlete to remove any earrings, glasses, and so on that may interfere with the placement of the halter.
3. Lay the athlete on the treatment table in the supine position.
4. Place a pillow or two under the athlete's knees.
5. Position the unit so that the force of pull runs with the midline of the athlete's body (i.e., so that the head is not laterally flexed).
6. Secure the halter to the cervical region according to the manufacturer's instructions. Normally the pressure points are the occipital processes and, to a lesser degree, the chin.
7. Connect the halter to the spreader bar.
8. Align the unit so that the angle of pull places the cervical spine in approximately 25 degrees of flexion.

Initiation of the Treatment

1. Remove any slack in the pulley cable.
2. Reset all controls to zero and turn unit ON.

Occiput: The posterior base of the skull.

3. Adjust the RATIO to the appropriate on/off sequence, normally a 3:1 or 4:1 ratio.
4. Adjust the TENSION to approximately 10 percent of the athlete's body weight. If this is the athlete's first exposure to intermittent cervical traction, or if the athlete is displaying apprehension about the treatment, the TENSION can be initiated at its lowest value.
5. Instruct the athlete what to expect during the treatment and to inform you if any discomfort is experienced. Explain that the force of the pull is felt at the occiput and not in the chin.
6. Set the appropriate treatment DURATION and initiate the treatment.
7. Allow the unit to cycle through its first tension cycle. The TENSION may be gradually increased during subsequent cycles. If pain is experienced at any time during the treatment, decrease the amount of force or discontinue the treatment.
8. Instruct the athlete to remain relaxed during both the on and off cycles.
9. If the pressure placed on the mandible causes discomfort in the teeth or temporomandibular joint, the athlete may bite down on gauze or a mouthpiece to dissipate the force.

Termination of the Treatment

1. If the traction unit does not automatically do so, gradually reduce the TENSION over a period of three or four cycles.
2. Gain some slack in the cable and turn the unit off.
3. Remove the SPREADER BAR and HALTER.
4. Question the athlete regarding any perceived benefit or complications derived from the treatment.
5. Record the pertinent information (tension, duration, duty cycle) in the athlete's file.

Duration and Frequency of Treatment

The duration of cervical traction can range into hours, but it is most commonly given for periods of 10 to 20 minutes. Cervical traction applied for a herniated disk has a duration of 5 to 10 minutes.

Precautions

- Cervical traction should never be attempted on conditions that have not been evaluated by a physician.
- The athlete must be closely monitored throughout the treatment and the treatment should be immediately discontinued if symptoms increase or if pain or paresthesia is experienced.

Indications

- Cervical or lumbar muscle spasm
- Certain degenerative disc diseases
- Herniated or protruding intervertebral disc
- Nerve root compression
- Osteoarthritis

- Capsulitis of the vertebral joints
- Pathology of the anterior or posterior longitudinal ligaments

Contraindications

- Unstable spine
- Vertebral fractures
- Extruded disc fragmentation
- Spinal cord compression
- Conditions in which vertebral flexion is contraindicated
- Conditions which worsen following traction treatments
- Osteoporosis

Biofeedback

The process of biofeedback involves "tapping into" the body's physiological processes. This activity is amplified by the biofeedback unit and converted into auditory and/or visual signals. It is important to note that biofeedback does not monitor the actual response, but rather, the conditions associated with response. For instance, when biofeedback is used to monitor muscular contractions, it is the electrical activity associated with the contraction being measured, not the actual force of the contraction. In athletic training, biofeedback is most often used as an adjunct to muscle reeducation or to encourage the relaxation of a muscle group.

Biofeedback units operate on one (or sometimes more) of four biophysical principles. **Electromyographic** (EMG) units measure the amount of electrical activity in skeletal muscle through the use of either implanted or surface-mounted electrodes. **Peripheral temperature** units measure changes in the temperature of the distal extremities, most commonly the fingers or toes. Increased temperature caused by increased blood flow indicates systemic relaxation while decreased temperature denotes stress, fear, or anxiety. The relative size of blood vessels is also the basis for **photoplethysmography**, which measures the amount of light reflected by subcutaneous tissues. The body's production of sweat is used in **galvanic skin response** biofeedback. Microcurrents are applied to the body (generally the fingers and palm) and the amount of electrical resistance is monitored. Sweaty skin contains more salt and is therefore a better conductor than dry skin.

Singularly, or in combination, these responses can be used to assist in developing the strength of muscular contractions, facilitating muscular relaxation, controlling blood pressure and heart rate, and decreasing the physical manifestation of emotional stress. It also forms the basis of lie detection tests.

Since the EMG technique of biofeedback using superficial electrodes is most prevalent in athletic training, it will be the focus of this text. Conceptually, the tasks of any biofeedback unit are:[41]

1. Monitoring the physiological process.

Osteoporosis: A porous condition resulting in softening of bone. Most commonly seen (but not exclusively) in postmenopausal women.

2. Objectively measuring the process.
3. Converting what is being monitored into feedback that optimizes the desired effects.

The electronic and physiological mechanisms associated with biofeedback will be covered in the next section. At this point a clarification must be made between "monitoring" and "measuring" the electrical activity. **Monitoring** infers the determination of whether neuromuscular activity is present and, if so, whether it is increasing or decreasing. **Measuring** the activity involves placing an objective scale on the monitored readout.

Consider the two analog meters depicted in Figure 5–13. The meter in Figure 5–13A would show that activity is taking place, and we could tell if it is increasing, decreasing, or holding steady by observing the relative position of the needle. By placing a scale on the meter in Figure 5–13B, the degree of activity, and therefore the degree of change, can be objectively measured. The scale on a biofeedback unit may use the number of microvolts as the measure, or there can be a simple 0 to 10 scale. Because of the lack of a standard biofeedback scale, measures made on a unit of one brand cannot be compared to measurements on a unit of another brand.[41] Also, placement of skin electrodes from treatment to treatment will effect the measurement's reliability.

The meter is only one form of "meaningful information" that biofeedback units can provide. Most units can convert the signals into sound waves. This is advantageous because it does not require that visual attention be focused on

(A)

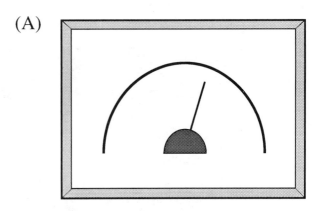

(B)

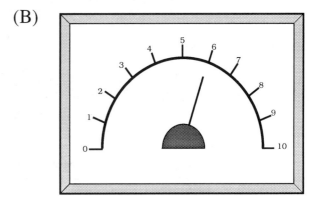

Figure 5–13. Measuring vs. monitoring of biofeedback. Meter (A) indicates if activity is occurring while meter (B) places objective measures through the use of a numeric scale.

the unit. The pitch of the sound increases and decreases based on the amount of neuromuscular activity.

BIOPHYSICAL PROCESSES AND ELECTRICAL INTEGRATION

Application of EMG biofeedback involves the use of three electrodes positioned over the muscle or muscle group that is the focus of the session (Fig. 5–14). As motor units are recruited into the contraction, the amount of electrical activity within the muscle increases. These signals are then picked up by the electrodes, amplified, and converted into visual and auditory signals.

Although this process seems rather simple, it is complicated by the presence of other electrical activity in our environment. As you will recall from Chapter 2, we are always being bombarded by electromagnetic energy. A small portion of this energy is absorbed by the body and is consequently detected by the biofeedback unit. This unwanted energy, known as "noise," must be filtered out before the meaningful activity can be used.

Referring to Figure 5–14, you will notice that the electrodes on either end are white and the one in the middle is black. This black electrode serves as a point of reference for a very small current passed between the two white "active" electrodes. This results in two sources supplying input to a **differential amplifier** within the unit. Here, the meaningful information is separated from the useless noise.

Since the extraneous noise is produced by electromagnetic sources, it occurs at a constant frequency and is detectable anywhere in the body. The differential

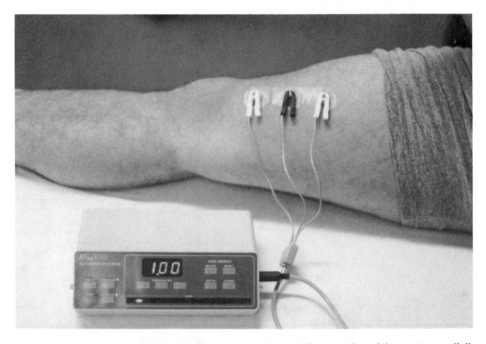

Figure 5–14. Biofeedback electrode placement over the oblique portion of the vastus medialis.
Note the two white "active" electrodes and the black "reference" electrode. (The AT 33 Biofeedback Unit, courtesy of the Autogenic Corp.)

amplifier compares the input from two sources and eliminates any activity that is common to both. In theory, the remaining activity represents neuromuscular activity. However, the integrity of the final signal is dependent on the quality of the unit and the number of filters used.

EFFECT ON THE INJURY RESPONSE CYCLE

Biofeedback itself does not affect the injury response process. Unlike other modalities presented in this text, this device assists voluntary functions to produce the desired results. Because of this, the effectiveness of biofeedback is judged on a case-by-case basis. Clearly, however, proper use of this unit does facilitate muscle re-education or promote relaxation and increase range of motion. In turn, these effects can lead to a reduction in pain.

Neuromuscular Effects

Biofeedback is most often incorporated into the athlete's treatment and rehabilitation program following surgery or long-term immobilization. After surgical intervention, edema, pain, and decreased input from joint receptors make voluntary muscle contraction difficult, if not impossible. The use of biofeedback shapes the response that enables the central nervous system to re-establish sensory-motor loops "forgotten" by the athlete.[42,43] Upon reaching the brain, afferent stimuli, in this case sound or visual cues, stimulate cerebral areas that normally receive proprioceptive information. These artificial signals, combined with the visual cue of actually watching the muscle contract, assist in opening a neural loop that sends efferent signals to the appropriate muscle(s).

Biofeedback is used to augment the input lost from these receptors, by providing other types of information. The normal proprioceptive, and perhaps kinesthetic, input is amplified through the use of sound, light, or meters. This concept not only applies to restoring the function of an injured body part, but it is also applicable to increasing the strength of healthy muscle.[44]

The cognitive process of neuromuscular relaxation is similar to that of evoking muscle contractions. However, rather than attempting to re-establish neural loops, these pathways are inhibited. The goal of relaxation therapy is to decrease the number of motor impulses being relayed to the spasming muscle. This technique is best used with cases of subconscious *muscle guarding*.

The use of relaxation biofeedback does not significantly increase flexibility in healthy individuals when compared with standard flexibility exercises. However, athletes combining flexibility with biofeedback displayed a greater retention of improvement than those training without the aid of biofeedback.[45]

It is best to try regaining deficits first through voluntary contractions. If this method is ineffective, biofeedback is then introduced. Dramatic results can be seen following a single treatment bout.

Pain Reduction

The primary benefit in the reduction of pain stems from restoring normal function of the body part. Re-educating muscle removes the unwanted stress

---

Muscle Guarding: A voluntary or subconscious contraction of a muscle to protect an injured area.

associated with abnormal biomechanics. Facilitating reduction of muscle spasm reduces the amount of mechanical pressure placed on nociceptors. Although its mechanism is beyond the scope of this book, biofeedback has also been successfully used in the reduction of myofascial pain, and the pain associated with migraine and tension headaches, as well as in general stress reduction.

CLINICAL APPLICATION OF BIOFEEDBACK

Instrumentation

Biofeedback units range from the very simple to the ultracomplex. These may be found in clinical models or portable, "take-home" units.

Sensitivity range: Provides coarse adjustments on the threshold necessary to acquire feedback.

Tuner: Allows for fine adjustments on the threshold required to obtain feedback.

Output: Determines the type of feedback available to the athlete. Visual feedback appears by way of a meter or bar graph. The audio output is normally adjustable between various frequencies. Advanced units allow for a computer interface that stores the athlete's results.

Statistics: Better biofeedback units will calculate statistics of the athlete's muscular activity for assessing the athlete's rehabilitation progress. Measures such as the mean, maximum, and standard deviation provide quantitative information for evaluating the athlete's progression.

Setup and Application

Preparation of the Athlete

1. Remove any dirt, oil, or makeup in the area where the electrodes are to be applied, by wiping the skin with alcohol. These substances will impede the conduction of the bioelectric signals.
2. Very sensitive biofeedback units may require that the electrode site be mildly abraided with an emery cloth.
3. Apply a suitable conductive gel to the electrodes.
4. Secure the electrodes over the belly of the muscle targeted in this therapy. Note that the active electrodes must be applied over the target muscle. The reference electrode may be secured anywhere on the body, but by convention it is normally placed between the two active electrodes (see Fig. 5–14).
5. Plug the common electrode lead(s) into the INPUT jack(s) on the unit.
6. Turn the unit ON.
7. Adjust the OUTPUT to the desired mode of feedback (visual, audio, or both).

Facilitation of Isometric Muscle Contractions

1. Instruct the athlete to relax the body part as much as possible.
2. Adjust the SENSITIVITY RANGE to the lowest value that does not provide feedback.
3. Place the body part in the desired position.

4. Instruct the athlete to maximally contract the muscle and keep the meter (be it visual or audio) peaked.
5. Hold the isometric contraction for 6 seconds.
6. Complete relaxation should be obtained prior to the next contraction. Instruct the athlete to completely relax the muscle so that the meter resets to the baseline.
7. Have the athlete repeat the contractions as indicated. If the muscle group is severely atrophied, the number of contractions is normally limited to 10 to 15 contractions because of fatigue.
8. By decreasing the sensitivity, the athlete will have to elicit a stronger contraction to receive feedback.
9. If the athlete is unable to evoke a contraction, two strategies can be implemented: (1) have the athlete contract the muscle on the opposite limb, then attempt to contract the involved muscle, or (2) apply the biofeedback unit to the opposite limb so that the athlete will "learn" the biofeedback technique. Other strategies include:
   ○ Have the athlete watch and/or touch the contracting muscle.
   ○ Contracting surrounding or opposing muscles.
   ○ Contract the proximal portion of the muscle to facilitate neuromuscular activity in the distal motor units.

Termination of the Procedure

1. Remove the electrodes and wipe away any excess gel.
2. To avoid dependency on biofeedback, it is recommended that the athlete perform additional sets of contractions without the aid of the unit to "remember" how to perform the contraction.

Duration and Frequency of the Treatment

Biofeedback can be performed daily as needed by the athlete either in the athletic training room or at home. Be aware of any muscle soreness that may occur after exercise and adjust the treatment protocol accordingly.

Precautions

- Do not exceed the prescribed range of motion.
- Avoid undue muscle tension that may affect grafts, and so on.

Indications

- To facilitate muscular contractions
- To regain neuromuscular control
- To decrease muscle spasm
- To promote systemic relaxation

Contraindications

- Conditions where muscular contractions would insult the tissues

Massage

Massage, the systematic manipulation of the body's tissues, is one of the oldest healing techniques still used in modern medicine. Dating back at least to the ancient Olympics, massage has been present in most cultures. Regional variations have all contributed to the different forms of massage used today and it is this diverse background that leads to inconsistencies in application protocols.

Because it is a time-consuming task, and it requires the full attention of the athletic trainer, the popularity of massage as a therapeutic technique has faded. Still, massage is a very effective treatment method for promoting local and systemic relaxation or invigoration, increasing local blood flow, and encouraging venous return.

Since massage is a skill-based technique, and since the possibility of abuse is high, many states provide for licensure of massage therapists. Most other healing professions, such as physical therapy and athletic training, incorporate massage techniques into their schooling.

MASSAGE STROKES

There are several different types of massage strokes, and each may be varied by adding more or less pressure, using different parts of the hand, or changing the direction of the stroke. These elements may then be sequenced to produce different effects. The following sections describe the basic elements of each stroke and discuss how they can be varied.

Effleurage

Effleurage, the stroking of the skin, is performed with the palm of the hand to stimulate deep tissues, or with the finger tips to stimulate sensory nerves (Fig. 5–15). This stroke is categorized as being either superficial or deep. Superficial stroking may either follow the contour of the body itself or it may relate to the direction of the underlying muscles. Deep stroking should follow the course of veins and lymph vessels to force fluids in these vessels back towards the heart.

The strokes may be performed slowly to promote relaxation or rapidly to encourage blood flow and stimulate the tissues. In either case, the strokes are done in a rhythmic manner. Ideally, at least one hand should be in contact with the skin at any given point in time. This may be achieved by stroking the skin in one direction and lightly gliding the hands back to the starting point. Another method involves staggering the strokes. The stroke of one hand begins just before the other hand leaves the surface of the skin.

Light effleurage is generally done at both the beginning and end of the massage. During the initial stages of the treatment, effleurage relaxes the athlete and serves to indicate the areas that will be massaged. At the conclusion of the treatment, this stroke serves to "calm down" any nerves that may have become irritated during the massage.

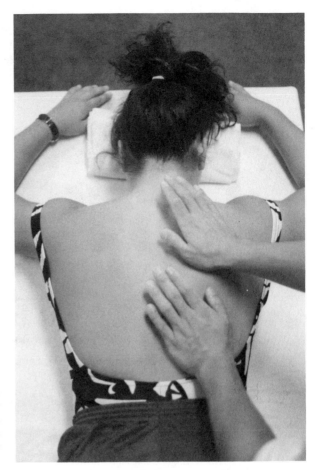

Figure 5–15. Effleurage (stroking) of the spinal erector group. The deep pressure is applied with the palm of the hands and runs the length of the muscle group.

Petrissage

This method of massage involves the lifting and kneading of the skin, subcutaneous tissue, and muscle with the fingers or hand (Fig. 5–16). The skin is gently lifted between the thumb and fingers or the fingers and palm and gently rolled and kneaded in the hand. For this reason, petrissage is often performed without the use of a lubricant. This process stretches and separates muscle fiber, fascia, and scar tissue.

Friction

The goal of friction massage is to mobilize muscle and separate adhesions in muscle, tendon fibers, or scar tissue that restrict movement and cause pain.[46] There are two basic types of friction massage: circular and transverse. Circular friction massage is applied with the thumbs working in circular motion. In transverse friction massage, the thumbs stroke the tissue from opposite directions. When treating a large muscle mass, the elbow can be used in place of the thumb (Fig. 5–17). In each case, sufficient force is applied so that the pressure will reach deep into the tissues. Begin lightly and gradually progress to firmer, deeper strokes. To achieve the optimal effects of friction massage, the muscle should be placed in a relaxed position.

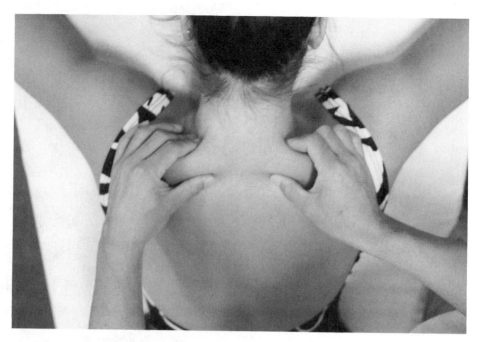

Figure 5–16. Petrissage (kneading) of the trapezius muscle groups. The skin and underlying tissue is lifted and rolled in the hand.

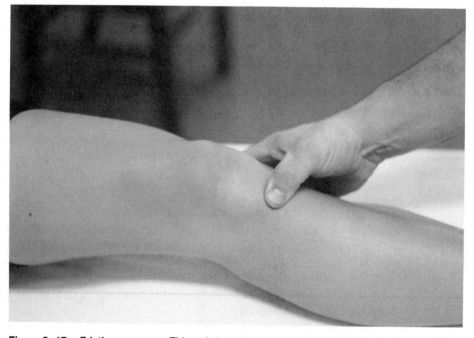

Figure 5–17. Friction massage. This technique is used to isolate deep tissue, such as scar tissue.

This method of massage is to be avoided in conditions where the underlying tissues would be further injured by the pressure, such as acute injuries. Friction massage differs from the other massage strokes in that this is not necessarily pleasing to the athlete. Indeed, many times friction massage is painful, especially when trigger points are the target of the treatment. Friction massage can be followed by a stretching routine to further facilitate the range of motion.

Tapotement

Tapotement involves the gentle tapping or pounding of the skin. The most common form of tapotement uses the ulnar side of the wrist to contact the skin, in a manner similar to a "karate chop" (Fig. 5–18). This stroke is performed with the wrist and fingers limp so that the hand more or less "slaps" the skin. In an alternate form of tapotement, a cupped hand is used.

A tapotement variation that promotes relaxation and desensitization of irritated nerve endings is found in the form of "raindrops." The fingers lightly touch the skin in an alternating manner, as if you were typing on a keyboard.

Vibration

This method involves the rapid shaking of the tissue. Although a skilled masseuse is quite capable of achieving therapeutic effects manually, a mechanical vibrator is oftentimes used by less-skilled individuals.

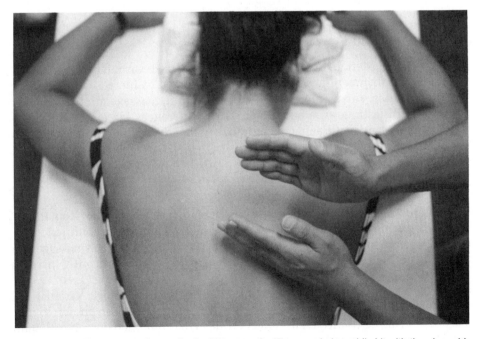

Figure 5–18. Tapotement (pounding) of the muscle. The muscle is rapidly hit with the ulnar side of the hand.

MASSAGE MEDIA

Most massages will incorporate some type of medium to decrease the friction between the athlete's skin and the hand; however, massage can be given without any medium being used. Lubricants, including massage lotion, peanut oil, powder, and even counterirritants, allow the hands to glide smoothly over the skin and focus the effects on the underlying muscle. If the massage is being given over hairy areas, lubricants are needed to keep from pulling the hair.

Massage may be given without the use of a lubricant. In strokes such as petrissage, lubricants can interfere with the lifting and kneading of the skin. Additionally, friction assists in mobilizing the skin over the underlying tissues, making the use of lubricants contraindicated with this style of massage.

EFFECT ON THE INJURY RESPONSE CYCLE

Massage has been said to evoke a number of responses within the body. Many of these reputed effects, such as the mobilization of adipose tissue and increased muscle tone, have never been substantiated. This section will attempt to separate fact from fiction.

In general, the same massage stroke can produce various responses, depending on the amount of pressure applied and the speed of the stroke. Light, slow stroking of the skin results in systemic relaxation of the athlete. Fast, deep strokes cause an increase in blood flow to the area, and the athlete tends to feel invigorated.

It is difficult to differentiate between the physiological and the psychological effects of massage. Athletes who *think* that massage will improve their performance or assist in the healing process, often will see improvement simply through the power of suggestion.

Changes in Blood Flow

Deep, friction, or vigorous massage can evoke vascular changes similar to those of inflammation. The treated area is marked by increased blood flow, histamine release, and an increased temperature. But, massage prior to submaximal treadmill testing revealed no significant differences in cardiac output, blood pressure, and lactic acid concentration compared with a group receiving no massage prior to testing.[47]

Neuromuscular Changes

Petrissage has been shown to decrease neuromuscular excitability, but only during the duration of the massage, and the effects are confined to the muscle(s) being massaged.[48,49,50] A study examining the effects of massage prior to competition concluded that this technique does not significantly increase the stride frequency of sprinters.[51]

A massage routine, consisting of deep effleurage, circular friction, and transverse friction applied to the hamstrings has been shown to increase hamstring flexibility.[52] This effect is due to the combined decrease in neuromuscular excitability (relaxation) and stretching of muscle and scar tissue.

Massage is less effective in decreasing muscular recovery time following exercise.[53,54] Massaging muscles between exercise bouts, be it a sprinter's legs between races or a pitcher's shoulder between innings, does little to reduce muscular fatigue.

Reduction of Edema

When performed properly, massage can increase venous and lymphatic flow that assists in the removal edema.[55] Manual or mechanical massage (see Intermittent Compression Pump) forces fluids within the vessels to move towards the heart.

The key to reducing edema is to first mobilize the proximal area of edema before attempting to move the distal areas (Fig. 5–19). This procedure, known as "uncorking the bottle," can be visualized as removing a traffic jam. Cars at the back of the pack cannot move forward until the car at the front of the line moves.

The step-by-step application of this method of massage is presented in the section on setup and application in this unit.

Pain Control

Pain reduction through the application of massage is no doubt the result of several different mechanisms. Mechanical pain is reduced through interrupting muscle spasm and reducing edema. Chemical pain is diminished by increasing blood flow and encouraging the removal of cellular wastes. However, simply touching the athlete can also reduce the pain by activating cutaneous receptors.

Gentle massage activates sensory nerves and therefore inhibits pain through

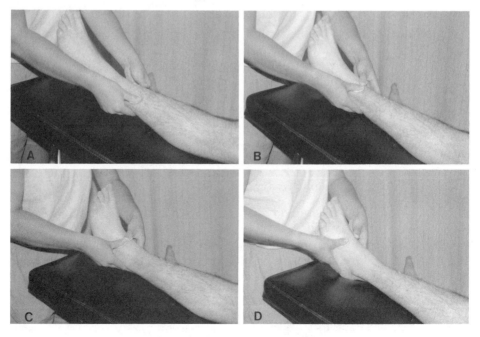

Figure 5–19. Massage for edema reduction. "Uncorking the bottle" involves mobilizing the proximal edema and progressively working distally.

the gate mechanism. Massage has also been shown to activate the autonomic nervous system and *Pacinian receptors*, both of which assist in hindering nociceptive impulses.[55] However, massage has not been shown to significantly affect serum levels of endogenous opiates such as β-endorphin when compared to a control group.[56]

CLINICAL APPLICATION OF MASSAGE

Setup and Application

General Considerations

1. The position of the athlete relative to the athletic trainer is important to both parties. The athletic trainer should stand in a place that requires little or no repositioning. Likewise, long strokes, such as those applied to the back or hamstrings should be performed through little steps, rather than bending of the back. The athlete should be positioned so that the muscles being massaged are in a relaxed position. If an extremity is being massaged to reduce edema, it should be elevated.
2. If a massage medium is being used, warm it slightly so that it is not uncomfortable when it is applied (i.e., not too hot or too cold).
3. The athlete must be draped so that modesty is assured.

"Classical Massage"

1. The area may be preheated with moist heat to promote relaxation of the musculature.
2. A pillow may be placed under the ankles and a small pad, such as a folded towel, placed under the abdomen to assist in the relaxation of the lumbar musculature.
3. If applicable, apply the massage medium on the body part(s) to be treated.
4. Follow the application of the medium with a light, slow effleurage.
5. Gradually build up to deeper effleurage.
6. Begin petrissage strokes.
7. Where, and if, applicable, apply deep friction massage.
8. Apply tapotement to the back and extremities (if treated).
9. Reapply petrissage and deep effleurage.
10. End the treatment with light effleurage.

Massage for Edema Reduction

1. Elevate the body part to be treated using an incline board, pillow, or other device.
2. Cover the entire surface to be treated with a lubricating massage lotion.
3. Position yourself distal to the limb. For example, if the ankle is being massaged, stand so that you see the bottom of the athlete's foot.

Pacinian Receptors: Receptors located deep in the skin which relay information regarding pressure and vibration. Within the joints, they assist in relaying proprioceptive information.

4. Begin by making long, slow, strokes toward the heart, starting proximal to the injured area. Every fourth or fifth stroke, move the starting point of the massage slightly distal.
5. Continue stroking longitudinally, with the starting point gradually being moved distally.
6. When the distal portion of the edematous area is reached, begin working back to the original starting point.

Termination of the Treatment

1. If a lubricant was used, remove it with a towel.

Duration and Frequency of Treatment

Massage for relaxation or invigoration may be given as needed. The duration of the massage ranges from a few minutes up to an hour. Massage for edema reduction is given once a day for an average duration of 5 to 10 minutes. Friction massage to tendons is performed once a day for 5 minutes or as needed.

Precautions

- Massage may increase the inflammatory response when used early in the acute or subacute stage of the injury response cycle.

Indications

- To increase venous return
- To break the pain-spasm pain cycle
- To evoke systemic relaxation
- To improve or stimulate local blood flow

Contraindications

- Sites where fractures have failed to heal
- Acute sprains or strains
- Skin conditions or lesions

Intermittent Compression Units

These devices use mechanical pressure to encourage venous and lymphatic drainage from the extremities. Intermittent compression units consist of a nylon appliance designed to fit the body part (e.g., foot and/or ankle, half leg, full leg) that is connected to the unit through a series of hoses (Fig. 5–20). The compression is then formed by the flow of air or cold water into the appliance.

Intermittent cold compression units are ideal for the treatment of acute injuries because they provide cold and compression while the limb is elevated (ICE). However, this device should not be used until the possibility of a fracture

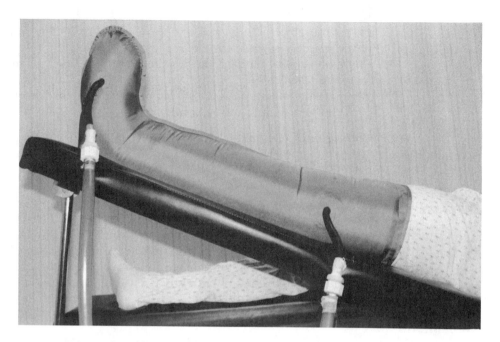

Figure 5–20. Intermittent compression applied to the lower extremity. Elevating the extremity assists in venous return. The amount of pressure applied to the extremity should not exceed the athlete's diastolic blood pressure.

or *compartment syndrome* has been ruled out by a physician. In subacute conditions, intermittent compression is used to reduce edema and remove ecchymosis from the area.

EFFECT ON THE INJURY RESPONSE CYCLE

The movement of fluids out of the extremity is caused by the formation of a number of pressure gradients. By applying external compression, the gradient between the tissue hydrostatic pressure and the capillary filtration pressure is reduced, thus encouraging the reabsorption of interstitial fluids. Since the tissues are being compressed, a second pressure gradient is formed between the distal portion of the extremity (high pressure) and the proximal portion (low pressure). This gradient forces the fluids to move from the area of high pressure to an area of lower pressure. If the extremity is elevated during this treatment, both of the aforementioned pressures are increased by gravity, speeding venous drainage.

The compression applied to the tissue is either circumferential or sequential. **Circumferential compression** simultaneously applies an equal amount of pressure to all parts of the extremity. This pressure builds up to a level determined by the operator and holds the pressure at this level for a preset time. The pressure then drops and the process repeats. Through this cycle, fluids are forced up the venous and lymphatic return systems. **Sequential compression** increases the distal to proximal gradient through the sequential filling of pres-

---

Compartment Syndrome: A condition where nerves, blood vessels, or tendons are constricted within a confined space (e.g., the anterior compartment of the lower leg).

sure chambers within the appliance. The most distal compartment will inflate, followed by the next compartment, and so on, until pressure is applied to the length of the appliance (Fig. 5–21). This method massages the fluids through the venous and lymphatic systems.

Both circumferential and sequential compression units have been shown to significantly reduce the amount of edema in an injured body part. During the treatment of lower leg edema, low pressure (35 to 55 mm Hg) increases the venous flow velocity 175 percent. When this pressure is increased to the range of 90 to 100 mm Hg, the venous flow accelerated to 336 percent of resting values.[58] By removing extracellular debris, the fresh blood flow to the area has been shown to significantly increase following the treatment.[59]

CLINICAL APPLICATION OF INTERMITTENT COMPRESSION

Instrumentation

Power: Turns the unit on or off.

Temperature: With cold compression units, this regulates the temperature of the fluid flowing through a refrigeration device to the appliance. Some portable cold compression units use ice cubes for this purpose. The temperature of the fluid is displayed in the TEMPERATURE GAUGE.

Pressure: Adjusts the amount of compression in millimeters of mercury (mm Hg) applied to the extremity. This value must not exceed the athlete's *diastolic blood pressure.*

On/off time: Controls the proportion of the time that the compression is on and off. This control may be a single switch with selectable duty cycles, or the ON and OFF times may be adjusted individually.

Pump: Turns on the pressure to the appliance.

Drain: Removes the pressure and deflates the appliance.

Setup and Application

Preparation for the Treatment

1. Determine the athlete's diastolic blood pressure.
2. Cover the area to be treated with Stockinette or similar material.
3. Select the appropriate size of appliance for the extremity being treated.
4. Insert the injured limb into the appliance.
5. For best results, elevate the limb. (On some fluid-filled units, it is easier to allow the appliance to initially fill and then elevate the body part.)
6. Connect the appliance to the compression unit. Note that these units have an input and exhaust tubes. The hoses must be properly connected to the appliance and the unit.

Initiation of the Treatment

1. If the intermittent compression unit uses a cold fluid, select the TEMPERATURE to be used, generally between 50 and 55°F.
2. Select the maximal PRESSURE for the treatment. *This pressure must*

Diastolic Blood Pressure: The lowest level of pressure in the arteries. For example, when a blood pressure reading is given as 120/80, 80 represents the diastolic value.

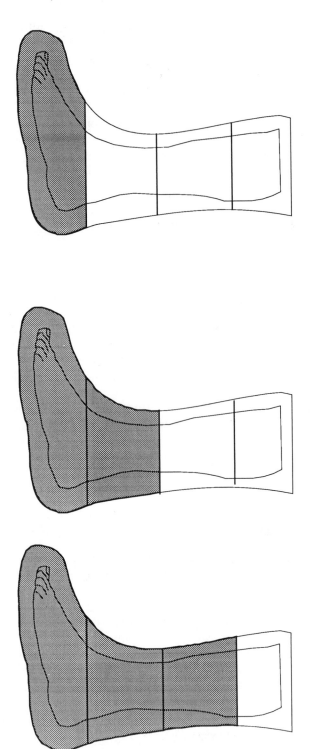

Figure 5-21. Sequential compression. Compartments within the appliance fill distal to proximal.

not exceed the athlete's diastolic blood pressure. Normal pressure ranges are 40 to 60 mm Hg for the upper extremity and 60 to 100 mm Hg for the lower extremity.

3. Select the ON and OFF times. Normally a 3:1 duty cycle (e.g., 45 seconds on, 15 seconds off) is used.
4. Select the appropriate treatment TIME.
5. Inform the athlete about the sensations to be expected during the treatment. Instruct the athlete to contact you if any unusual sensations, such as pain or a "tingling" feeling, are experienced during the treatment.
6. Encourage the athlete to perform gentle range of motion exercises during the off cycle, if appropriate.

Termination of the Treatment

1. Reduce ON time or select the DRAIN mode to remove the air or fluid from the appliance.
2. Gently remove the body part from the appliance.
3. If applicable, apply an open basket weave and cover with an elastic wrap.

Duration and Frequency of Treatment

Intermittent compression can be applied once or twice a day for 20 minutes to several hours. If the unit uses cold fluid, the temperature is increased as the treatment duration increases.

Indications

- Posttraumatic edema
- Postsurgical edema
- Primary and secondary lymphedema

Contraindications

- In acute conditions where the possibility of a fracture has not been eliminated.
- Conditions where the pressure would further damage the structures (e.g., compartment syndromes).
- Peripheral vascular disease

Summary

The modalities presented in this chapter transcend many different categories. Ultrasound can produce both thermal and nonthermal changes within the tissues. Because of this, pulsed ultrasound—producing nonthermal effects—can be used in acute conditions while continuous ultrasound is reserved for conditions that are more chronic.

Continuous passive motion, cervical traction, and biofeedback fill a gap

---

Lymphedema: Swelling of the lymph nodes due to blockage of the vessels.

between therapeutic modalities and therapeutic exercise. By applying mechanical forces to the body, positive stresses are introduced, serving to deter unwanted effects of the injury response process.

Massage and intermittent compression utilize mechanical pressure to elicit involuntary responses from the body. Massage is capable of producing local and systemic relaxation or invigoration and is also useful in reducing edema. However, massage also includes a psychological component. Intermittent compression assists in reducing the amount of edema in a limb and thus restoring circulation. When combined with a cold fluid, this modality is useful in the immediate treatment of an injury by providing rest, ice, compression, and elevation simultaneously.

Like most modalities presented in this text, mechanical modalities should be an adjunct to the athlete's rehabilitation progression. In Chapter 6, we will see how these modalities are incorporated into the athlete's rehabilitation scheme.

CHAPTER QUIZ

• •

1. When applying ultrasound with a metered output of 4.0 watts and an indicated beam nonfunctionality ratio (BNR) of 4.0, the highest intensity in the beam is:
   A. 4.0 watts
   B. 8.0 watts
   C. 16 watts
   D. 32 watts.

2. Which of the following is not a contraindication of ultrasound:
   A. Scar tissue
   B. Infection
   C. Warts
   D. Trigger points.

3. The spreading of an ultrasound beam is due to:
   A. Attenuation
   B. Collimation
   C. Thermal synthesis
   D. Divergence.

4. A metered reading of 2 watts per square centimeter passing through a sound head having an effective radiating area of 10 square centimeters produces an output of _____ total watts.
   A. 5 watts
   B. 10 watts
   C. 15 watts
   D. 20 watts

5. Reflection of ultrasonic energy occurs least between:
   A. Water and soft tissue
   B. Soft tissue and fat
   C. Soft tissue and bone
   D. Soft tissue and air.

6. All of the following are nonthermal (mechanical) effects of ultrasound except:
   A. Increased extensibility of collagen-rich structures
   B. Increased blood flow
   C. Synthesis of protein
   D. Increased cell membrane permeability.

7. All of the following effects have been attributed to continuous passive motion except:
   A. Increased nutrition to the meniscus
   B. Increased nutrition of the articular cartilage
   C. Increased tensile strength of tendons and allografts
   D. Increased nutrition to the anterior cruciate.

8. Intermittent cervical traction can be useful in relieving the pain associated with intervertebral disc herniations. This reduction of pain occurs by reducing the bulge of the _____ through the _____.
   A. Fiberous pulposus/nucleus pulposus
   B. Annulus fibrosis/nucleus pulposus

    C. Nucleus pulposus/annulus fibrosis

    D. Nucleus pulposus/fibrous pulposus

9. When applying intermittent compression to an extremity, the pressure in the appliance should not exceed:

    A. The athlete's diastolic blood pressure

    B. The athlete's systolic blood pressure

    C. The difference between the athlete's diastolic and systolic blood pressure

    D. The athlete's resting heart rate.

10. Electromyographic biofeedback measures:

    A. The amount of tension produced by a muscle group

    B. The amount of electrical activity with a muscle

    C. The amount of myelin activity within a muscle

    D. All of the above.

11. The effectiveness of cervical traction is dependent upon many factors including the amount of tractive force applied. Other factors include:

    A.

    B.

    C.

    D.

12. List two reasons why separation of the vertebral column occurs at a lower percentage of the athlete's body weight in the reclining position than in the sitting position.

    A.

    B.

13. Match the following massage strokes to method of delivery:

    A. Petrissage   ____ Pounding of the skin

    B. Tapotement   ____ Kneading of the skin

    C. Effleurage   ____ Stroking of the skin

14. When applying massage to remove edema from a limb, the strokes begin _____ and are progressively worked _____.

REFERENCES

1. Ziskin, MC, McDiarmid, T, and Michlovitz, SL: Therapeutic ultrasound. In Michlovitz, S (ed): Thermal Agents in Rehabilitation, ed 2. FA Davis, Philadelphia, 1990, pp 134–169.
2. ter Haar, G: Basic physics of therapeutic ultrasound. Physiotherapy 73:110, 1987.
3. Ferguson, BH: A Practitioner's Guide to the Ultrasonic Therapy Equipment Standard. U.S. Department of Health and Human Services, Public Health Service, Food and Drug Administration, Rockville, MD, 1985.
4. Dyson, M: Mechanisms involved in therapeutic ultrasound. Physiotherapy 73:116, 1987.
5. Kitchen, SS and Partridge, CJ: A review of therapeutic ultrasound. Part 1: Background, physiological effects and hazards. Physiotherapy 76:593, 1990.
6. Williams, R: Production and transmission of ultrasound. Physiotherapy 73:113, 1987.
7. Weinberger, A and Lev, A: Temperature elevation of connective tissue by physical modalities. Critical Reviews in Physical and Rehabilitation Medicine 3:121, 1991.
8. Baker, RJ and Bell, GW: The effect of therapeutic modalities on blood flow in the human calf. JOSPT 13:23, 1991.
9. Kitchen, SS and Partridge, CJ: A review of

therapeutic ultrasound. Part 2: The efficacy of ultrasound. Physiotherapy 76:595, 1990.

10. Young, SR and Dyson, M: Macrophage responsiveness to therapeutic ultrasound. Ultrasound Med Biol 16:809, 1990.

11. Jackson, BA, Schwane, JA, and Starcher, BC: Effect of ultrasound therapy on the repair of achilles tendon injuries in rats. Med Sci Sports Exerc 23:171, 1991.

12. Enwemeka, CS: The effect of therapeutic ultrasound on tendon healing: A biomechanical study. Am J Phys Med Rehabil 68:283, 1989.

13. Downing, DS and Weinstein, A: Ultrasound therapy of subacromial bursitis. A double blind trial. Phys Ther 66:194, 1986.

14. Davick, JP, Martin, RK, and Albright, JP: Distribution and deposition of tritiated cortisol using phonophoresis. Phys Ther 68:1672, 1988.

15. Henley, EJ: Transcutaneous drug delivery: Iontophoresis, phonophoresis. Physical and Rehabilitation Medicine 2:139, 1991.

16. Quillen, WS: Phonophoresis: A review of the literature and technique. Athletic Training 15:109, 1980.

17. Ciccone, CD, Leggin, BG, and Callamaro, JJ: Effects of ultrasound and trolamine salicylate phonophoresis on delayed-onset muscle soreness. Phys Ther 71:666, 1991.

18. Oziomek, RS, et al: Effect of phonophoresis on serum salicylate levels. Med Sci Sports Exerc 23:397, 1991.

19. Cameron, MH and Monroe, LG: Relative transmission of ultrasound by media customarily used for phonophoresis. Phys Ther 72:142, 1992.

20. Bensen, HAE, McElnay, JC, and Harland, R: Use of ultrasound to enhance percutaneous absorption of benzydamine. Phys Ther 69:113, 1989.

21. McDiarmind, T and Burns, PN: Clinical application of therapeutic ultrasound. Physiotherapy 73:155, 1987.

22. Salter, RB: The biologic concept of continuous passive motion of synovial joints. The first 18 years of basic research. Clin Orthop May:12, 1989.

23. McCarthy, MR, et al: The clinical use of continuous passive motion in physical therapy. JOSPT 15:132, 1992.

24. O'Donoghue, PC, et al: Clinical use of continuous passive motion in athletic training. Athletic Training 26:200, 1991.

25. Diehm, SL: The power of CPM: Healing through motion. Patient Care 8:34, 1989.

26. Namba, RS, et al: Continuous passive motion versus immobilization. The effect on post-traumatic joint stiffness. Clin Orthop Jun:218, 1991.

27. Gershuni, DH, Hargens, AR, and Danzig, LA: Regional nutrition and cellularity of the meniscus. Implications for tear and repair. Sports Med 5:322, 1988.

28. Kim, HKL, Moran, ME, and Salter, RB: The potential for regeneration of articular cartilage in defects created by chondral shaving and subchondral abrasion. An experimental investigation in rabbits. J Bone Joint Surg (am), 73:1301, 1991.

29. Skyhar, MJ, et al: Nutrition of the anterior cruciate ligament. Effects of continuous passive motion. Am J Sports Med 13:415, 1985.

30. Giudice, ML: Effects of continuous passive motion and elevation on hand edema. Am J Occup Ther 44:914, 1990.

31. Mullaji, AB and Shahane, MN: Continuous passive motion for prevention and rehabilitation of knee stiffness: A clinical evaluation. J Postgrad Med 35:204, 1989.

32. Drez, D, et al: In vivo measurement of anterior tibial translation using continuous passive motion devices. Am J Sports Med 19:381, 1991.

33. Takai, S, et al: The effects of frequency and duration of controlled passive mobilization on tendon healing. J Orthop Res 9:705, 1991.

34. Graham, G and Loomer, RL: Anterior compartment syndrome in a patient with fracture of the tibial plateau treated by continuous passive motion and anticoagulants. Report of a case. Clin Orthop May:197, 1985.

35. Walker, GL: Goodley polyaxial cervical traction. A new approach to a traditional treatment. Phys Ther 66:1255, 1986.

36. LaBan, MM, Macy, JA, and Meerschaert, JR: Intermittent cervical traction: A progenitor of lumbar radicular pain. Arch Phys Med Rehabil 73:295, 1992.

37. Harris, PR: Cervical traction: Review of literature and treatment guidelines. Phys Ther 57:910, 1977.

38. Jette, DU, Falkel, JE, and Trombly, C: Effect of intermittent, supine cervical traction on the myoelectric activity of the upper trapezius muscle in subjects with neck pain. Phys Ther 65:1173, 1985.

39. Murphy, MJ: Effects of cervical traction on muscle activity. JOSPT 13:220, 1991.

40. DeLacerda, FG: Effect of angle of traction pull on upper trapezius muscle activity. JOSPT 1:205, 1980.

41. Peek, CJ: A primer of biofeedback instrumentation. In Schwartz, MS (ed): Biofeedback: A Practitioner's Guide. Guilford Press, New York, 1987.

42. Draper, V: Electromyographic biofeedback and recovery of quadriceps femoris muscle

function following anterior cruciate ligament reconstruction. Phys Ther 70:25, 1990.

43. Wolf, SL: Neurophysiological factors in electromyographic feedback for neuromotor disturbances. In Basmajian, JV (ed): Biofeedback: Principles and Practice for Clinicians. Williams & Wilkins, Baltimore, 1983.

44. Croce, RV: The effects of EMG biofeedback on strength acquisition. Biofeedback Self Regul 11:299, 1986.

45. Cummings, MS, Wilson, VE, and Bird, EI: Flexibility development in sprinters using EMG biofeedback and relaxation training. Biofeedback Self Regul 9:395, 1984.

46. Cyriax, JH: Clinical applications of massage. In Rogoff, JB (ed): Manipulation, Traction, and Massage, ed 2. Williams & Wilkins, Baltimore, 1980.

47. Boone, T, Cooper, R, and Thompson, WR: A physiologic evaluation of the sports massage. Athletic Training 26:51, 1991.

48. Morelli, M, Seaborne, DE, and Sullivan, J: Changes in H-reflex amplitude during massage of triceps surae in healthy subjects. JOSPT 12:55, 1990.

49. Sullivan, SJ, et al: Effects of massage on alpha motoneuron excitability. Phys Ther 71:555, 1991.

50. Morelli, M, Seaborne, DE, and Sullivan, SJ: H-reflex modulation during manual muscle massage of human triceps surae. Arch Phys Med Rehabil 72:915, 1991.

51. Harmer, PA: The effect of pre-performance massage on stride frequency in sprinters. Athletic Training 26:55, 1991.

52. Crosman, LJ, Chateauvert, SR, and Wesiberg, J: The effects of massage to the hamstring muscle group on range of motion. JOSPT 6:168, 1984.

53. Cafarelli, E, et al: Vibratory massage and short-term recovery from muscular fatigue. Int J Sports Med 11:474, 1990.

54. Crosman, LJ, Chateauvert, SR, and Wesiberg, J: The effects of massage to the hamstring muscle group on range of motion. JOSPT 6:168, 1984.

55. Naliboff, BD and Tachiki, KH: Autonomic and skeletal muscle response to nonelectrical cutaneous stimulation. Percept Mot Skills 72:575, 1991.

56. Day, JA, Mason, RR, and Chesrown, SE: Effect of massage on serum level of β-endorphin and β-lipotropin in healthy adults. Phys Ther 67:926, 1987.

57. Muhe, E: Intermittent sequential high-pressure compression of the leg. A new method of preventing deep vein thrombosis. Am J Surg 147:781, 1984.

58. Muhe, E: Intermittent sequential high-pressure compression of the leg. A new method of preventing deep vein thrombosis. Am J Surg 147:781, 1984.

59. Olavi, A, Kolari, PJ, and Esa, A: Edema and lower leg perfusion in patients with post-traumatic dysfunction. Acupunct Electrother Res 16:7, 1991.

60. Bischko, JJ: Use of the laser beam in acupuncture. Acupunct Electrother Res 5:29, 1980.

61. Kitchen, SS and Partridge, CJ: A review of low level laser therapy. Part I: Background, physiological effects and hazards. Physiotherapy 77:161, 1991.

62. Greathouse, DG, Currier, DP, and Gilmore, RL: Effects of clinical infrared laser on superficial radial nerve conduction. Phys Ther 65:1184, 1985.

63. King, CE, et al: Effect of helium-neon laser auriculotherapy on experimental pain threshold. Phys Ther 70:24, 1990.

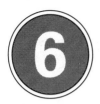

The Problem-Solving Approach

JEFF RYAN, PT, ATC

This chapter relates the use of therapeutic modalities to their proper and timely application during the treatment and rehabilitation program. Using the problem-solving approach, the student is presented with a series of case studies that reinforce the decision-making process.

The problem-solving approach (PSA) is a specific rehabilitation strategy used in planning the treatment and rehabilitation program. This method allows for successful treatment of an injury by utilizing the athletic trainer's knowledge of basic sciences, pathomechanics, and the principles underlying therapeutic exercise and modalities. The PSA is the antithesis of the "cookbook" approach, where all injuries of the same type are treated in the same way by following specific guidelines (e.g., all inversion ankle sprains following the same protocol). Using the PSA allows for the entry-level, as well as the highly experienced, athletic trainer to treat any athletic injury in a safe and timely manner. This allows for an orderly transition through the rehabilitation process to the return to full activity.

The first part of this chapter will take the athletic trainer through the PSA, focusing on its individual components. The chapter will end with examples of applying the PSA to selected athletic injuries using many of the therapeutic modalities discussed in this text. Therapeutic exercise will be mentioned whenever necessary for complete understanding, but it will not be the focus of the problems addressed.

The PSA is composed of four components: (1) recognition of problems, (2) prioritization of problems, (3) goal setting (short-term and long-term goals), and (4) treatment planning. Utilization of this approach allows the athletic trainer to successfully address all aspects of an athlete's injury. The problem-solving approach guides the treatment of the injured athlete based on the known physiological effects of the modalities and exercises on the problem(s) encountered from the injury.

Recognition of Problems

The successful treatment of any injured athlete begins with a thorough evaluation to determine the problems that must be addressed. The evaluation needs to be complete and properly performed so that all conditions keeping the athlete from returning to successful activity are identified.

The problems should be identified in an objective and measurable manner whenever possible. Objectivity makes it possible to determine the extent of the problem and provides baseline data used in gauging the success of the treatment plan. With re-evaluation of the athlete, current data is compared with baseline data to determine whether improvement has occurred or if changes in the treatment plan are needed due to lack of improvement.

Table 6–1 lists common evaluative tools used in the determination of these problems. The table presents the problems being assessed, common methods of measurement, and the information gained from each of the evaluative tools. While performing an evaluation, it is important to consider whether there would be a contraindication to the use of any specific evaluative tool due to a specific pathologic condition (e.g., manual muscle test to a rotator cuff surgically repaired 1 week ago). In this case it becomes important to note any portion of the evaluation that was not completed, so that it can be performed at a time when it is not contraindicated (e.g., manual muscle test to a rotator cuff repaired 8 weeks ago).

The findings of this portion of the PSA should be documented in the athlete's medical file. This baseline data will be needed later to demonstrate progression through the rehabilitation process. Commonly accepted medical shorthand is presented in Appendix C.

Prioritization of Problems

Once the problems specific to the injury have been determined, they should be prioritized before considering the treatment plan. Prioritizing the problems assists in planning the rehabilitation program by: (1) establishing a logical order of treatment, (2) defining the focus of self-treatment, and (3) allocating the athletic trainer's time.

A logical order of treatment is essential to the overall success of the rehabilitation program. Certain problems must be addressed before others. A logical prioritization of the problems will aid in the formation of the treatment progression. A good example of this is the athlete who cannot bear weight due to pain. The problem of pain must take higher priority than the problem of a decreased weight-bearing status. The treatment plan should be prioritized to

Table 6-1 **TOOLS USED IN THE EVALUATION OF ATHLETIC INJURIES**

Tool	How Measured	Information Gained
Subjective information	Active listening and note taking on the subjective information offered by the athlete.	(A) Injury mechanism, (B) inflammation based on reports of pain, swelling, warmth, etc., (C) functional limitations, and (D) treatment considerations based on previous successful or unsuccessful protocol.
Range of motion	Measured goniometrically or as a percentage of full movement in the case of the spine.	Ability to move with reference to specific motions.
Swelling and/or edema	Measured circumferentially with a tape measure around specific landmarks or by *volumetric measurement* in the case of a distal extremity.	Indicates the presence of swelling or edema.
Strength	Measured by manual muscle test using a grading scale, a hand-held *dynamometer*, or an isokinetic device.	Indicates strength deficits of a muscle or group of muscles. Can also determine injury to a muscle or tendon by eliciting pain associated with contraction of that muscle or muscle group.
Weight-bearing status	Measured as full, partial, or non–weight bearing. Can also be described as a percentage of full weight bearing.	Ability of the athlete to bear weight within the limitations of pain, weakness, and/or lack of range of motion.
Atrophy or hypertrophy	Measured circumferentially with a tape measure.	Determines the decrease or increase of tissue mass. Note that there is little correlation between limb girth and strength.
Pain	Pain rating scale of 0 to 10, with 0 being no pain at all and 10 being the worst pain imaginable.	Presence of pain with a specific functional activity (squatting), movement (shoulder flexion), special test (valgus stress to the elbow), or at rest. Ratings can be utilized within a single athlete but cannot be compared with those of other athletes.
Deep tendon reflex	Graded in an orthopedic population as 0 = none, 1 = *hyporeflexia*, 2 = normal.	Determination of the functional level of the reflex arc.
Sensation	Determined in the athlete by light touch to bilateral areas of the body having the same dermatomal or specific nerve distributions.	Assesses the function of the sensory nervous system.
Joint mobilization	Evaluation of the accessory motions found in joints. Graded as hypomobile, normal, or hypermobile.	Determines the presence of adequate accessory motion needed to produce normal physiological motion.
Balance and proprioception	Ability to stand on one leg with eyes closed for a 20-second time period. Compared with the uninjured limb.	Provides a gross determination of the function of the proprioceptive receptors in a joint.

Volumetric Measurement: Determination of the size of a body part by measuring the amount of water it displaces.

Dynamometer: A device used for measuring muscular strength.

Hyporeflexia: Diminished function of the reflexes.

Table 6-1 **TOOLS USED IN THE EVALUATION OF ATHLETIC INJURIES**
Continued

Tool	How Measured	Information Gained
Flexibility	Assessment of muscle length by fixing one end of the unit and moving the other end to the maximal length. Can sometimes be measured goniometrically, but can also be graded as normal or tight, based on normative findings.	Determination of whether a muscle or muscle group is functioning at a normal length or if it is producing abnormal stresses due to tightness.
Biomechanical assessment	Can detect biomechanical problems such as differences in limb length or foot motion, deformity, etc.	Determines the causes of abnormal stresses placed on the body due to inherent biomechanical problems. Sometimes the effects of these problems can be decreased or eliminated by the use of an orthotic device.
Special tests	Including tests that elicit pain in the presence of pathology; laxity in ligaments, and tests the integrity of structures, etc.	Determination of the clinical function and degree of pathology.
Function	Measured as the capability of an athlete to perform activities of daily living as well as sport-specific functions.	Determines the amount of function the athlete has with regard to a specific injury.
Posture	Determined by inspection and observation of posture and comparison with normative information.	Assesses abnormal stresses put on tissues by poor postural control or habits. Such stresses can cause pain or paraesthesia.

first address the pain. Once this is controlled, an increased weight-bearing status will follow. If the weight-bearing status is treated without first addressing the pain, the pain will most likely increase and prolong the rehabilitation time.

It is an idealization to think that the successful return of the athlete is due to the tireless treatment undergone by the athlete in the athletic training room. In reality, no athlete returns to full activity in a safe and timely manner unless that athlete has remained fully involved in the treatment and has complied with the instructions of the athletic trainer and physician. The most important time in the athlete's rehabilitation is the time spent **between** treatments with the athletic trainer.

Consider the following hypothetical situation: Two athletes have exactly the same injury, and receive exactly the same treatments by the same athletic trainer. However, athlete 1 is compliant with the instructions for treatment outside of the athletic training room and athlete 2 is noncompliant with these instructions. Given these exact situations, and the best care possible in the athletic training room, athlete 1 will return to competition more quickly than athlete 2. This is due to compliance during the time between treatments.

Since self-treatment time is so important, it must be utilized to address the athlete's problems. After the problems have been prioritized, it is easier to choose the modalities or exercises that the athlete will be instructed to use for self-treatment. In general, the more an athlete is given to do during self-treatment, the less chance there is that the treatment will actually be performed.

To obtain greater compliance it is a good idea to give the athlete no more than three modalities or exercises in his or her self-treatment.

In almost any profession, time and resources must be allocated so that tasks are performed efficiently. In many situations the athletic trainer is faced with too many injured athletes, in too small a treatment area, and without enough time to properly treat every athlete. One way to continue to be successful is to allocate time and resources efficiently. Prioritizing problems allows the athletic trainer to decide which treatment needs the personal attention of the athletic trainer versus that which the athlete can perform independently.

As an athlete's condition improves the athlete's problems will call for less hands-on intervention by the athletic trainer and more independence of the athlete in the treatment. With constant re-evaluation of the athlete's problems, and the priority of those problems, the athletic trainer can more optimally allocate his or her time and resources.

Goal Setting

The athletic trainer is accountable for all that is done in the treatment of the injured athlete. The setting of short-term and long-term goals allows the athletic trainer to test the efficacy of the treatment plan. At timely intervals a re-evaluation of the athlete is performed to determine the present status of the athlete's condition. In comparing the results of the re-evaluation with the goals that have been set, it can be determined if the treatment plan has been effective, if it can be progressed, or if it needs to be changed due to lack of progress.

Short-term and long-term goals should be determined for every treatment plan. Short-term goals are usually established for a one-week to two-week period that allows the athletic trainer to determine the success of the treatment plan as it now stands. Short-term goals are redefined at the time of every re-evaluation so that accommodations for change and progress can be made in the treatment plan.

Long-term goals provide direction to the treatment plan. The long-term goals determine what must be accomplished so that the athlete returns successfully to full athletic competition. The long-term goals determine the overall efficacy of the rehabilitation program.

There are other important reasons for setting goals during the rehabilitation process. Providing motivation to the rehabilitating athlete is one of the most important reasons for goal-setting. Goal-setting provides the athlete with incentive to attain a certain physical condition in a defined amount of time. Another important reason for setting goals is to provide realistic timetables for the athlete, coach, and sometimes the parents of the athlete. A realistic idea of the time that is needed to rehabilitate the athlete can prevent unnecessary pressure on the rehabilitation staff, as well as the athlete, to return the athlete to full activity in less than a safe physical condition.

Goals should be realistic, but more importantly, goals need to be as objective as possible. Upon the initial evaluation of the athlete, an attempt should be made to define the athlete's problems in objective, measurable terms. To keep treatment programs accountable, goals must be set in an objective, measurable manner whenever possible. Objective goals provide direction to the treatment plan. It is very unlikely that the objective measurements attained on re-evaluation will be exactly what had been set in the goals; however, objective measurements should be in the direction and within the general area that has been set in the goals. This would signify progress toward a successful resolution and a return to safe, full activity.

Treatment Planning

Once the problems of the injured athlete have been determined and prioritized, and short-term and long-term goals have been set, the planning of the treatment follows naturally. The planning of the treatment is the application of the athletic trainer's knowledge of the physiological effects of therapeutic modalities and exercise, in resolving problems and achieving the goals for the athlete's rehabilitation. The treatment is planned in the same logical order that has been followed in the PSA, allowing all problems to be addressed in the treatment plan.

The treatment plan should be as specific as possible so that continuity of care can be established in the case that more than one athletic trainer is treating the athlete. The slightest changes in the parameters of a modality can have drastically different physiological effects. A lack in continuity of treatment is a pitfall that may delay the successful return of the athlete. One measure that helps in avoiding this pitfall is good documentation in the evaluation and treatment of all athletic injuries.

CLINICAL APPLICATIONS

The case presentations will encompass an opening scene that provides information about the athlete and the evaluation of the athlete. The PSA will then be applied to each case to demonstrate how a treatment plan can be established utilizing modalities and therapeutic exercise. The theory behind the priority of the problems as well as the choice of the treatment plan will be explained.

Case Presentation 1

Opening Scene

A 20-year-old wrestler injured his neck during practice yesterday. He reports that he was "slammed" and landed on his head and right shoulder so that his head was bent to the left, but continued to wrestle. He woke up this morning around 4:00 AM with severe neck pain and stiffness. A warm morning shower provided temporary relief for about 30 minutes. He denies any pain or paresthesia in his extremities. He has no past medical history of cervical injury. He was referred to the team orthopedist and returned with a diagnosis of severe cervical muscle strain. The physician has ruled out any head injury or cervical fracture.

The athlete has returned from the doctor in a soft cervical collar which is to be worn for comfort and has instructions from the doctor for evaluating and treating the pain and spasm of the cervical musculature.

The evaluation findings are:

Observation:	Guarded posture	
Range of motion:	Flexion	30%
	Extension	20%
	Right rotation	20%
	Left rotation	30%
	Right side bending	20%
	Left side bending	10%
	(All motion is limited by pain.)	
Manual muscle test:	No grades can be given due to pain.	
	Cervical flexion—minimal pain.	
	Cervical extension—moderate pain.	
	Left upper trapezius—minimal pain.	
	Right upper trapezius—extreme pain.	
Flexibility:	Right upper trapezius—not tested due to pain.	
	Left upper trapezius—not tested due to pain.	
	Right sternocleidomastoid—not tested due to pain.	
	Left sternocleidomastoid—not tested due to pain.	
Pain rating:	Rating with left side bending is 7/10.	
	Reports constant pain of varying intensity with all activities of daily living.	
Palpation:	Increased tone of right upper trapezius due to muscular spasm.	
	Point tenderness of right upper trapezius.	
Upper quarter screen:	Deep tendon reflexes—all 2/2.	
	Sensation—intact for light touch.	
	Manual muscle test—5/5 throughout.	

Problems

1. Decreased cervical range of motion.
2. Muscular spasm of the right upper trapezius.
3. Pain of a 7/10 rating with left side bending.
4. Inability to assess strength and flexibility of the cervical musculature due to pain.
5. Inability to perform athletic activities.
6. Must wear soft cervical collar for comfort.

Prioritization of Problems

1. Pain of a 7/10 rating with left side bending.
2. Muscle spasm of the right upper trapezius.
3. Decreased cervical range of motion.
4. Inability to assess strength and flexibility of the cervical musculature due to pain.

5. Must wear soft cervical collar for comfort.
6. Inability to function in wrestling.

Explanation

Pain is given the highest priority because of its severity and its effect on the other evaluative findings. The increased afferent input to the central nervous system has triggered an efferent reflexive response resulting in muscular spasm to guard the area against further injury. While the spasm may be limiting the cervical range of motion, the pain caused by the initial mechanical trauma to nerve endings and the chemical irritation of the nerve endings are also causing decreased range of motion. Many of the evaluative techniques could not be performed because of pain. *Weaning* of the soft collar should coincide with decreased pain and increased range of motion. The inability to perform movement is very important, but the other problems must be controlled before return to activity can be addressed.

Short-term Goals (1 week)

1. Pain rating of 3/10 with left side bending.
2. Intermittent muscular spasm of the right upper trapezius.
3. Cervical range of motion:

Flexion	70%
Extension	50%
Right rotation	50%
Left rotation	70%
Right side bending	60%
Left side bending	50%

4. Assess strength and flexibility.
5. Pain-free activities of daily living 90% of time.
6. Use of the soft collar at night only.

Long-term Goals (2 weeks)

1. Elimination of pain.
2. Elimination of muscular spasm.
3. Full cervical range of motion.
4. A 5/5 rating of cervical muscle strength and normal flexibility of the upper trapezius and sternocleidomastoid.
5. Independence from the soft collar.
6. Return to full activity.

Plan

1. Ice bag application to upper trapezius with the athlete in the supine position for 20 minutes.

Weaning: Decreasing the dependence on a substance or device by gradually reducing its use.

THEORY:

> The supine position will decrease the amount of electromyographic activity in the cervical musculature by reason of the head's supported position. Cold application will decrease pain by increasing the pain threshold and decreasing the nerve conduction velocity. The cold application will also decrease the muscle spasm by decreasing the muscle spindle sensitivity to stretch. Ice is used to decrease the metabolic rate of the injured and surrounding tissues, thereby decreasing the chance of secondary hypoxic injury to those tissues.

Plan

> 2. Utilization of sensory-level electrical stimulation to the trapezius musculature with a pulse rate of 50 to 100 pulses per second (pps) and a pulse duration of 30 to 200 milliseconds (msec). Can be given concurrently with the ice application.

THEORY:

> The electrical stimulation could be delivered with a TENS, a high-voltage stimulator, or a neuromuscular stimulator, providing that the unit has the capability of adjusting the pulse rate and pulse width to levels that would produce comfortable sensory-level stimulation without muscular contraction. The stimulation is utilized to decrease pain by creating a counterirritant effect.

Plan

> 3. Phonophoresis with 10 percent hydrocortisone to the right upper trapezius. This procedure is only applied with a prescription from a physician. The phonophoresis is performed with 1-MHz pulsed ultrasound at 0.75 to 1 watts per square centimeter for a period of 5 minutes with an ultrasound head of 5 square centimeters.

THEORY:

> Pulsed ultrasound at lower intensity can decrease pain and increase cellular permeability allowing for the transport of medication and nutrients into the injured tissues. The 1-MHz frequency will allow for greater depth of penetration of the ultrasound beam. The 5-minute treatment time is needed to adequately cover the involved area, based on the effective radiating area of the ultrasound head.

Plan

> 4. Moist heat application for 15 minutes. To be utilized after the pain and spasm begin to decrease and range of motion begins to improve.

THEORY:

> Once the inflammatory response and the pain-spasm pain cycle have been reduced, moist heat can be applied prior to exercise. The heat would be utilized prior to exercise to promote relaxation, increase tissue temperature, and

decrease pain as an analgesic and increasing the threshold of pain receptors. Ice would still be utilized following exercise to lower the metabolic rate and to decrease pain.

Plan

5. Range of motion, flexibility, and strengthening exercises.

THEORY:

Exercise would be added to the program as tolerated by the athlete. Range of motion and flexibility exercises would initially be performed in a supine position to decrease the electrical activity in the muscles so that there would be less resistance to stretching of the involved tissues. Isotonic strengthening exercises would be performed pain free. These exercises would be progressed to manual resistance through the full range of motion.

Plan

6. Cardiovascular exercise.

THEORY:

Cardiovascular exercise with a bicycle would be utilized early to maintain the athlete at an optimal cardiovascular condition. The athlete could progress to using a stair climber or cross-country ski machine. Lastly the athlete could progress to using an upper body *ergometer* as the levels of cervical pain and spasm decrease.

Plan

7. Progressive return to wrestling.

THEORY:

The athlete would progress first through individual wrestling drills and then to one-on-one drills. After successful completion of these, he could progress to scrimmaging and then match competition.

Case Presentation 2

Opening Scene

A 16-year-old female soccer player reports to the athletic training room with complaints of recurrent right knee pain. Reporting pain "along the inside of my kneecap," she has experienced the pain every season and has been treated in the past with rest, ice, and therapeutic exercise consisting of straight leg raising and knee extension exercises in the terminal 30 degrees of range of motion.

Ergometer: A device used to measure the amount of work performed by the legs or arms.

She has been evaluated by an orthopedic surgeon. Her x-rays show no abnormalities and the doctor has diagnosed patellofemoral pain syndrome. The athlete has been referred back to you for evaluation and treatment of her condition.

The evaluation findings are:

Subjective: Athlete reports pain after 15 minutes of sitting with her knee flexed. She also reports pain while going up and down stairs, with more pain experienced while going down the steps.

Biomechanics: Leg length is equal.

Static standing: Feet assume a bilaterally pronated position.

Gait: Excessive pronation that begins early in the gait cycle.

Range of motion: Left—0° of extension to 145° of flexion.
Right—5° of extension to 135° of flexion.

Girth:

	Left	Right
Joint line:	13.0 in	13.5 in
Superior patellar border:	13.5 in	14.0 in

Patellar mobility: The right patella has a decreased medial glide and is tilted laterally indicating a tight lateral *retinaculum*.

Patellar tracking: The patella shows excessive lateral tracking as compared to the contralateral side. This occurs on quadriceps contraction with both open and closed kinetic chain exercises.

Quadriceps tone: Quadriceps tone is decreased when compared with the contralateral side.

Strength: All hip groups—5/5 bilaterally.
Quadriceps—pain with test, no grade given on the right.
5/5 on the left.
Hamstrings—5/5 bilaterally.

Flexibility: Hip flexors—normal bilaterally.
Adductors—normal bilaterally.
Quadriceps—tight on the right leg; prone knee flexion to 130°.
Hamstrings—slightly tight bilaterally; with hip flexed to 90°, the knee extends to $-10°$ of full extension.
Iliotibial band—tight on the right leg; positive Ober test.
Gastrocnemius—tight bilaterally; only capable of 5° of dorsiflexion.
Soleus—tight bilaterally; only capable of 5° of dorsiflexion.

Pain rating: Rating is 5/10 for walking downstairs.

Special tests: All negative.

Problems

1. Pain of 5/10 on going downstairs.
2. Range of motion is $-5°$ of extension to 130° of flexion.
3. Joint line and superior patellar girth measurements are increased by 0.5 inch due to swelling.
4. Excessive pronation of feet.
5. Tight lateral retinaculum.

Retinaculum: A fibrous membrane that holds an organ or body part in place.

6. Decreased muscular tone (neuromuscular control) of quadriceps mechanism.
7. Lateral tracking of patella.
8. Decreased flexibility of the quadriceps, hamstrings, iliotibial band, gastrocnemius, and soleus.
9. Cannot grade manual muscle test of quadriceps due to pain.
10. Inability to function in soccer.

Prioritization of Problems

1. Excessive pronation of feet.
2. Tight lateral retinaculum.
3. Laterally tracking patella.
4. Joint line and superior patellar girth measurements increased by 0.5 inch due to swelling.
5. Decreased quadriceps tone (neuromuscular control) of quadriceps mechanism.
6. Pain of 5/10 on going downstairs.
7. Decreased flexibility of the quadriceps, hamstrings, iliotibial band, gastrocnemius, and soleus.
8. Range of motion is $-5°$ of extension to $130°$ of flexion.
9. Cannot grade manual muscle test of quadriceps due to pain.
10. Inability to function in soccer.

Explanation

The first focus of treatment must be with the biomechanical problems. The excessive *pronation* and tight lateral retinaculum are mechanical problems leading to abnormal stresses being placed on the patellofemoral joint. The abnormal stresses are causing the athlete's pain, swelling, and quadriceps insufficiency which then lead to the laterally tracking patella. The first steps in correcting the pain and dysfunction must be correction of the causes of these problems.

The swelling present within the joint can inhibit the quadriceps muscle activity. Prior to addressing the neuromuscular control and strength problems, swelling must be minimized or eliminated. Pain appears to be low on the priority list but it will be greatly decreased as the problems due to abnormal biomechanics and swelling are addressed. Flexibility may be a mechanical problem leading to patellofemoral dysfunction but probably has less of a causal relationship than the pronation, tight retinaculum, and muscular insufficiency. The range of motion will more than likely increase as all of the above-mentioned problems are addressed.

As always, anything that cannot be assessed in the evaluation should be listed as a problem, because it is information that should be obtained during the complete assessment of the athlete. Decreased athletic activity is listed last because it represents the sum of the other problems. Solving the other problems will prepare the athlete to return to soccer activity.

Pronation: An inward flattening and tilting of the foot, resulting in the lowering of the medial longitudinal arch.

Short-term Goals (2 weeks)

1. Correct pronation with *orthotics*.
2. Increase medial glide of the patella to normal.
3. Decrease lateral tracking of the patella with the use of tape.
4. Decrease joint line and superior patellar girth to a 0.25-inch positive deviation from normal.
5. Improve quadriceps tone to a grade of fair.
6. Decrease pain to a rating of 2/5 when going downstairs.
7. Increase grades of flexibility as follows:

   Quadriceps—prone knee flexion to 140°.
   Hamstrings—hip flexion at 90° with knee extension to $-5°$.
   Iliotibial band—negative Ober test.
   Gastrocnemius—dorsiflexion to 10°.
   Soleus—dorsiflexion to 10°.

8. Increase range of motion to 0° of extension and 140° of flexion.
9. Assess quadriceps strength.
10. Maintain physical conditioning for athletic activity.

Long-term Goals (4–6 weeks)

1. Normal tracking of patella without tape.
2. Bilaterally equal girth at joint line and superior patella.
3. Normal quadriceps tone.
4. Pain-free activity of all kinds.
5. Normal flexibility in all lower extremity musculature.
6. Bilaterally equal range of motion.
7. Normal quadriceps strength.
8. Return to full activity.

Plan

1. Correction of pronation with orthotics and a reduction in abnormal patellar stresses with taping.

THEORY:

The causal mechanical stresses must be eliminated prior to proceeding with the other forms of treatment.

Plan

2. Continuous 3-MHz ultrasound to the lateral retinaculum, intensity to tolerance with a sound head of 5 square centimeters for 5 minutes, applied concurrently with a medial glide to the patella for 3 to 4 minutes.

Orthotics: The use of orthopedic devices for correcting deformity or malalignment.

THEORY:

> Continuous ultrasound is utilized to heat the tissues before and during stretch to increase the extensibility of the tissues. An intensity to tolerance is utilized to achieve the maximal amount of heating. A 3-MHz sound head allows concentration of the ultrasound in the tissues approximately 1 centimeter deep. Five minutes is usually needed to adequately cover this treatment area based on the effective radiating area of this ultrasound head. A possible increase in swelling from deep heating of the retinacular structures is not a problem since the swelling is usually not related to these structures.

Plan

> 3. Use of neuromuscular stimulation to the quadriceps. Electrode placement is at the femoral triangle and distal quadriceps, with the vastus medialis oblique being the targeted muscle group.
>
> Treatment parameters:
> A frequency of 50 Hz with a carrier frequency of 2500 Hz.
> A pulse width of 225 to 250 milliseconds.
> An on/off time of 12/8 seconds with a ramp of 3 seconds.
> Total stimulation time of 10 minutes.
> Intensity to tolerance. Stimulation should be concurrent with quadriceps isometric exercises.

THEORY:

> The parameters are optimal for comfort and recruitment at the neuromuscular junction. On/off time (duty cycle) is less than the 15/50 reported in most studies for optimal strengthening because most patients will not tolerate the electrical stimulation intensities needed for strengthening to occur. Patients can tolerate the shorter off times without fatigue and can utilize the stimulation as an adjunct to quadriceps setting exercises. A total stimulation time of 10 minutes will allow 30 repetitions.

Plan

> 4. Biofeedback over the vastus medialis oblique with exercise. Utilized in a step-up mode at the intensity level barely achievable by the patient.

THEORY:

> True neuromuscular re-education must come from a voluntary contraction of the muscle and not solely from the involuntary contraction found with electrical stimulation. Portable biofeedback units allow isolation over the vastus medialis oblique during a wide range of exercise including, but not limited to, the following: quadriceps setting, adductor setting, straight leg raise with hip flexion, straight leg raise with hip adduction, pain-free isotonics in concentric and eccentric motions, and closed kinetic chain exercises, such as quadriceps setting, mini squats, and leg presses.

Plan

5. Ice following exercise for 20 minutes.

THEORY:

Cryotherapy will decrease the metabolic needs of the tissues. It will also help to moderate pain through analgesia and by decreasing the pain threshold.

Plan

6. Patellar mobilization with medial joint glides.

THEORY:

Patellar medial joint glides will be needed in addition to those performed with the ultrasound. Self-mobilization should also be taught to the athlete.

Plan

7. Range of motion, flexibility, and strengthening exercises.

THEORY:

Exercise would be added to the program as tolerated by the athlete. Range of motion exercises will be performed with heel slides. Flexibility exercises for tight musculature will be performed with contract/relax stretching as well as using a self-stretch by the athlete. Strengthening exercises are performed as listed above with the biofeedback unit but can also be performed without the use of biofeedback.

Plan

8. Cardiovascular exercise.

THEORY:

Cardiovascular exercise would be utilized early on to maintain the cardiovascular conditioning of the athlete, so that she returns to her soccer activity in optimal cardiovascular condition.

Plan

9. Progressive return to activity.

THEORY:

The athlete would progress first through jogging and running and then on to agility drills. Lastly, sport-specific drills would be utilized before return to full scrimmage and game conditions.

Case Presentation 3

Opening Scene

A 21-year-old All-American quaterback sprains his left ankle 1 week before a bowl game to determine the national championship. The ankle is immediately x-rayed and evaluated by the team orthopedist, who has diagnosed a grade 2 lateral ankle sprain. The physician orders the ankle immobilized in a removable walker boot and prescribes an aggressive rehabilitation program. The athlete is to be non–weight bearing for 2 days and is then to progress to full weight bearing and practicing by day 4.

The evaluation findings are:

Subjective:	Pain on weight bearing that has a 4/10 rating.	
	A constant dull ache that has a 1/10 rating.	

Range of motion:		Left	Right
	Dorsiflexion	0°	12°
	Plantarflexion	16°	37°

Weight-bearing status: Non–weight bearing.

Swelling and/or edema:		Left	Right
	Around heel	16.0 in	15.0 in
	Base of 5th metatarsal	12.5 in	12.0 in

Strength:	Not tested due to pain.
Proprioception:	Not tested due to non–weight-bearing status.
Flexibility:	Not tested due to pain and decreased range of motion.
Special tests:	Not tested due to pain.
Palpation:	Pain at the anterior talofibular ligament. *Pitting edema* throughout the ankle and foot.

Problems

1. Pain rating of 4/10 with weight bearing, and 2/10 resting.
2. Decreased weight-bearing status.
3. Increased swelling at the ankle and foot.
4. Decreased range of motion of the ankle.
5. Inability to test strength, flexibility, or proprioception, or to perform special tests.
6. Inability to participate in football.

Prioritization of Problems

1. Increased swelling at ankle and foot.
2. Pain rating of 6/10 with weight bearing, and 2/10 resting.
3. Decreased range of motion of the ankle.
4. Decreased weight-bearing status.
5. Inability to participate in football.

Pitting Edema: An exudate-rich form of edema that is characterized by being easily indented by pressure (hence, "pitting").

6. Inability to test strength, flexibility, or proprioception, or to perform special tests.

Explanation

Most of the problems are due to the increased swelling in the joint. The swelling increases pain, decreases range of motion, and decreases the ability to bear weight. Addressing the swelling will enable you to move toward a resolution of this athlete's problems. The pain must be addressed early to improve the range of motion and weight-bearing ability. Addressing either range of motion or weight bearing without addressing the swelling and pain will result in a poor outcome. As the range of motion and weight-bearing status are improved the athlete will move closer to the goal of returning to full competition in 1 week. The assessment of strength, flexibility, and proprioception, and the special tests are irrelevant in this athlete due to time constraints. In such a short period there is not enough time to address all of these.

Short-term Goals (2 days)

1. Decrease pain to a 2/10 rating with full weight bearing, and a 0/10 rating with a partial weight bearing of 50%. Pain will have a 0/10 rating at rest.
2. Increase ambulation to 50% weight bearing.
3. Decrease swelling to a 0.5-inch difference around the heel and 0.25-inch difference at the base of the 5th metatarsal.
4. Increase range of motion to 5° of dorsiflexion and 22° of plantarflexion.
5. Maintain cardiovascular conditioning.

Long-term Goals (1 week)

1. Pain rating of 0/10 to 1/10 for full weight-bearing athletic activities with tape support.
2. Full weight-bearing status.
3. Decrease swelling to 0.25-inch difference around the heel and no difference at the base of the 5th metatarsal.
4. Increase range of motion to 10° of dorsiflexion and 30° of plantarflexion.
5. Return to full activity with minimal pain and dysfunction while taped.
6. Completely rehabilitate the athlete's ankle after the bowl game.

Plan

1. Intermittent compression with elevation utilized for 30 minutes every hour for the first 4 days. Ice added under the compression with every other treatment. Treatment to continue with a compression unit at night. Pressure setting of 60 mm/Hg with an on/off cycle of 30 seconds on and 15 seconds off.

THEORY:

> Intermittent compression with elevation will aid lymphatic return of edema. This process helps to decongest the area and allow nutrients and oxygen to get to the damaged tissues and surrounding areas. Ice is utilized to decrease the metabolic rate of the tissues and to limit the effects of secondary hypoxia. It is also an analgesic, decreasing pain and increasing the pain threshold.

Plan

> 2. Massage using slow effleurage strokes from the toes to the lower leg to "milk" edema proximally. The effleurage strokes would be preceded by "uncorking" the leg proximal to the ankle.

THEORY:

> The injured area is congested with edematous fluid that increases pain and may prolong the healing process. Massage using effleurage strokes will aid the lymphatic system in transporting fluid proximally. Movement of fluid out of the injured area will decrease pain and help to improve range of motion.

Plan

> 3. Cryokinetic progression begun on the day 2 postinjury to promote weight bearing and increase the range of motion.

THEORY:

> Cryokinetics can be effective in returning the athlete to functional activity by promoting increases in range of motion and weight-bearing status while decreasing pain and limiting harmful stresses.

Plan

> 4. Therapeutic exercise began on the day 2 postinjury to promote increased range of motion and to aid in the lymphatic return through utilization of the muscle pump.

THEORY:

> The athlete will need specific exercises to promote increased range of motion to achieve functional limits. This must be done in conjunction with cryokinetics as well as cryotherapy.

Plan

> 5. Maintain cardiovascular condition.

THEORY:

> Maintenance of cardiovascular condition must be achieved so that the athlete is ready to return to function cardiovascularly as well as musculoskeletally.

Plan

6. Progressive return to activity over last 3 days prior to competition.

THEORY:

The capabilities of the injured ankle to withstand progressively more difficult stresses must be adequately addressed to allow the athlete to return in a safe manner. Progression would include jogging, running, and progressively harder agility and sport-specific drills, to tax the injured area. The final progression would lead to participation in a scrimmage under game conditions.

Summary

The problem-solving approach promotes the successful treatment of athletic injuries by utilizing the athletic trainer's knowledge of modalities and therapeutic exercise in an individualized, interactive approach to treatment and rehabilitation. It has been presented as a model for both the student athletic trainer and the certified athletic trainer, as it enables an athletic trainer of any experience level to evaluate any injury and begin a successful treatment regimen.

This model is based on a thorough evaluation that leads to determination of the athlete's problems, prioritization of the problems, setting of short-term and long-term goals, and a plan of treatment. The model's main purpose is to develop completeness in the use of therapeutic modalities and exercise when treating athletic injuries. The approach is designed to promote treatment that enables the injured athlete to return to competition in the quickest and safest manner possible.

The solutions of these case studies are not the only acceptable approaches in the management of these injuries. There are many possible methods by which each of these cases could be managed. The essence of this chapter has been to illustrate the decision-making process and emphasize the need for proper planning and implementation of the program.

Administrative Considerations in the Application of Therapeutic Modalities

This chapter discusses some of the administrative considerations associated with the application of therapeutic modalities. The focus of the chapter is to make the student aware that proper procedure and planning can reduce an athletic trainer's exposure to liability.

As the athletic trainer's knowledge, ability, and scope of employment increase, so do requirements of the *standard of practice* and the potential for liability.[1] Proper planning and the following of accepted procedure can reduce much of the liability faced by the athlete trainer. Through identifying potentially hazardous situations and initiating steps to avoid them, as well as administering therapy in a safe and proper manner, athletic trainers can assure that they and the athletes are working in a safe environment.

Standard of Practice: The criteria against which an individual's performance is measured. The National Athletic Trainers' Association Board of Certification establishes the Standards for Direct Service.

Liability and the Athletic Trainer

The treatment and rehabilitation of athletic injuries is but one small fragment of the athletic trainer's daily routine. It is, however, a primary cause for concern when dealing with liability issues. In the treatment and rehabilitation process, the athletic trainer's legal duty is to **prevent further injury or harm to the injured party** by performing the tasks at hand in a professionally accepted manner. Courts have ruled that reasonable facilities and equipment, as well as qualified personnel, are necessary to provide proper medical coverage to athletes.[2]

Fortunately, litigation against athletic trainers is still a rare occurrence. Between 1960 and 1989 a total of nine lawsuits were brought against certified athletic trainers, but a much greater number of cases have been brought against team physicians.[3] As the scope of practice of the athletic trainer expands, the likelihood of liability suits will become greater.

In the treatment and rehabilitation of athletic injuries, the athletic trainer must be intimately familiar with the indications and contraindications of the devices being used. Athletic trainers are expected to recognize those physical conditions that prohibit the use of various therapeutic modalities and forms of therapeutic exercise. Additionally, to ensure the proper application of therapeutic modalities, athletic trainers must know the characteristics, maintenance requirements, and safety considerations of the devices being used, and must document their adherence to these standards. In most states, it is also the duty of the athletic trainer to apply therapeutic modalities with the consent of, and under the direction of a physician.

Furthermore, it is the duty of the athletic trainer, team physician, or family physician to inform the athlete about the severity and consequences of the injury being treated, while the athlete has the right to refuse any treatment and seek a second medical opinion from an outside source.

The first six chapters of this text address the preceding concerns. The remainder of this chapter will discuss those organizational factors that may expose athletic trainers to liability during the treatment of athletic injuries, and some methods for avoiding that legal risk.

It is important to note that this chapter deals primarily with the treatment and rehabilitation phases of the athletic trainer's duties. It does not represent all aspects of liability that an athletic trainer may be exposed to in the day-to-day operation of an athletic training room and the coverage of practices and games.

TORT LAW

The United States judicial system is composed of several types of laws. Most legal actions regarding the practice of athletic training are tried under tort law, but action could also be taken under statutory law or common law (see Box 7–1). A **tort** is broadly defined as a civil wrong for which the court will provide a remedy for damages that have been suffered. The tort action most commonly seen in the athletic training profession is **negligence**. In a tort case, the *plaintiff*

Plaintiff: A person who is the complaining party in a lawsuit.

Box **7–1**	COMMON LAW AND STATUTORY LAWS

Common laws having evolved from customs and early "unwritten laws" are most generally used to recover money for damages suffered by the plaintiff. Court rulings on common law issues are based on *precedents*, that are legally binding in the state where they were set. However, if no precedent exists in particular states, precedents set in other states can serve as a guide in the court's decision. Common laws can be overruled if there are changes in social attitudes, and tend to evolve and expand based on court decisions. Cases are tried on common law principles unless statute law governs.

Statutory laws are initiated, amended, or repealed by action of the state or federal legislature. Based on a hierarchy, federal law usually has priority over state laws, which in turn, has priority over local laws. If a state or community enacts a statutory law, it cannot conflict with preceding federal laws. Many common laws have evolved into statutory law.

---

claims that the action of the defendant has caused harm, and compensation is sought to cover damages.

As described by Pozgar,[4] "The basic purpose of tort laws is to keep peace between individuals by supplying a substitute for vengeance and to find fault for a wrongdoing, and encourage adherence to the law." In past times disagreements were settled by more archaic means, such as duels with swords or guns. This style of freelance justice did not conform with the standards of a civilized society. Courts were therefore established to allow an impartial party to weigh the facts and arrive at a reasonable settlement. In court, it is the plaintiff's duty to prove that the defendant acted in a negligent manner and that damages resulted from negligence by the accused.

Torts may be classified as being either **intentional torts** (Table 7–1), **negligent torts** (Table 7–2), or strict liability. What distinguishes between the first two types of torts is "intent." The intent to cause harm is present in intentional torts, but not in negligent torts. Intent not only implies that the act was the result of a conscious effort, but also that the perpetrator was aware that harm would result from the act. In strict liability, the defendant is held liable in the absence of any intent which the law finds wrongful, usually for reasons of policy.

Table 7–1 INTENTIONAL TORTS

Assault:	A deliberate verbal threat accompanied by the ability to do physical harm to another.
Battery:	An intentional touching without consent.
False imprisonment:	Unlawful imprisonment by either physical or psychological force.
Defamation of character:	Communication to a third party that causes harm to an individual. If this communication is spoken, it is **slander**. If it is written, **libel**.
Fraud:	Intentional misrepresentation of oneself.
Invasion of privacy:	People have a right to be left alone. Public figures (such as athletes) have fewer rights in this regard than do ordinary citizens.

Precedent: A previous ruling that serves as a guide in future legal actions.

Table 7–2 **NEGLIGENT TORTS**

Malfeasance:	The performance of an unlawful or improper act.
Misfeasance:	The improper performance of an otherwise lawful act.
Nonfeasance:	The failure to act when there is a duty to act.
Malpractice:	Negligence on the part of a professional person serving in the line of duty.
Gross negligence:	Total disregard for the safety of others.

TYPES OF TORTS

Battery

A very common form of an intentional tort is that of **battery**. A person who touches another without permission has potentially committed the act of battery. In the strictest sense of the law, a person must want to be touched before another can lay a hand on that person. Obviously, not every unwanted touching may be considered battery. If you have ever ridden on a subway during rush hour, you realize that inadvertent touching is sometimes unavoidable. It is the willful touching of one person by another that requires permission. This consent, known as **consensual touching**, must be established before an athletic trainer can treat an athlete. Otherwise, the athletic trainer could have committed an act of battery. It is much easier to prove a claim of battery than a claim of negligence because battery does not require proof of misconduct.

Negligence

While it may still cause harm, negligence implies the lack of malice and forethought found in intentional torts. **Ordinary negligence** is the failure to act as a reasonable and prudent person would act under similar circumstances (see Box 7–2). **Gross negligence** is the total failure to provide elements that would normally be deemed proper in a given situation.

For the courts to find a person guilty of negligence, a clear relationship between the alleged act of negligence and the harm suffered by the individual must be established (Table 7–3). A court must first establish if the defendant had a **duty** to the plaintiff. Then, if a duty exists, the court asks, "Did the defendant **breach** this obligation?" The **breach of duty** is established by comparing the actions of the defendant against those that a reasonable and prudent person would have taken under similar circumstances. If the defendant was not obliged to respond, or if the defendant acted reasonably and prudently, no negligence can be found.

The amount of care which one is expected to exercise changes with the circumstances. As the danger or risk increases, the care which must be exercised by the person increases. Traditionally, those who deal with potentially dangerous devices, such as many of the therapeutic modalities discussed in this text, must exercise greater care. Also, those who accept unusual responsibilities must utilize special care.

If the defendant was obliged to respond, but failed to act in a reasonable and prudent manner, the courts must determine if the plaintiff actually suffered **harm**. The plaintiff must prove that physical injury, financial loss, mental anguish, or an invasion of a personal right occurred. If no harm was suffered, no damages will be awarded.

The final link in determining negligence is that of **causation**. A direct

---

Box (7-2) SO WHO IS THIS REASONABLE AND PRUDENT PERSON?

When a charge of negligence is brought upon an individual, the person's actions are measured against those that a reasonable and prudent person would have performed in the same situation. So where is this reasonable and prudent person found?

The reasonable and prudent person is a fictional person who is created by the court. Variables such as the defendant's age, gender, physical condition, education, and mental capacity are factored together to detemine what actions would be considered reasonable.[4] Since the criteria for determining reasonable and prudent behavior would change from situation to situation, and since juries are not qualified to determine what the proper standard of care would be in a given situation, a mechanism must exist to create a reasonable and prudent person for any type of case that may arise.

Through the testimony of expert witnesses, a standard of care is established that describes what actions should be expected of an individual in a given situation. In the case of athletic training, the standard of care is determined through the standard of practice (Appendix D), if the state in which the case is heard does not have licensure for athletic trainers. In those states having licensure, the standard of care is based in part on the licensure law as well as on the standard of practice. However, if the athletic trainer exceeds the accepted scope of practice and ventures into another field, then the athletic trainer may be held to the reasonable standard of care for that profession. For example, if an athletic trainer devises custom-fit mouthpieces, he or she may be held to the standard of care of a dentist, rather than an athletic trainer.

---

relationship between the actions of the defendant and the harm suffered by the plaintiff must be established. For example, if an athletic trainer fails to properly stabilize the neck of an athlete suffering a fracture of a cervical vertebra and the athlete is subsequently paralyzed, a court could potentially rule that the athletic trainer's actions contributed to the athlete's paralysis. The plaintiff must prove that each of the four elements of negligence existed. If one of these elements fails to exist, damages will not be awarded (Fig. 7–1)

If a negligent act has been committed, the accused's supervisors may also be found guilty of negligence through the *doctrine* of **respondeat superior** or

Table 7–3 **ELEMENTS OF NEGLIGENCE**

Duty to use due care:	There must be an established duty between the two parties involved. If no duty to due care exists, negligence cannot have occurred.
Breach of duty:	Did the charged party depart from the duty implied? This element relies on the reasonable and prudent doctrine.
Harm:	Did the defendant suffer an injury because of the actions (or lack of action) on the part of the plaintiff? Note that injury does not necessarily imply physical harm. Injury may also take the form of psychological or financial harm. If no injury occurred, no damages will be awarded.
Causation:	The breach of duty must be the immediate cause of the injury suffered. There must be a close and reasonable relationship between the defendant's conduct and the claimed damages.

Doctrine: A statement of fundamental government policy.

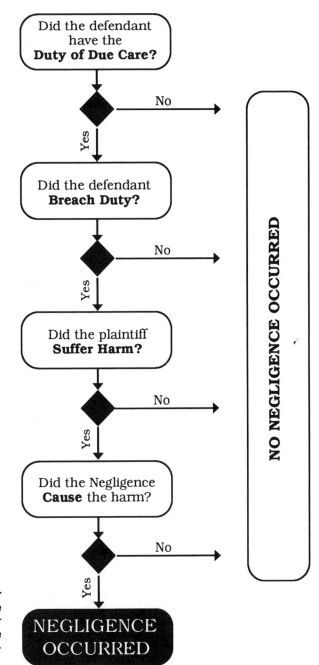

Figure 7–1. Flow chart for determining negligence. The plaintiff must prove that all four conditions were met before the defendant is found guilty of negligence.

vicarious liability. Supervisors can be found guilty of negligence because of the acts of their employees, or due to their own negligent failure to supervise. Many institutions will hire team physicians and athletic trainers as independent contractors to reduce this type of liability.

Negligent behavior occurs when an individual departs from the standard of care imposed by society.[4] If the athletic trainer, or a student serving under the direction of the certified staff, performs unnecessary or detrimental acts, he or she could be found liable for failure to use due care under the law of negligence.[2] The action of a student athletic trainer that results in an injury could cause legal action not only against the student, but also against the supervising athletic trainer who could be sued on the grounds of vicarious liability.[5]

Negligence may be classified into two types on the basis of behavior: omission and commission. **Omission** occurs when an individual fails to respond to a given situation when a response is necessary to limit or reduce harm. Consider the following example: an athlete goes to the athletic trainer with complaints of an injury. If the athletic trainer fails to evaluate, treat, or refer the injury, an act of omission may have occurred. In this case, the negligent act stems from the athletic trainer's failure to properly respond to an injury.

Commission occurs when an individual acts on a situation, but does not perform at the level that a reasonable and prudent person would. In athletic training, an act of commission could occur if the athletic trainer treats lower leg pain with ultrasound, and the injury turns out to be a fracture. In this example, negligence occurred because the athletic trainer responded to an injury, but he responded with an improper technique.

Invasion of Privacy and/or Breach of Confidentiality

If an athletic trainer releases medical information without the athlete's consent, it may be a libelous act through **defamation of character**. When this occurs by way of the spoken word it is termed **slander**; if this occurs through print, it is termed **libel**. For example, if, during a television interview after a game, an athletic trainer states an athlete's heat exhaustion was the result of steroid use, a case for slander could be made, especially if the reputed steroid use cannot be proven.

Those people in the public eye, such as athletes, have a lesser right to privacy than "private" figures. However, athletic trainers must maintain a high standard of practice and protect the athlete from being exposed to a breach of confidentiality with regard to their medical records. This becomes especially important when dealing with recruiters and visiting professional scouts.

Scope of Practice

In determining the scope of practice for athletic trainers, a differentiation between national **certification** and state **licensure** must be made. Certification granted by the National Athletic Trainers' Association Board of Certification, Inc. (NATABOC) indicates that an individual has met minimal educational standards and displayed competency on a three-part standardized examination. While national certification indicates that a person has met certain educational requirements and displayed knowledge and skill in selected tasks, it is state legislation that defines the parameters within which an athletic trainer must function.

States regulate the practice of athletic training through processes such as licensure, registration, or certification. In this text the term licensure will be used to describe the process of state regulation.

Currently there are 20 states requiring licensure for athletic trainers, and many other states have legislation pending[6] (Table 7–4). As a part of the licens-

Table 7–4 **STATES REQUIRING LICENSURE, REGISTRATION, OR CERTIFICATION TO PRACTICE ATHLETIC TRAINING**

Delaware	New Mexico
Georgia	North Dakota
Idaho	Ohio
Illinois	Oklahoma
Kentucky	Pennsylvania
Louisiana	Rhode Island
Massachusetts	South Carolina
Mississippi	South Dakota
Missouri	Tennessee
Nebraska	Texas
New Jersey	

Source: For information on how to become licensed or an up-to-date list of states regulating the practice of athletic training, contact:
The National Athletic Trainers' Association,
2952 Stemmons
Dallas, TX 75247.

ing process, the state sets the educational requirements that must be met to obtain a license. To date, every state having licensure, with the exception of Texas, requires NATABOC certification to obtain a license.

The process of creating a licensure law sets the legal bounds within which an athletic trainer may operate within that state. Because of this, and the fact that athletic training is still a relatively young profession, the scope of practice varies greatly from state to state. A common feature of these laws is the precept that athletic trainers treat athletes under the supervision and direction of a physician.

The role of the athletic trainer in nontraditional settings (e.g., private, for-profit, sports medicine centers) is a topic of great debate in local, state, and national forums. And while athletic trainers are allowed to function relatively freely in clinics in one state, in other states athletic trainers cannot even function as physical therapy aides in for-profit clinics.[7] In states where licensure laws for athletic trainers restrict the function of athletic trainer in the nontraditional setting, or in those states that have no licensure law, athletic trainers who are applying therapeutic modalities may find themselves in violation of the *physical therapy practice act.*

It is important that athletic trainers are knowledgeable about the laws governing the practice of athletic training in the state where they are working. Newly certified athletic trainers, or certified athletic trainers moving into a new state, should consult the state's Allied Health Board or the state athletic training organization regarding these regulations.

It is the duty of the athletic trainer to follow the advice and direction of a physician when using therapeutic modalities. Many of these devices, such as ultrasound and electrical stimulation, require a physician's prescription before they can be legally applied (see section on standing operating procedures in this chapter).

Physical Therapy Practice Act: State legislation that governs the practice of physical therapy procedures.

Record Keeping

Although it is an extremely important task, record keeping is not mandated by law.[2] This fact notwithstanding, athletic trainers should feel an obligation to keep records because of the wide range of purposes they serve (Table 7–5). Medical records serve as a communication tool between the various parties providing care to the athlete. This documentation becomes invaluable during the planning and evaluation of the rehabilitation program by providing a method of determining the effectiveness of various treatment and rehabilitation protocols (see Chapter 6). Medical records also describe the quantity and quality of athletic training room activity. The many functions that medical records serve also provide accountability for the athletic trainer and for the services provided by the department.

The process of record keeping is time-consuming. In a crowded athletic training room, it is tempting to make "mental notes" of what treatments were given and then record them later. Unfortunately, this method leads to inconsistent and inaccurate record keeping. The best practice is to record the information immediately after treatment is given. Although this may slightly extend the time between treatments, it increases the reliability and validity of the record-keeping process.

In the event of a lawsuit against the athletic trainer and/or the institution, well-documented records can assist in proving that the athletic trainer and medical staff exercised reasonable care in the management of the injury. If the case comes to trial, the medical staff may use the records to refresh their memories when testifying about a case. Furthermore, the actual documents may be admitted as evidence in the trial.[8]

CONFIDENTIALITY OF MEDICAL RECORDS

All medical records maintained by the athletic trainer are confidential documents. Before these records are released to an outside individual (for example, a doctor, college recruiter, or professional scout), written permission must be obtained from the athlete explicitly stating to whom the information is being released and for what purpose it will be used (Fig. 7–2). Additionally, if this information is being released for an athlete potentially earning a college athletic scholarship or professional sports contract, the form should have a disclaimer stating that the information found in the medical records will be used as a part of the decision-making process and may either aid or hinder the athlete's cause.[2] If the athlete is under 18 years of age, this document must also be signed by

Table 7–5 **PURPOSE OF MEDICAL RECORDS**

Serve as a communication tool between athletic trainers and physicians
Document treatment and/or rehabilitation progression
Assist in the continuity of care given
Provide a basis for developing future treatment and/or rehabilitation plans
Serve as a legal document to show that the medical staff provided reasonable care
Provide a data base for research

NATIONAL FOOTBALL LEAGUE
PROFESSIONAL ATHLETIC TRAINERS SOCIETY

MEDICAL AND INJURY HISTORY QUESTIONNAIRE

Player's Name _____   School _____

Athletic Trainer _____   Office Phone _____

Team Physician _____   Office Phone _____

RELEASE OF INFORMATION AUTHORIZATION

    I,_____ give my consent for the team physician,
                  (PLAYER'S NAME)

athletic trainers, or other medical personnel of _____to release such
                                            (NAME OF SCHOOL)

information regarding my medical history, record of injury, record of serious illness,·

and rehabilitation results as may be requested by a representative of the National

Football League, any National Football League team's medical staff, National Football

Scouting, Inc., Blesto, Inc. or National Invitational Camp, Inc.

    I understand that such representative has made representations to the team

physician, athletic trainers, or other medical personnel of_____
                                            (NAME OF SCHOOL)

that the purpose of this request for my medical information is to assist that organization

represented in making a determination as to offering me employment.

    This information is normally confidential and, except as provided in this Release,

will not be otherwise released by any of the parties in charge of the information. This

release remains valid until revoked by me in writing.

_____   _____
      (PLAYER'S SIGNATURE)   (DATE)

Figure 7–2. Release of medical information permission form. If the athlete is under the age of 18, this form would require the signature of the athlete's parents or guardian. (From The Professional Football Athletic Trainers' Society, with permission.)

the athlete's parents or *legal guardian*. Athletes under 18 years of age cannot legally waive any rights. Accordingly, the athlete's waiver is of no legal significance unless it is signed by the parents.

The ideal operating procedure is to have the athlete (and parents, if applicable) sign an authorization form each time the records are released. This procedure provides a paper trail indicating that the athlete was aware of when, and to whom, the records were released. An alternative method would be to have the athlete sign an authorization form at the beginning of each season. In this scenario, the athletic trainer should note to whom the information was released, and for what purpose it was used.

The athlete should be allowed to review his or her medical records on request.[1] Any time a copy of the athlete's medical records is removed from the athletic training room, the date the records were sent, the purpose of the release, and the date of return should be documented.

Storage of Medical Records

Medical records must be maintained throughout the athlete's career and/or *matriculation*. Records of current athletes should be stored in a manner that makes them easily accessible to the athletic training staff and team physicians, yet protects them from unauthorized access. With these criteria in mind, the logical place to store current records would be in the athletic trainer's office or physician's examining room. Storage of records in the public portion of the athletic training room is not recommended unless the information is kept under lock and key.

Upon the athlete's graduation, or from the time when the athlete is no longer participating in athletics, the records must be stored until the state's *statute of limitation* expires. These records should be stored in a logical manner (such as by the year of graduation) in a cool, dry environment that is relatively safe from environmental influences such as floods or leaky roofs. As with current medical records, "dead files" should be stored in a secure area with limited access. The decision of when to destroy medical records is based on both the state's statute of limitations and the policy of the individual institution as determined by an attorney.

COMPUTERIZATION OF MEDICAL RECORDS

Once a novelty in the athletic training room, computers are rapidly becoming an indispensable item. In addition to serving as a data reduction device for isokinetic units, word processors for correspondence, and spreadsheets for inventory control, computers are also beginning to serve a major role in the management of medical records. Either with desktop personal computers or

---

Legal Guardian: An individual who is legally responsible for the care of an infant or minor.
Matriculation: The time spent in a college or university pursuing a degree.
Statute of Limitations: A legal time limit allowed for the filing of a lawsuit.

centralized *mainframe computers*, the record-keeping process is expedited by the rapid entry and recall of data.

A single piece of technology has been able to tie the various functions and advantages of comprehensive medical record keeping together into a single unit. Besides simply keeping track of individual pieces of information, most computer record-keeping software can produce information such as injury frequency statistics and modality usage. Such records can assist the athletic trainer in obtaining equipment, supplies, and additional personnel by substantiating the amount of service provided by the athletic training staff.

Several methods can be used to develop a computer-based medical records system. Individual institutions may develop customized systems using various data-base software packages or commercially prepared injury-reporting programs (Fig. 7–3). Each option has its inherent advantages and disadvantages. If an institution develops a system from scratch, it will meet the exact needs of the athletic training staff. However, programming such a system generally requires the assistance of a computer programmer or someone experienced in this area, and can prove to be a time-consuming process. If a preprogrammed injury-reporting program is purchased, it may be immediately ready for use, but the institution is limited to the reporting constraints of the software.

In general, computers provide an efficient manner of storing and retrieving large amounts of information; but computers are not without their perils. As with paper records, the confidentiality of the records must be maintained.

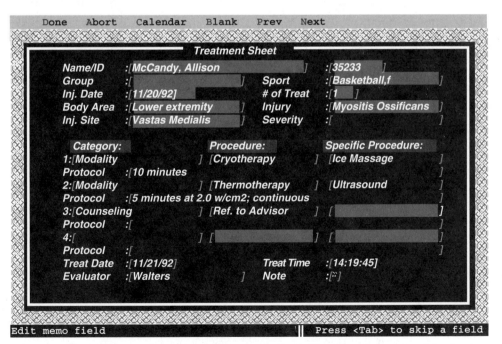

Figure 7–3. A computer-based treatment record. (SportsWare™ courtesy of Computer Sports Medicine, Inc., Waltham, MA.)

Mainframe Computer: A centrally located computer that serves a large number of remote terminals.

Computer-based records should be protected from unauthorized access through password or *turnkey systems*. The second peril is unique to computers. A spilled cup of coffee, a misplaced diskette, or a "crashed" hard disk can lead to the immediate loss of a large amount of data. For this reason, regular backups and *hard copies* should be made of all medical records stored on the computer. This may be accomplished through the use of multiple floppy disks or tape backups.

Certainly the future holds some exciting options for the use of computers in athletic training. With the development of *CD-ROM*, optical scanners, and voice-recognition systems, the total record-keeping system will someday be entirely computer based. With these pieces of technology, doctor's notes, *magnetic resonance images* (MRIs), and even video images of game or practice footage displaying the mechanism of the injury, or segments of the surgery video, can be entered into the athlete's computer record.

DOCUMENTATION

The complete process of record keeping is beyond the scope of this text. However, certain documents within the record-keeping system directly relate to the athletic trainer's application and evaluation of the effectiveness of therapeutic modalities.

Chapter 6 dealt with the problem-solving approach in the application of therapeutic modalities. The purpose of this section is to detail the legal requirements of the record-keeping process with the problem-solving approach in mind. Appendix C presents accepted medical shorthand that assists in record keeping.

Medical History and Preparticipation Physical Examination

In addition to identifying pre-existing injuries and evaluating conditions that predispose the athlete to new injuries, the athlete's **medical history** should identify conditions that contraindicate the use of certain therapeutic modalities. The information gained through the medical history should be annually updated through the **preparticipation physical examination**. Obvious examples of this type of information could be cold allergy or circulatory insufficiency. Other less obvious details could be that the athlete is taking tetracycline, which may decrease the athlete's tolerance to laser or infrared therapy.

Turnkey System: A system designed to prevent unauthorized access. Some software packages require that a specially coded floppy disk be inserted before the user can gain access to the program or copy data.

Hard Copy: A printed version of computer data.

CD-ROM: Compact disc—read only memory. A device that reads computer data through the use of lasers.

Magnetic Resonance Image (MRI): A view of the body's internal structures obtained through the use of magnetic and radio fields.

Consent Forms

This form is designed to prevent the charge of battery being brought upon the medical staff, by providing documentation that authorizes the athletic training staff to treat the athlete's injuries. If the athlete is under 18 years of age, this form must also be signed by the athlete's parent or legal guardian.

The consent form is not comprehensive. For example, an additional consent form is required before an athlete undergoes surgery. Additionally, athletes still possess the legal right to refuse treatment.

Although the consent form is designed to provide the athletic trainer with immunity from charges of battery, it does not provide protection from negligence or malpractice because this right cannot be waived prior to the act being committed. The athletic trainer still must provide assurance that the modality is being properly applied at the appropriate phase in the healing process.

Injury Reports

The purpose of the initial injury report is to describe the injury or illness suffered by the athlete. The content of this report should be sufficiently detailed so that the physician or athletic training staff can read it and gain a firm understanding of the athlete's condition. The basic elements of an athletic injury report are presented in Table 7–6. The scope of this report may be expanded, depending on the information required by individual leagues, states, institutions, or insurance companies.

A common question raised is, "What injuries should be documented?" Unfortunately, there is no common answer. Standards could include: (1) any injury or illness that alters the athlete's daily activity, (2) an injury or illness that requires evaluation by an athletic trainer or physician, (3) any condition that requires extraordinary attention. Each institution should use standardized criteria in determining which injuries are considered reportable to ensure standardization of reports.

Items related to the injury report, such as physician referrals, surgical notes, and the treatment and rehabilitation progression should be linked to the initial injury report. The injury report should be signed by the athletic trainer and, if applicable, the team physician. Each subsequent entry should be signed and dated.

Table 7–6 **COMPONENTS OF AN ATHLETIC INJURY REPORT**

Who:	In addition to the athlete's name, a form of permanent identification such as the student ID number or social security number should be used.
When:	The date that the injury occurred. Also, the dates of any subsequent referrals should be noted.
Where:	The place, sport, and activity that the athlete was involved in at the time of the injury. An injury report should also be filed for injuries or illnesses not related to athletics.
What:	The specific injury suffered by the athlete, including the specific structures traumatized. This document should contain both the **athletic trainer's evaluation** and the **physician's diagnosis** of the injury. The injury report must also describe how the injury was initially and subsequently managed.
How:	The mechanism of injury and any predisposing factors leading to the onset of injury.
Why:	While the remaining components of this list are subjective, explaining why an injury occurred is an objective determination.

Referral Forms

The use of a referral form allows for feedback from the physician regarding the athlete's participation status and treatment prescription.[9] When matched with the treatment and rehabilitation records, this document can provide proof that the athletic trainer was meeting the prescribed treatment protocol.

Treatment and/or Rehabilitation Records

All treatments given by the athletic training staff should be documented in the athlete's medical files. These treatments may be classified as being either therapeutic or prophylactic. Therapeutic treatments are given for an existing injury, as a part of the rehabilitation process. Prophylactic treatments are given to minimize accumulation of microtrauma, such as ice packs being applied to a pitcher's shoulder following practice.

Therapeutic treatments are related to the initial and follow-up injury reports and should reflect the plans established through the problem-solving approach (Chapter 6). The information that should be collected in the treatment record is presented in Table 7–7. This documentation should be complete so that the effectiveness of the treatment plan can be evaluated. Additionally, the treatment records should show not only compliance with the treatment plan, but also noncompliance. Any missed treatment session should be noted in the athlete's record.

Facilities

The design of the athletic training facility must guarantee that athletes receive treatment in the safest environment possible. Ensuring safety is an ongoing process involving thorough planning, evaluation, and maintenance. Injury sustained through improper or unsafe facilities can result in charges of negligence being brought against the athletic training staff and the institution.

ELECTRICAL SAFETY

In the athletic training room, athletes are exposed to both electricity and water. When used in the proper manner, this combination can produce many therapeutic effects. However, electricity is an inherently dangerous form of energy, and the presence of water increases the potential for harm so that, as previously discussed, great care in the application of these devices must be taken to reduce liability exposure.

Table 7–7 **CONTENT OF A TREATMENT RECORD**

Athlete's name and identification number
The injury being treated
The date of the injury
The date and time of the treatment
The physical agents used in the treatment
The duration and parameters used with the modality (e.g., continuous ultrasound, 1.0 W/cm² for 5 minutes to the lateral epicondyle)
Any pertinent comments regarding the effectiveness of the treatment

Table 7–8 **CONSIDERATIONS FOR ELECTRICAL SAFETY**

All electrical modalities should be connected to a ground fault interrupter. Whirlpools and Jacuzzis must be connected to these devices.

Athletes must not turn whirlpools on or off while they are in the water. Ideally, the switches should be located so that they cannot be reached from the whirlpool.

Conduct annual inspections of electrical modalities to ensure that the current leakage is within acceptable levels.

There are several design considerations that must be addressed to ensure the safe operation of an athletic training facility, especially in the hydrotherapy area (Table 7–8). Failure to meet safety guidelines could result in the athletic trainer and the institution being found guilty of negligence.

Electrical current flow occurs because electrons are attempting to move from an area of high concentration to an area of low concentration. Always seeking the course of least resistance, the current tends to stay within the insulation of the path formed by the circuit. Despite the precautions used, and the quality of the manufacturing, some current leakage inevitably occurs within the unit. As a result of condensation, microscopic imperfections in the circuitry, or even dust, electrons can create their own path from the intended circuit to the *chassis*.

If you will recall the schematic diagram of an alternating current (see Fig. 4–4), only two leads are required to complete an electrical current. However, most outlets contain a third conductor that leads to a **ground**. As the name describes, the ground wire literally leads to the ground (or earth) through a rod buried in the soil or through the plumbing. Normally when current leaks into the chassis, it will follow the ground wire and return to the earth undetected.

If the unit is not properly grounded (for example, if the ground prong is removed from the plug), any leaked current must find an alternate route back to the ground. This alternate route can easily be formed by a person touching an ungrounded unit and grounded device at the same time, forming a **ground fault** (Fig. 7–4). In this case the current would leak from the chassis of the ungrounded device and flow through the person to the ground, as, for example, with an athlete sitting in a whirlpool that is not properly grounded. If, while in contact with the whirlpool, the athlete touches the faucet to add more water, a ground fault can be established between the whirlpool, the athlete, and the grounded plumbing system.

Ground Fault Interrupters

Because of the way in which electricity is used in the athletic training room, added precautions must be taken to assure the safety of the athletes and the operators. **Ground fault interrupters** (GFIs or GFCIs for ground fault circuit interrupters) are used to guard against hazardous currents by continuously monitoring the amount of current entering a circuit compared with the amount of current leaving it. If there is a discrepancy of more than 5 milliamperes, a ground fault has been detected and the GFI will terminate the flow of electricity to the unit in as little as 1/40 of a second.[10]

Ground fault interrupters must be distinguished from standard circuit

---

Chassis: The framework to which electronic components are attached.

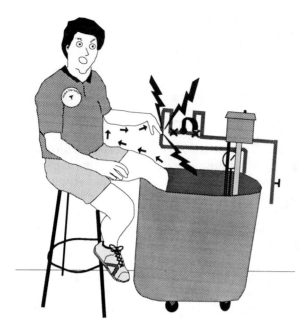

Figure 7–4.   A hazardous ground fault. If a fault occurs in an improperly grounded whirlpool, a path to the ground can be formed by the athlete touching plumbing. A ground fault interrupter would break the circuit before the current could cause harm to the athlete.

breakers. While GFIs stop the current flow at very low amperages, standard circuit breakers require a much larger discrepancy (up to 25 A) to be activated. This amount of amperage is quite sufficient to cause bodily harm to a person who comes in contact with it. Circuit breakers are not adequate for use in high-risk areas such as the athletic training room. The 1991 National Electric Code requires the use of GFIs in all health care facilities that use therapeutic pools.[11]

Ground fault interrupters may be housed in either the wall outlet or in the circuit breaker box. In either case, GFIs are easily recognizable by their TEST and RESET buttons (Fig. 7–5). Each GFI should be tested at regular intervals, with monthly intervals being considered ideal. Each testing date should be documented.

In the event that the GFI trips itself, disconnect the athlete from the unit,

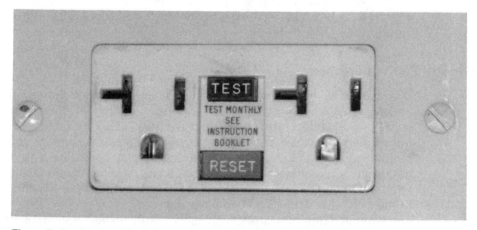

Figure 7–5.   A ground fault interrupter mounted in a standard outlet. Note that some ground fault interrupters may be mounted in the circuit breaker box. These devices should be tested at regular intervals.

and turn the power to the unit off. Check all connections and assure that a ground fault did not occur. Depress the RESET button on the GFI and reinitiate the treatment. If the GFI trips again, disconnect the unit and call for service.

Hydrotherapy Area

Of special safety concern is the hydrotherapy section of the athletic training room. It is here, perhaps more than in any other portion of the facility, that the greatest potential hazards exist. Of foremost concern is electrical safety. As described previously, all whirlpools (or similar devices) must be connected to a certified ground fault interrupter.

Ideally, the ON/OFF switches controlling the whirlpool motors should be located so that they cannot be reached by an athlete who is in the tub. If the whirlpool has this switch mounted on the motor, athletes are not to turn the unit on or off while in the water. It is a good practice to post signs stating rules for the use of these devices in the hydrotherapy area.

Whirlpool outlets should be located high enough above the floor to avoid any accidental contact with water. Likewise, whirlpool cords should be secured so that they do not touch the floor.

The hydrotherapy area itself should be in full view of the athletic training staff. Because of the noise associated with this modality, this area is normally "glassed off" from the rest of the athletic training room. The floor should be made of a nonslip surface and should be gently sloped towards one or more floor drains.

Operational Plans

Each institution should develop a policy and procedure manual that describes how the athletic training program will be administered. Such a document will reinforce the decision-making process and establish an orderly line of communication. When written rules are developed, their enforcement becomes easier because all parties know what the procedures are. However, failure to follow established guidelines also creates an area of additional legal exposure.

STANDARD OPERATING PROCEDURES

The standard operating procedures (SOP) should define the duties and function of each member of the athletic training and/or sports medicine staff. Job descriptions and an organizational chart should clarify the chain of command between individuals and departments (Fig. 7–6).

Standard operating procedures covers all facets of the athletic training program, including preseason physical examinations, insurance payments, communication with physicians and coaches, and emergency procedures. Of special concern in the treatment of athletic injuries are **standing orders**.

Serving as a "blanket prescription," standing orders describe the protocol to be used in the management of an injury before the athlete is seen by a physician. These orders may be further expanded to detail the sequence and methods to be used during the long-term treatment and rehabilitation process. In essence, these procedures recognize that the physician will not be present

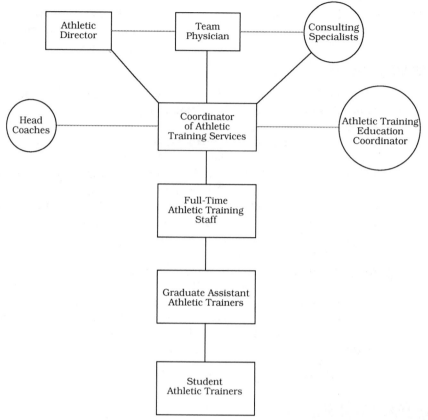

Figure 7–6. **An organizational chart**. Such a schematic describes the chain of command in providing athletic training services.

when every injury occurs and will not be in daily contact with the injured athlete. Standing orders may be superseded by the physician's specific treatment and rehabilitation orders.

PRODUCT MAINTENANCE

Knowingly using an unsafe therapeutic modality reflects negligent behavior on the part of the athletic trainer. All therapeutic equipment should be inspected and calibrated by a qualified service technician at the intervals recommended by the manufacturer, with these inspections documented on the unit. This process should become a part of the yearly operation of the athletic training program.

Proper care is the primary element in assuring the safe condition of equipment. Wear and tear of equipment through normal use is to be expected, and proper treatment of the equipment will keep this to a minimum. Logical precautions, such as avoiding spills into the equipment, proper positioning of electrical cords, and regular inspection of plugs, assist in maintaining the longevity of equipment.

If a defect is found in the plug or cord, the GFI continues to trip, or the unit fails to function properly, it should be unplugged and removed from the athletic training room. The unit should then be immediately serviced by a qualified technician.

BLOODBORNE PATHOGENS

The *Occupational Safety and Health Administration (OSHA)* has developed a series of rules requiring institutions to protect workers from bloodborne pathogens such as the *hepatitis B virus (HBV)* and the *human immunodeficiency virus (HIV).*[12] These rules apply to all individuals who are exposed to biological hazards, including blood, synovial fluid, and saliva, as a part of their daily routine. Employers must show evidence that several provisions have been made to protect employees from accidental contact with potential carrying agents.

The OSHA requirements mandate that each institution develop a written **exposure control plan**. The plan must consist of an exposure determination where employees in the group are classified by the risk of exposure to bloodborne pathogens. The first classification includes those job descriptions that place all employees at an exposure risk. The second classification contains those job descriptions where some, but not all, of the employees are at risk. By the nature of the athletic training profession, all practicing professionals could be considered at risk to exposure. This plan must contain a time line for implementation and must be reviewed by the institution on an annual basis. Updates must be made that reflect changes in job descriptions or revised procedures.

Athletic trainers may be exposed to bloodborne pathogens in many aspects of their daily routine. The treatment of acute injuries and postsurgical wounds, handling of mouthpieces, and handling of wound dressings all require extraordinary precautions.

To ensure the protection of the institution's employees, the employer must provide proof that safety measures are being met. Although not all-encompassing, measures that are most pertinent to athletic training include:

- **Observation of Universal Precautions**: All blood and body fluid should be treated as if it is known to be infectious. This requires that the athletic trainer take precautionary measures in the handling and cleanup of such material (Table 7–9).
- **Engineering and Work Practice Controls, Personal Protective Equipment, and Housekeeping**. The employer shall make provisions that the employees have access to, and use, protective equipment and procedures that reduce the risk of exposure. In athletic training, this may consist of the use of disposable rubber gloves, CPR mouth shields, and biohazard disposal containers. Of equal concern are uniforms, towels, and sheets that have become contaminated. Provisions must be made so that these

---

Occupational Safety and Health Administration (OSHA): A Federal agency responsible for assuring safe working conditions. This agency has enforcement powers and is capable of levying fines against employers.

Hepatitis B Virus (HBV): A virus that results in inflammation of the liver. Following a 2- to 6-week incubation period symptoms develop which include gastrointestinal and respiratory disturbances, jaundice, enlarged liver, muscle pain, and loss of weight.

Human Immunodeficiency Virus (HIV): The virus that causes acquired immune deficiency syndrome (AIDS).

Table 7–9 **UNIVERSAL PRECAUTIONS AGAINST BLOODBORNE PATHOGENS**

Protect skin and mucous membranes against blood and other fluids through the use of a barrier membrane such as rubber gloves.

If the skin comes into contact with a potential carrying agent, immediately wash the area with soap and water.

Contaminated surfaces, such as tables and countertops, should be cleansed with a 1:10 mixture of household bleach and water.

Dispose of all used needles in a proper manner.

Staff members who have open, draining sores or skin lesions should refrain from direct patient care until the condition clears.

Soiled linen or uniforms should be bagged and washed in hot water and detergent.

Source: Adapted from: Bloodborne pathogens: Rules and regulations. Federal Register 56:64175, 1991.

items are handled in a safe manner. Ideally, these items are washed separately.

- **Evaluation of Accidental Incidents of Exposure**. This is necessary when an athlete's bodily fluids come into contact with the athletic trainer's (or other employee's) eyes, mouth, broken skin, or other areas which may act as routes of infection. The goal of this process is to identify situations where accidental exposure occurs and institute plans to prevent their recurrence.

- **Implementation of an Employee Training Program**. This training program covers the content described by the OSHA standard. A training session is required for all workers who may come into contact with bloodborne pathogens prior to the time the employee is assigned to tasks where contact may occur. This means that student athletic trainers should undergo an in-service program prior to covering a sport or working in the athletic training room.

- **Long-term Record Keeping**. Employers must maintain records of employees who have occupational exposure to bloodborne pathogens. These records must contain records of the employee's vaccination status and postexposure follow-up examinations. These records are confidential and must be kept for 30 years after the employee leaves the company.

Summary

While the practice of athletic training contains many inherent risks, both legal and physical, the risks can be reduced through the proper management of the athletic training facility. Athletic trainers must work within the scope of the athletic training regulations of their state, stay educated and current in the use of therapeutic modalities, and be familiar with the legal aspects of health care.

Medical records should be maintained that will describe exactly how an athlete's injury was managed for future reference. The preparticipation medical exam, injury report, referral notes, and treatment and rehabilitation records should be meticulously maintained. The information from these records will not only assist the athletic trainer in the court of law, but will also provide useful information in evaluating the rehabilitation plan.

Each institution should develop and follow a policy and procedure manual that explicitly describes the duties of each member of the athletic training staff. Additionally, standard operating procedures should describe how injuries are to be managed in the team physician's absence. The safety of the athletes, as well as the athletic staff, must be assured through proper maintenance of equipment and protection against bloodborne pathogens.

The development of such a plan is not an overnight process. The policies and procedures should be continuously monitored and changes should be made when needed. Although there are no guarantees against liability, the identification of risk, and the development of plans, as well as common sense, all make the athletic training room a safer place to work.

CHAPTER QUIZ

. . . .

1. Precedents influence the rulings in certain court cases. In which of the following types of law do precedents have the strongest influence?
   A. Common law
   B. Statutory law
   C. Contract law
   D. Tort law

2. The type of law that must be initiated, amended or repealed by action of the state or federal legislature is:
   A. Common law
   B. Statutory law
   C. Contract law
   D. Tort law

3. If a student athletic trainer commits an act of negligence, the supervising athletic trainer could also be held liable under the doctrine of:
   A. Consensual touching
   B. Misfeasance
   C. Vicarious liability
   D. Contributory negligence

4. A consent to treatment form must be obtained from each athlete at the start of the season to prevent the charge of _____ from being brought against the athletic training staff.
   A. Negligence
   B. Malpractice
   C. Battery
   D. Slander

5. The failure of an athletic trainer to respond to an injury situation could be classified as:
   A. Omission
   B. Commission
   C. Malfeasance
   D. Misfeasance

6. The application of continuous ultrasound over the site of infection could be ruled a negligent act because it is potentially an act of:
   A. Malfeasance
   B. Misfeasance
   C. Nonfeasance
   D. Omission

REFERENCES

1. Hunter-Griffin, L: Athletic Training and Sports Medicine. Park Ridge, IL. The American Academy of Orthopaedic Surgeons, 1991, pp 40–67.
2. Drowatzky, JN: Legal duties and liability in athletic training. Athletic Training 20:10, 1985.
3. Leverenz, LJ and Helms, LB: Suing athletic trainers, I: A review of case law involving athletic trainers. Athletic Training 25:212, 1990.
4. Pozgar, GD: Legal Aspects of Health Care Administration, ed 3. Aspen Publications, Rockville, MD, 1987, pp 11–21.
5. Gieck, J, Lowe, J, and Kenna, K: Trainer malpractice: A sleeping giant. Athletic Training 19:41, 1984.
6. Morin, GE: An overview of selected state licensure athletic training laws. Athletic Training 27:162, 1992.
7. Governmental Affairs, NATA NEWS, 4:21, 1992.
8. Pozgar, GD: Legal Aspects of Health Care Administration, ed 3. Aspen Publications, Rockville, MD, 1987, p 216.
9. Gabriel, AJ: Medical communications—records for the professional athletic trainer. Athletic Training 16:68, 1981.
10. Porter, MM and Porter, JW: Electrical safety in the training room. Athletic Training 16, 1981.
11. Therapeutic pools and tubs in health care facilities. In: National Electric Code. National Fire Protection Association, Quincy, MA, 1991.
12. Bloodborne pathogens: Rules and regulations. Federal Register 56:64175, 1991.

Answers to Chapter Quizzes

· ·

Chapter 1

MULTIPLE CHOICE:

1. B	8. B
2. B	9. C
3. A	10. C
4. A	11. C
5. D	12. A
6. D	13. A
7. C	14. C

15. A: Mechanical deformation
    B: Chemical irritation

16.
Sign	Event
Heat	Increased blood flow; increase in rate of cell metabolism
Redness	Same as heat
Swelling	High concentration of proteins, gamma globulins, fibrinogen; leakage of fluids into the extracellular space
Pain	Mechanical and chemical irritation of nerve endings
Loss of function	Long-term result of the first four signs

17. Chemotaxis
18. Muscle contractions squeeze fluids up the venous return system.
    Respiration has a dual effect of squeezing the fluids and creating a siphon.
    Gravity influences fluids downward.
    The use of compression and elevation assist this process.
    Proteins can only be removed through the lymphatic system.

19. The list of valid responses is endless. Your answer should fit into one of the following categories:
    • Provide psychological comfort
    • Provide a distraction from the pain (talking, etc.)

Chapter 2

MULTIPLE CHOICE:

1. E.	6. D.
2. D.	7. B.
3. A.	8. B.
4. A.	9. C.
5. B.	10. D.

Chapter 3

MULTIPLE CHOICE:

1. B	4. D
2. D	5. D
3. B	6. C

7. By reducing the cell's need for oxygen.

8.

Step	Effect
Rest	Prevent further physical trauma
Ice	Decrease the cells' need for oxygen
Compression	Reduce pressure gradient, reduce hemorrhage, and limit the collection of edema
Elevation	Decrease local blood pressure and encourage venous and lymphatic return

9. Cold causes a vasoconstriction that limits the amount of warm blood entering the area. Heat application encourages blood flow, and cooled blood is constantly being delivered to the area.

10. As the percentage of surface area being exposed to the water increases, the percentage of the remaining unexposed tissues decreases. Thermoregulation must occur through this unexposed tissue.

Chapter 4

MULTIPLE CHOICE:

1. C
2. A
3. C
4. A
5. D
6. C
7. D
8. B

9. D
10. C
11. B
12. D
13. A
14. D
15. A
16. B

Chapter 5

MULTIPLE CHOICE:

1. C
2. B
3. D
4. D
5. B

6. A
7. D
8. C
9. A
10. B

11. A. The position of the neck
    B. The duration of the traction
    C. The angle of pull
    D. The position of the athlete
12. A. The cervical musculature is allowed to relax.
    B. The force of gravity is eliminated.
13. A. Petrissage   kneading of the skin
    B. Tapotement   pounding of the skin
    C. Effleurage   stroking of the skin
14. When applying massage to remove edema from a limb, the strokes begin **proximally** and are progressively worked **distally**.

Chapter 7

MULTIPLE CHOICE:

1. A
2. B
3. C
4. C

5. A
6. B

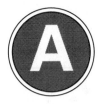

Trigger Points and Pain Patterns

∙ ∙

"Trigger points" are small areas of localized sensitivity and pain found in muscles and connective tissue. They may be produced by trauma, can be a result of chronic strain, or may be developed as a result of stress from daily activities or postural habits. Although the pain and sensitivity are localized, reports in the literature suggest that the discomfort may be referred to other parts of the body ("referred pain") through the autonomic nervous system.

These areas may be located by palpation, or with the aid of the eraser end of a pencil, or by means of electrical currents. It has been suggested that the combination of electrical stimulation and ultrasound is beneficial in both locating and treating the involved areas. A tetanizing current within the comfortable intensity range of the patient is normally used for both location and treatment, offering "massage-like" contraction to the muscles to which it is applied.[1,2] Successful treatments have been reported in both acute and chronic conditions.

Illustrations from Mettler Electronics Corporation, Anaheim, California, with permission.

REFERENCES

1. Travel, J and Rinzier, SH: The myofascial genesis of pain. Postgrad Med II(5), May, 1952.

2. Sola, AE: Myofascial trigger point pain in the neck and shoulder girdle. Northwest Medicine 54:980, 1955.

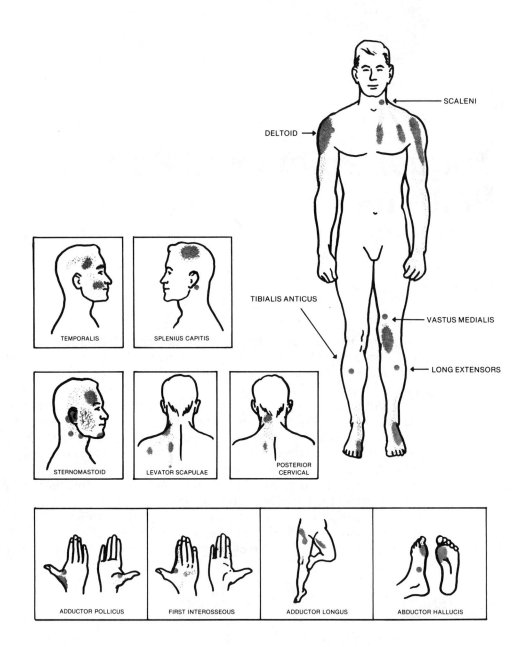

TEMPORALIS

SPLENIUS CAPITIS

STERNOMASTOID

LEVATOR SCAPULAE

POSTERIOR CERVICAL

SCALENI

DELTOID

TIBIALIS ANTICUS

VASTUS MEDIALIS

LONG EXTENSORS

ADDUCTOR POLLICUS

FIRST INTEROSSEOUS

ADDUCTOR LONGUS

ABDUCTOR HALLUCIS

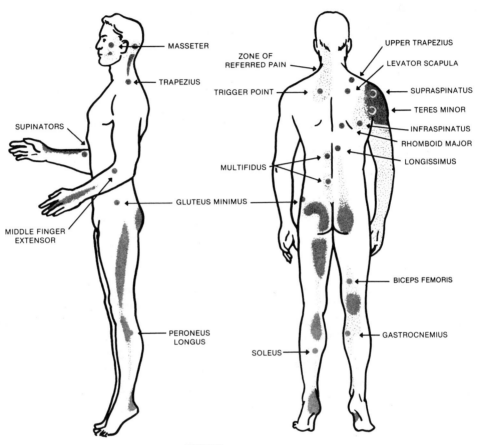

REFERENCES:
Travel, J. and Rinzier, S.H., "The Myofascial Genesis of Pain," POSTGRADUATE MEDICINE, Vol. II, No. 5, May, 1952.

Sola, A. E. "Myofascial Trigger Point Pain in the Neck and Shoulder Girdle," NORTHWEST MEDICINE, Vol. 54, pp. 980-984 September, 1955.

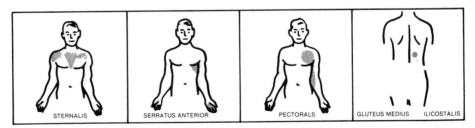

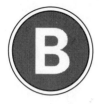

Motor Points

· ·

A motor point is the place in a muscle where the muscle is most easily excited with a minimum amount of electrical stimulation; the motor point is usually located near the center of the muscle mass, where the motor nerve enters the muscle. For each muscle, the motor point may vary from patient to patient, or even at different times for the same patient, depending on the pathology. The accompanying charts are guides to the motor points.

From Mettler Electronics Corporation, Anaheim, California, with permission.

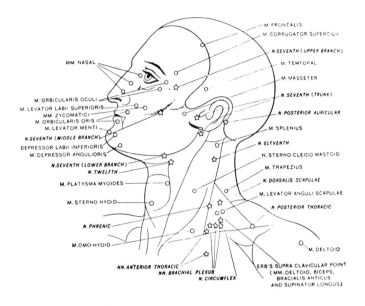

M. FRONTALIS
M. CORRUGATOR SUPERCILII
N. SEVENTH (UPPER BRANCH)
M. TEMFORAL
M. MASSETER
N. SEVENTH (TRUNK)
N. POSTERIOR AURICULAR
M. SPLENIUS
N. ELEVENTH
N. STERNO-CLEIDO-MASTOID
M. TRAPEZIUS
N. DORSALIS SCAPULAE
M. LEVATOR ANGULI SCAPULAE
N POSTERIOR THORACIC
M. DELTOID
ERB'S SUPRA CLAVICULAR POINT
(MM. DELTOID, BICEPS,
BRACIALIS ANTICUS
AND SUPINATOR LONGUS)

MM. NASAL
M. ORBICULARIS OCULI
M. LEVATOR LABII SUPERIORIS
MM. ZYCOMATICI
M. ORBICULARIS ORIS
M. LEVATOR MENTI
N. SEVENTH (MIDDLE BRANCH)
DEPRESSOR LABII INFERIORIS
M. DEPRESSOR ANGULIORIS
N. SEVENTH (LOWER BRANCH)
N. TWELFTH
M. PLATYSMA MYOIDES
M. STERNO HYOID
N. PHRENIC
M. OMO-HYOID
NN. ANTERIOR THORACIC
NN. BRACHIAL PLEXUS
N. CIRCUMFLEX

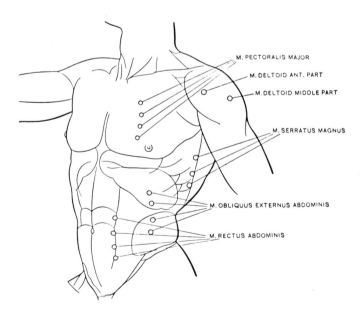

M. PECTORALIS MAJOR
M. DELTOID ANT. PART
M. DELTOID MIDDLE PART
M. SERRATUS MAGNUS
M. OBLIQUUS EXTERNUS ABDOMINIS
M. RECTUS ABDOMINIS

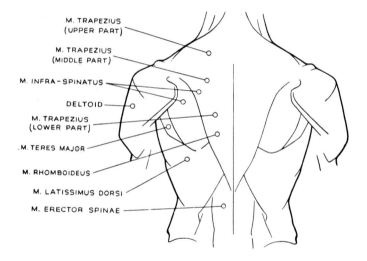

M. TRAPEZIUS
(UPPER PART)

M. TRAPEZIUS
(MIDDLE PART)

M. INFRA-SPINATUS

DELTOID

M. TRAPEZIUS
(LOWER PART)

.M. TERES MAJOR

M. RHOMBOIDEUS

M. LATISSIMUS DORSI

M. ERECTOR SPINAE

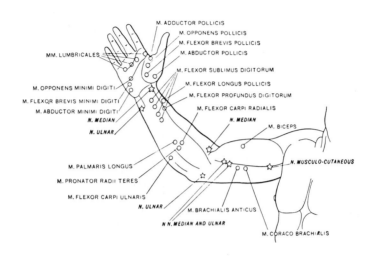

M. ADDUCTOR POLLICIS
M. OPPONENS POLLICIS
M. FLEXOR BREVIS POLLICIS
M. ABDUCTOR POLLICIS
MM. LUMBRICALES
M. FLEXOR SUBLIMUS DIGITORUM
M. FLEXOR LONGUS POLLICIS
M. OPPONENS MINIMI DIGITI
M. FLEXOR PROFUNDUS DIGITORUM
M. FLEXOR BREVIS MINIMI DIGITI
M. FLEXOR CARPI RADIALIS
M. ABDUCTOR MINIMI DIGITI
N. MEDIAN
N. MEDIAN
N. ULNAR
M. BICEPS
N. MUSCULO-CUTANEOUS
M. PALMARIS LONGUS
M. PRONATOR RADII TERES
M. FLEXOR CARPI ULNARIS
N. ULNAR
M. BRACHIALIS ANTICUS
N N. MEDIAN AND ULNAR
M. CORACO BRACHIALIS

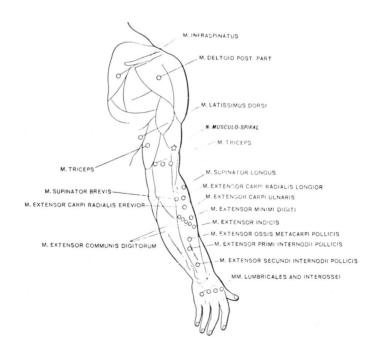

M. INFRASPINATUS
M. DELTOID POST. PART
M. LATISSIMUS DORSI
N. MUSCULO-SPIRAL
M. TRICEPS
M. TRICEPS
M. SUPINATOR LONGUS
M. EXTENSOR CARPI RADIALIS LONGIOR
M. SUPINATOR BREVIS
M. EXTENSOR CARPI ULNARIS
M. EXTENSOR CARPI RADIALIS EREVIOR
M. EXTENSOR MINIMI DIGITI
M. EXTENSOR INDICIS
M. EXTENSOR OSSIS METACARPI POLLICIS
M. EXTENSOR COMMUNIS DIGITORUM
M. EXTENSOR PRIMI INTERNODII POLLICIS
M. EXTENSOR SECUNDI INTERNODII POLLICIS
MM. LUMBRICALES AND INTEROSSEI

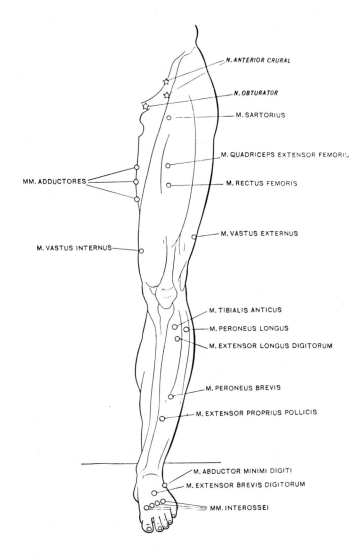

N. ANTERIOR CRURAL

N. OBTURATOR

M. SARTORIUS

M. QUADRICEPS EXTENSOR FEMORIS

M. RECTUS FEMORIS

MM. ADDUCTORES

M. VASTUS EXTERNUS

M. VASTUS INTERNUS

M. TIBIALIS ANTICUS

M. PERONEUS LONGUS

M. EXTENSOR LONGUS DIGITORUM

M. PERONEUS BREVIS

M. EXTENSOR PROPRIUS POLLICIS

M. ABDUCTOR MINIMI DIGITI

M. EXTENSOR BREVIS DIGITORUM

MM. INTEROSSEI

M = Muscle
N = Nerves

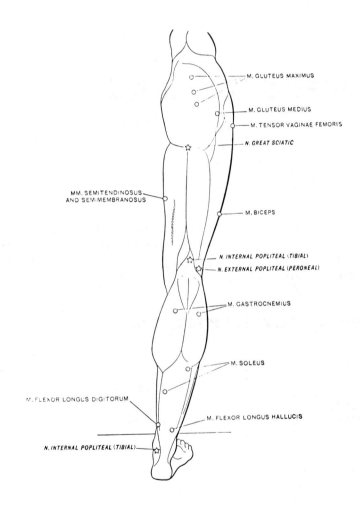

M. GLUTEUS MAXIMUS

M. GLUTEUS MEDIUS

M. TENSOR VAGINAE FEMORIS

N. GREAT SCIATIC

MM. SEMITENDINOSUS
AND SEMIMEMBRANOSUS

M. BICEPS

N. INTERNAL POPLITEAL (TIBIAL)

N. EXTERNAL POPLITEAL (PERONEAL)

M. GASTROCNEMIUS

M. SOLEUS

M. FLEXOR LONGUS DIGITORUM

M. FLEXOR LONGUS HALLUCIS

N. INTERNAL POPLITEAL (TIBIAL)

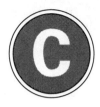

Medical Shorthand

· ·

The following is an abbreviated list of commonly accepted shorthand that may be used when documenting treatments. An excellent resource on medical note-taking and record keeping is *Writing S.O.A.P. Notes* by Ginge Kettenbach (F.A. Davis Company).

Therapeutic Modalities and/or Treatments

CWP	Cold Whirlpool
EMS	Electrical Muscle Stimulation
ES	Electrical Stimulation
HP	Hot Pack
HVPGS	High-Voltage Pulsed Electrogalvanic Stimulation
HVGS	High-Voltage Electrogalvanic Stimulation
HWP	Hot Whirlpool
I.C.E	Ice, Compression, Elevation
MENS	Microcurrent Electrical Neuromuscular Stimulation
MWD	Microwave Diathermy
RICE	Rest, Ice, Compression, Elevation
SWD	Shortwave Diathermy
TENS	Transcutaneous Electrical Nerve Stimulation
US	Ultrasound
UV	Ultraviolet
WP	Whirlpool

Dosage and/or Medication

Meds.	Medication
od	Once daily

pc	After meals
prn	Whenever necessary
q	Every
qd	Every day
qh	Every hour
qid	Four times a day
qn	Every night
tid	Three times a day
W/cm²	Watts per centimeter squared

Range of Motion and Exercise

ADL	Activities of Daily Living
AROM	Active Range of Motion
BR	Bed Rest
CWI	Crutch Walking Exercise
FWB	Full Weight Bearing
NWB	Non–Weight Bearing
PWB	Partial Weight Bearing
PNF	Proprioceptive Neuromuscular Facilitation
PRE	Progressive Resistance Exercises
PROM	Passive Range of Motion
ROM	Range of Motion
ROT	Rotate, Rotational
RROM	Resistive Range of Motion
SLR	Straight Leg Raise

Measurements and Time

+, pos.	Positive
−, neg.	Negative
<	Less than
=	Equals
>	Greater than
cm	Centimeter
F	Fair
ft.	Foot/Feet
G	Good
h, hr	Hour
hs	At bedtime
H & P	History and Physical
in.	Inch
lb.	Pounds
min.	Minutes
mo.	Month
N	Normal
P	Poor
sec.	Seconds
SOS	When necessary, if necessary
stat.	Immediately
UNK	Unknown
wk.	Week
wt.	Weight
WNL	Within Normal Limits
x	Number of times performed

y/o	Years old
yr.	Year

Body Area

Ⓛ	Left
Ⓡ	Right
ACJ	Acromioclavicular Joint
ACL	Anterior Cruciate Ligament
AIIS	Anterior Inferior Iliac Spine
AP	Anterior-Posterior
ASIS	Anterior Superior Iliac Spine
ATF	Anterior Talo-Fibular Ligament
CF	Calcaneofibular Ligament
CV	Cardiovascular
DIP	Distal Interphalangeal Joint
GH	Glenohumeral Joint
LCL	Lateral Collateral Ligament
LE	Lower Extremity
MCL	Medial Collateral Ligament
PCL	Posterior Cruciate Ligament
PIP	Proximal Interphalangeal Joint
PSIS	Posterior Superior Iliac Spine
PTF	Posterior Talo-Fibular Ligament
SCJ	Sternoclavicular Joint
UE	Upper Extremity

Personnel

DO	Doctor of Osteopathy
MD	Medical Doctor
PT	Physical Therapist/Physical Therapy
Pt., pt.	Patient

General Note Taking

$\bar{p}$	After
~	Approximately
$\bar{a}$,a	Before
Δ	Change
↓	Down, decreasing
♀	Female
♂	Male
1°	Primary
2°	Secondary
↑	Up, increasing
$\bar{c}$	With
$\bar{s}$	Without
c/o	Complains of
CC	Chief Complaint
D/C	Discontinue
Dx	Diagnosis
eval	Evaluation
Hx, hx	History

M&R	Measure and Record
P.H.	Past History
post-op	Following surgery
pre-op	Prior to surgery
R.O.	Rule Out
re:	Regarding, relating, pertaining
Rx	Treatment, prescription
Sx	Symptoms
vo	Verbal orders

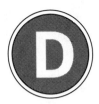

Standards for Athletic Training: Direct Service

· ·

STANDARD 1: DIRECTION

The athletic trainer renders service or treatment under the direction of a physician or dentist.

STANDARD 2: INJURY AND ONGOING CARE SERVICES

All services should be documented in writing by the athletic trainer and shall become part of the athlete's permanent records.

STANDARD 3: DOCUMENTATION

The athletic trainer shall accept responsibility for recording details of the athlete's health status. Documentation shall include:
1. Athlete's name and any other identifying information.
2. Referral source (doctor, dentist).
3. Date, initial assessment, results, and data base.
4. Program plan and estimated length.
5. Program methods, results, and revisions.

(Courtesy of the National Athletic Trainers' Association Board of Certification, Inc., Dallas, TX.)

6. Date of discontinuation and summary.
7. Athletic trainer's signature.

STANDARD 4: CONFIDENTIALITY

The athletic trainer shall maintain confidentiality as determined by law and shall accept responsibility for communicating assessment results, program plans, and progress with other persons involved in the athlete's program.

STANDARD 5: INITIAL ASSESSMENT

Prior to treatment, the athletic trainer shall assess the athlete's level of functioning. The athlete's input shall be considered an integral part of the initial assessment.

STANDARD 6: PROGRAM PLANNING

The athletic training program objectives shall include long- and short-term goals and an appraisal of those goals which the athlete can realistically be expected to achieve from the program. Assessment measures to determine effectiveness of the program shall be incorporated into the plan.

STANDARD 7: PROGRAM DISCONTINUATION

The athletic trainer, with collaboration of the physician or dentist, shall recommend discontinuation of the athletic training service when the athlete has received optimal benefit of the program. The athletic trainer, at the time of the discontinuation, shall note the final assessment of the athlete's status.

Book Glossary

· ·

A-Fibers: A class of nerves responsible for transmitting sensory impulses.

Absolute Refractory Period: Used for recharging the electrical potential, this is the period following a nerve's depolarization during which a subsequent depolarization cannot occur.

Absolute Zero: Theoretically the lowest possible temperature, equal to $-273°C$ or $-460°F$. At this point, all atomic and molecular motion ceases.

Absorption: The process of a medium collecting thermal energy and changing it to kinetic energy.

Acclimatization: The process of becoming physiologically adapted to an environment.

Accommodation: The decrease in a nerve's action potential frequency over time when exposed to an unchanging depolarization stimulus.

Acoustical Interface: A surface where two materials of different densities meet.

Acoustical Spectrum: Energy transmitted through mechanical waves.

Actin: A contractile muscle protein.

Action Potential: The change in electrical potential of a nerve or muscle fiber when stimulated.

Acupuncture Point: Points on the skin theorized to control systemic functions. These points lie along 12 main channels, 8 secondary channels, and a network of subchannels.

Acute: Of short onset. The period after an injury when the local inflammatory response is still active.

Aerobic: Requiring the presence of oxygen.

Afferent: Carrying impulses toward a central structure, for example, the brain.

Alarm Stage: First step in the general adaptation syndrome where the body readies its defensive systems.

Allograft: A replacement or augmentation of a biological structure with a synthetic one.

Alternating Current: The uninterrupted flow of electrodes marked by a change in the direction and magnitude of the movement.

Amino Acids: Building blocks of protein.

Amperage: The rate of flow of an electrical current. One ampere is equal to the rate of flow of 1 coulomb per second.

Amplitude: The maximum departure of a wave from the baseline.

Amplitude Ramp: The gradual rise or fall in amplitude of a pulse train.

Anaerobic: Able to survive in the absence of oxygen. Anaerobic systems derive their energy through the breakdown of adenosine triphosphate (ATP) into adenosine diphosphate (ADP).

Analgesia: Absence of the sense of pain.

Analgesic: A pain-reducing substance.

Analog: A readout on a continuously variable scale. A clock with hands is a type of analog display.

Anesthesia: A loss of, or decrease in, sensation.

Angstrom (Å): A distance equal to 10^{-10} meter, or one billionth of a meter.

Annulus Fibrosis: The dense, inflexible outer layering of an intervertebral disc.

Anode: The positive pole of an electrical circuit. It has a low concentration of electrons and is the opposite of the cathode.

Antibiotic: A substance that inhibits the growth of, or kills, microorganisms.

Arndt-Schultz Principle: For energy to affect the body it must be absorbed by the tissues at a level sufficient to stimulate a physiological response.

Arteriole: A small artery leading to a capillary at its distal end.

Arthroplasty: Surgical reconstruction or replacement of an articular joint.

Assault: A deliberate verbal threat accompanied by the ability to inflict physical harm to another.

Asymmetric: Lacking symmetry (e.g., two) halves are of unequal size and/or shape.

Attenuation: The decrease in a wave's intensity resulting from the absorption, reflection, and refraction of energy.

Average Current: The average amplitude of a current. When the current can be represented by a sine wave, the average current is calculated by multiplying the amplitude by 0.637.

Axon: The stem of a nerve.

Axonotmesis: Damage to nerve tissue without physical severing of the nerve.

Bacteria: A microscopic organism.

Battery: An intentional touching of another person without his or her consent.

Beam Nonuniformity Ratio (BNR): The ratio between the highest intensity in an ultrasonic beam and the output reported on the meter.

Beta-endorphin: A neurohormone similar to morphine.

Bilateral: On both sides of the body.

Biphasic Current: A pulsed current possessing two phases, each of which occurs on opposite sides of the baseline.

Bipolar Stimulation: Electrical stimulation using electrodes of equal surface area. The resultant current density under each electrode is equal.

Breach of Duty: A departure from the implied duty based on the reasonable and prudent doctrine.

C-Fibers: A class of nerves that primarily transmit pain impulses.

Calorie: The amount of energy needed to raise the temperature of 1 gram of water by 1°C.

Capacitance: The ability to store an electrical charge by means of an electrostatic field.

Capillary Filtration Pressure: The pressure that moves the contents of a capillary outwards to the tissues.

Cardinal Signs of Inflammation: Heat, redness, swelling, pain, and loss of function of the area; used as a gauge in determining the extent of the inflammatory process.

Carotid Sinus: An enlargement of the carotid artery near the branch of the internal carotid artery, located distal to the inferior arch of the mandible. Receptors at this site monitor and assist in the regulation of blood pressure.

Catalyst: A substance that accelerates a chemical reaction.

Cathode: The negative pole of an electrical circuit. It has a high concentration of electrons and carries the opposite charge to the anode.

Causation: This implies that the breach of duty directly leads to the suffering of harm by an individual.

Cavitation: The formation of microscopic bubbles. It occurs during ultrasound application.

CD-ROM: Compact disc—read only memory. A device that reads computer data through the use of lasers.

Certification (Athletic Training): Indicates that an individual has met the minimal criteria on a three-part examination. It is granted by the National Athletic Trainers' Association Board of Certification, Inc.

Change of State: Transformation from one physical state to another (e.g., ice to water).

Channel (Electrical): An electrical circuit, consisting of two poles, that operates independently of other circuits.

Chassis: The framework to which electronic components are attached.

Chemosensitive Receptors: Nerves that are excited by chemical stimulation.

Chemotaxis: Movement of living protoplasm toward or away from a chemical stimulus.

Chronic: Continuing for a long period; with injury, extending past the primary hemorrhage and inflammation cycle.

Circumferential Compression: Compression applied in a manner that provides an even pressure around the circumference of the body part.

Coagulation: The process of blood clotting.

Cold-induced Vasodilation: An unsubstantiated theory suggesting that cold application results in a net increase in the cross-sectional size of blood vessels.

Collagen: A protein-based connective tissue.

Collateral Compression: A form of compression that provides pressure on only two sides of the body part.

Collimated: Possessing a beam of parallel rays or waves which form a column of energy.

Commission: Response to a situation in a manner that is not reasonable and prudent.

Compartment Syndrome: A condition where nerves, blood vessels, or tendons are constricted within a confined space (e.g., the anterior compartment of the lower leg).

Compression: An external force applied to the

body (e.g., an elastic wrap) that serves to decrease the pressure gradient between the blood vessels and tissue.

Conduction (Thermal): Transfer of heat between two touching bodies.

Conductor (Electrical): A material having the ability to transmit electricity. Conductors have many free electrons and provide relatively little resistance to electrical flow. Within the body, tissues having a high water content are considered to be conductors.

Connective Tissue: Supports and connects other tissue types.

Consensual Touching: The person being touched has agreed to be touched. Consensual agreements negate the charge of battery.

Constructive Interference: Two waves that are perfectly synchronized combine to produce a single wave of greater amplitude.

Continuous Interference: Two waves slightly out of phase interact to produce a single wave whose amplitude and/or frequency varies.

Contracture: A condition resulting from the loss of a tissue's ability to lengthen.

Contraindicate: To make inadvisable.

Contralateral: Pertaining to the opposite side of the body. The left side is contralateral to the right.

Convection: The cooling of one object and the subsequent heating of another by the circulation of a fluid, usually air or water.

Convergent: Tending toward a common point, as when two input routes are reduced to one output route.

Conversion: Transformation of high-frequency electrical or mechanical energy into heat.

Cortisol: A cortisonelike substance produced in the body.

Cosine Law: As an angle deviates away from 90 degrees, the effective energy is reduced by the multiple of the cosine of the angle: Effective energy = Energy × Cosine of the angle. A deviation of ± 10 degrees is considered to be within acceptable limits for therapeutic treatments.

Coulomb: The net charge produced by 6.25 × 10^{18} electrons.

Coulomb's Law: Like charges repel and unlike charges attract.

Counterirritant: A substance causing irritation of superficial sensory nerves so as to reduce the transmission of pain from underlying nerves.

Cryokinetics: The use of cold modalities to improve a joint's range of motion through decreasing the element of pain.

Cryotherapy: The application of therapeutic cold agents to living tissue.

Cyanosis (Cyanotic): A blue-gray discoloration of the skin caused by a lack of oxygen.

Defamation of Character: Communication to a third party of information that causes harm to an individual.

Dendrite: Synaptic connections of a nerve arising from the body (soma).

Denervation: Lack of a proper nerve supply to, for example, an area or muscle group.

Dependent Position: An arrangement where the body part is placed lower than the heart, increasing the intravascular pressure.

Dermal Ulcer: A slow-healing, or nonhealing, break in the skin.

Dermatome: A segmental skin area supplied by a single nerve root.

Destructive Interference: Two waves that are exactly out of phase interact so as to cancel each other out.

Diagnosis: A physician's determination of the nature and scope of an injury or illness.

Diastolic Blood Pressure: The lowest level of pressure in the arteries. For example, when a blood pressure reading is given as 120/80, 80 represents the diastolic value.

Diathermy: A classification of therapeutic modality that uses magnetic fields to heat subcutaneous tissues.

Dipole: A pair of equal and opposite charges separated by a distance.

Direct Current: The uninterrupted flow of electrons in a single direction.

Divergence: The spreading of a beam or wave.

Doctrine: A statement of fundamental government policy.

Due Care: An established responsibility for an individual to respond to a given situation.

Duty Cycle: The ratio between the pulse duration and the pulse interval: Duty cycle = Pulse duration / (Pulse duration + Pulse interval).

Dynamometer: A device used for measuring muscular strength.

Ecchymosis: A blue-black discoloration of the skin caused by movement of blood into the tissues. In the latter stages, the color may appear as a greenish-brown or yellow.

Edema: An excessive accumulation of serous fluids.

Effective Radiating Area (ERA): The portion of

a transducer's surface that emits ultrasonic energy.

Efferent: Carrying impulses away from a central structure. Nerves leaving the central nervous system are efferent nerves.

Efficacy: The ability of a modality or treatment regime to produce the intended effects.

Electromagnetic Field: The lines of force created by positive and negative poles.

Electromagnetic Radiation: Energy found on the electromagnetic spectrum capable of traveling at the speed of light and exhibiting both electrical and magnetic properties.

Electromagnetic Spectrum: A continuum ordered by the wavelength or frequency of energy produced.

Electromyogram: A recording of the electrical charges associated with the contraction of a muscle.

Electron: A negatively charged atomic particle.

Electro-osmotic: Pertaining to the movement of ions as a result of electrical charges. Positive ions moving away from the positive pole toward the negative pole; negative ions moving away from the negative pole toward the positive pole.

Electrostatic Field: A field created by static electricity.

Endogenous Opiates: Pain-inhibiting substances produced in the brain. These include endorphins and enkephalins.

Endorphin: A morphinelike substance produced by the body. Endorphins are thought to increase the pain threshold by binding to receptor sites.

Endothelial Cells: Flat cells lining the blood and lymphatic vessels, and the heart.

Enkephalin: A substance released by the body which reduces the perception of pain by bonding to pain receptor sites.

Epiphyseal Plates: Growth plates of bones.

Epithelial Tissue: Tissue that forms the outer skin and lines the body's cavities. This type of tissue has a high potential to regenerate.

Ergometer: A device used to measure the amount of work performed by the legs or arms.

Evaluation: The athletic trainer's impression of the nature and scope of an injury.

Evaporation: The change of state from a liquid to a gas.

Exhaustion Stage: The third and final stage in the general adaptation syndrome. It is during this stage that cell death occurs.

External Fixation: A fracture-setting technique incorporating the use of metal rods that extend through the skin and are attached to a device outside of the body.

Extracellular: Outside the cell membrane.

Exudate: Fluid that collects in a cavity and has a high concentration of cells, protein, and other solid matter.

False Imprisonment: Unlawful keeping of a person by either physical or psychological force.

Far Infrared: The portion of infrared light located between 1,500 and 12,500 nm.

Far Ultraviolet: The portion of ultraviolet light located between 180 and 290 nm.

Farad: A measure of the storage capability of capacitors. One farad stores a charge of 1 coulomb when 1 volt is applied.

Fibrin: A filamentous protein formed by the action of thrombin on fibrinogen.

Fibrinogen: A protein present in the blood plasma and essential for the clotting of blood.

Fibrosis: An abnormally large formation of inelastic fibrous tissue.

Fibrositis: Inflammation of connective tissue. Most commonly occurring in muscular tissue.

Flux: A residual electromagnetic field created by two unlike charges.

Focal Compression: Applies direct pressure to soft tissue surrounded by prominent structures.

Foramen: An opening (e.g., in a bone) to allow the passage of blood vessels or nerves.

Fraud: Intentional misrepresentation of oneself and/or one's credentials.

Frequency: The number of times an event occurs in one second; measured in Hertz, cycles per second, or pulses per second.

Galvanic Current: An uninterrupted low-voltage direct current.

Galvanic Effect: The migration of ions as the result of the application of an uninterrupted low-voltage direct current.

Gamma Globulin: An infection-fighting blood protein.

General Adaptation Syndrome: A theory stating that the body has a common mechanism for adapting to stress. The three stages of this response are alarm, resistance, and exhaustion.

Golgi Tendon Organ: A sensory nerve ending found in tendons and aponeuroses.

Granulation Tissue: A delicate tissue composed of fibroblasts, collagen, and capillaries formed during the revascularization phase of wound healing.

Granuloma: A hard mass of fibrous tissue.

Gross Negligence: The total failure to provide

what would normally be deemed proper in a given situation.

Grotthus-Draper, Law of: There is an inverse relationship between the amount of penetration and absorption. The more energy that is absorbed by the superficial tissues, the less that remains to be transmitted to underlying tissues.

Ground: An electrical connection that provides a path for leaked current to safely return to the earth.

Ground Fault: A disruption in the normal electrical circuitry where the current exits from the normal circuit.

Ground Fault Interrupter: Discontinues the current flow when a ground fault is detected.

Habituation: A function of the central nervous system that filters out nonmeaningful information.

Hard Copy: A printed version of computer data.

Harm: Legally, harm suffered by a person includes physical injury, mental anguish, or financial loss.

Hematoma: A mass of blood confined to a limited area, resulting from the subcutaneous leakage of blood.

Hemorrhage: Bleeding from veins, arteries, or capillaries.

Henry: A measure of inductance. One henry induces an electromagnetic force of 1 volt when the current changes at a rate of 1 ampere per second.

Heparin: An inflammatory mediator produced by the mast cells of the liver. It inhibits the clotting process by preventing the transformation of prothrombin into thrombin.

Hepatitis B Virus (HBV): A virus that results in inflammation of the liver. Following a 2- to 6-week incubation period symptoms develop which include gastrointestinal and respiratory disturbances, jaundice, enlarged liver, muscle pain, and loss of weight.

Hertz (Hz): The number of cycles per second.

High TENS: The application of transcutaneous electrical nerve stimulation possessing high-frequency, short-duration pulses, and applied at sensory-level intensity.

Histamine: A blood-thinning chemical released from damaged tissue during the inflammatory process.

Homeostasis: State of equilibrium in the body and its systems which provides a stable internal environment.

Human Immunodeficiency Virus (HIV): The virus

that causes acquired immune deficiency syndrome (AIDS).

Hunting Response: A vascular response to cold application marked by a series of vasoconstrictions and vasodilations. This response has only been shown to occur in limited body areas.

Hydrocortisone: An anti-inflammatory drug that closely resembles cortisol.

Hydrostatic: Relating to the pressure of liquids in equilibrium or to the pressure they exert.

Hydrostatic Pressure: The pressure of blood within the capillary.

Hyperemia: A red discoloration of the skin caused by increased blood flow. The skin will turn white when pressure is applied.

Hyperthermia: Increased core temperature.

Hypertrophy: To develop an increase in bulk, for example in the cross-sectional area of muscle.

Hyporeflexia: Diminished function of the reflexes.

Hypothalamus: The body's thermoregulatory center.

Hypothermia: Decreased core temperature.

Hypoxia: Lack of an adequate supply of oxygen.

Immediate Treatment: Used in the initial management of athletic injuries, immediate treatment is composed of four components: rest, ice, compression, and elevation.

Impedance: The resistance to flow of an alternating current due to inductance and capacitance.

Impedance Plethysmography: A determination of blood flow based on the amount of electrical resistance in the area.

Inductance: The ability of material to store an electrical charge by means of an electromagnetic field. Inductance is negligible in biological systems.

Infection: A disease state produced by the invasion of a contaminating organism.

Inflammation: Tissue reaction to an injury.

Infrared Light: Energy possessing a wavelength between 770 and 12,500 nm. Infrared light is invisible to the human eye.

Injury Potential: Disruption of a tissue's normal electrical balance as a result of injury.

Innervate: A nerve impulse of enough magnitude to elicit a contraction.

Interpulse Interval: The elapsed period of time between the conclusion of one pulse and the start of the next pulse.

Interstitial: Between the tissues.

Intra-articular: Within a joint.

Intracellular: Within the membrane of a cell.

Intrapulse Interval: A period of time within a discrete pulse that the current is not flowing. The duration of the intrapulse interval cannot exceed the duration of the interpulse interval.

Invasion of Privacy: Infringement on the right to be left alone. Public figures have less rights in this regard than do "ordinary" citizens.

Inverse Square Law: The intensity of the energy striking the tissues is proportional to the square of the distance between the source of the energy and the tissues: Energy received = Energy at the source ÷ Distance from the source squared.

Ion: An atom, or group of atoms, that has a net charge other than zero.

Iontophoresis: Introduction of ions into the body through the use of an electrical current.

Ischemia: Local and temporary deficiency of blood supply due to obstruction of circulation to a part.

Isoelectric Point: The point where positive and negative electrical potentials are equal.

IUD: Intrauterine device. A plastic coil inserted within the uterus to prevent pregnancy. Older models were made of metal.

Joule: Basic unit of work in the International System of Units. One joule equals 0.74 foot-pounds of work. Joules = Coulombs × Volts.

Kinetic Energy: The energy an object possesses by virtue of its motion.

Kinins: A group of polypeptides that dilate arterioles, serve as strong chemotactics, and produce pain. They are primarily involved in the inflammatory process in the early stages of vascular response.

Labile Cells: Cells located in the skin, intestinal tract, and blood and possessing good regenerative abilities.

Lactic Acid: A cellular waste product produced by muscular contraction or cell metabolism. A fatiguing carbohydrate.

Laminectomy: Surgical removal of the lamina from a vertebra.

Legal Guardian: An individual who is legally responsible for the care of an infant or minor.

Leukocytes: White blood cells that serve as scavengers.

Leukotrienes: Fatty acids that cause smooth muscle contraction, increase vascular permeability, and attract neutrophils.

Licensure (Athletic Training): A state-legislated regulation of athletic training that determines the scope of practice for that state. The licensing process, which may also include registration and certification, sets the educational standards needed to practice within that state.

Lordosis: The forward curvature of the cervical and lumbar spine.

Low TENS: The application of transcutaneous electrical nerve stimulation using low-frequency, long-duration pulses, and applied with motor-level intensity.

Luminous Infrared: See near infrared.

Lymphatic Return: A return process similar to that of the venous network, but specializing in the removal of interstitial fluids.

Lymphedema: Swelling of the lymph nodes due to blockage of the vessels.

Macrophage: A cell having the ability to devour particles; a phagocyte.

Magnetic Resonance Image (MRI): A view of the body's internal structures obtained through the use of magnetic and radio fields.

Mainframe Computer: A centrally located computer that serves a large number of remote terminals.

Malfeasance: The performance of an unlawful or improper act.

Malpractice: Negligence on the part of a professional person serving in the line of duty.

Margination: Platelets and leukocytes, normally flowing in the bloodstream, begin to tumble along the walls of the vessel.

Master Points: According to the theory of acupuncture, these points connect skin areas to deeper energy channels. Stimulating master points results in systemic changes.

Matriculation: The time spent in a college or university pursuing a degree.

McGill Pain Questionnaire: One of many pain scales, this device uses a choice of words in describing the type, magnitude, and location of the pain.

Mechanosensitive Receptors: Nerve endings that are sensitive to mechanical pressure.

Mediators: Chemicals that act through indirect means.

Medium: A material used to promote the transfer of energy. An object—or substance—that permits the transmission of energy through it.

Meniscectomy: The surgical removal of the knee's meniscal cartilage.

Meridians: In acupuncture, meridians are primary pathways through which the body's energy flows.

Metabolism: The sum of physical and chemical reactions taking place within the body.

Metabolite: A by-product of metabolism.

Mho: The measure of a material's electrical conductance; the mathematical reciprocal of electrical resistance.

Microstreaming: Localized flow of fluids resulting from cavitation.

Misfeasance: The improper performance of an otherwise lawful act.

Modality: The application of a form of energy to the body which elicits an involuntary response.

Modulation: Regulation or adjustment.

Monophasic Current: A unidirectional pulse characterized by one discrete pulse.

Monopolar Stimulation: The application of electrical stimulation where the current density under one set of electrodes (the active electrodes) is much greater than the other electrode (the dispersive electrodes). All neuromuscular effects occur under the active electrode(s).

Motor Nerve: A nerve that provides impulses to muscles.

Motor Point: An area on the skin used to stimulate motor nerves.

Motor Unit: A group of skeletal muscle fibers that are innervated by a single motor nerve.

Mottling: A blotchy discoloration of the skin.

Muscular Tissue: Comprised of smooth (found in the internal organs) cardiac and skeletal muscle, this tissue has the ability to actively shorten and passively lengthen.

Muscle Guarding: A voluntary or subconscious contraction of a muscle to protect an injured area.

Muscle Spindle: An organ located within the muscular tissue that detects the rate and magnitude of a muscle contraction.

Myelin: A fatty layering around nerves.

Myelinated: Having a fatlike outer coating (myelin). This coating serves as insulation for nerves.

Myocardial: Pertaining to the middle layer of the heart walls.

Myosin: Noncontractile muscle protein.

Myositis Ossificans: Calcification of muscular tissues.

Myositis: Inflammation of muscular tissue.

Nanometer: One billionth (10^{-9}) of a meter.

Nanosecond: One billionth (10^{-9}) of a second.

Near Field: The portion of an ultrasonic beam close to the sound head.

Near Infrared: The range of infrared light that is closest to visible light, with wavelengths ranging between 770 and 1500 nm. Also known as luminous infrared.

Near Ultraviolet: The range of light with wavelengths between 290 and 390 nm. The portion of the ultraviolet spectrum located closest to visible light.

Necrosin: Increases the permeability of a cell membrane.

Necrosis: Cell death.

Negligence: Departure from the standard of care. See also omission and commission.

Neoprene: A synthetic rubber material.

Nervous Tissue: Possesses the ability to conduct chemo-electrical impulses.

Neutron: An electrically neutral particle found in the center of an atom.

Neurapraxia: A temporary loss of function in a peripheral nerve.

Neurological: Pertaining to the nervous system.

Neuron, First Order: Sensory neuron arising from a spinal nerve and having its body in a dorsal root ganglion.

Neuron, Second Order: A nerve having its body located in the spinal cord. It connects first and third order neurons.

Neuron, Third Order: A nerve having its cell body located in the thalamus and extending into the cerebral cortex.

Nociceptive Stimulus: Impulse giving rise to the sensation of pain.

Nociceptors: Nerves that transmit pain impulses.

Nonfeasance: The failure to act when there is a duty to act.

Nonunion Fracture: Fractures that fail to spontaneously heal within a normal time frame.

Noxious: Harmful, injurious.

Noxious-level Stimulation: Brief, intense electrical stimulation (above the threshold of pain) that is thought to activate the release of endogenous opiates.

Nucleus Pulposus: The gelatinous middle of an intervertebral disc.

Numbness: Lack of sensation in a body part.

Occiput: The posterior base of the skull.

Occupational Safety and Health Administration (OSHA): A Federal agency responsible for assuring safe working conditions. This agency has enforcement powers and is capable of levying fines against employers.

Ohm: Unit of electrical resistance required to develop 0.24 calories of heat when 1 ampere of current is applied for 1 second.

Ohm's Law: Current is directly proportional to resistance: Amperage = Voltage/Resistance ($I = V/R$).

Omission: The failure to respond to a situation when actions are necessary to limit or reduce harm.

Ordinary Negligence: The failure to act as a reasonable and prudent person would act under similar circumstances.

Orthotics: The use of orthopedic devices for correcting deformity or malalignment.

Osteoarthritis: Degeneration of a joint's articular surface.

Osteoblast: A cell concerned with the formation of new bone.

Osteoclast: A cell that absorps and removes unwanted bone.

Osteogenesis: Healing of fracture sites through the formation of callus, followed by the deposition of collagen and bone salts.

Osteoporosis: A porous condition resulting in softening of bone. Most commonly seen (but not exclusively) in postmenopausal women.

Overload Principle: For strength gains to occur, the body must be subjected to more stress than it is accustomed to. This is accomplished by increasing the load, frequency, or duration of the exercise.

Pacinian Receptors: Receptors located deep in the skin which relay information regarding pressure and vibration. Within the joints, they assist in relaying proprioceptive information.

Pallor: Lack of color in the skin.

Parallel Circuit: An electrical circuit in which electrons have more than route to follow.

Pathology: Deviations from the normal that characterize disease or injury.

Pavementing: Platelets adhere to the vessel walls in multiple layers to form a patch over the injury site.

Peak-to-peak Value: The sum of the maximum deviation above and below the baseline.

Penetration: Depth at which energy absorption takes place.

Periosteal Pain: A deep-seated ache resulting from an overly intense application of ultrasonic energy, which irritates the periosteum.

Periosteum: The outer layering of bone other than the articulating surfaces. The periosteum is highly vascular and highly sensitive.

Peripheral Vascular Disease: Actually a syndrome describing an insufficiency of arteries and/or veins for maintaining proper circulation (also known as PVD).

pH: (**p**otential of **H**ydrogen) A measure of acidity or alkalinity (bases). A neutral solution has a pH of 7. Acids have a pH of less than 7; bases greater than 7.

Phagocytosis: The ingestion and digestion of bacteria and particles by phagocytes.

Phase Duration: The amount of time required for a phase to complete its shape.

Phase: Individual sections of a single pulse that remain on one side of the baseline for a period of time.

Phonophoresis: The introduction of medication into the body through the use of ultrasonic energy.

Photon: A unit of light energy that has zero mass, no electric charge, and an indefinite life span.

Physical Therapy Practice Act: State legislation that governs the practice of physical therapy procedures.

Piezoelectric Crystal: A crystal that produces positive and negative electrical charges when it is compressed or expanded.

Pitting Edema: An exudate-rich form of edema that is characterized by being easily indented by pressure (hence, "pitting").

Placebo: A substance of no objective curative value and given to a patient to satisfy a need for treatment or used as a control in an experimental study. Interestingly, this word stems from the Latin for "I shall please."

Plaintiff: A person who is the complaining party in a lawsuit.

Platelet: A free-flowing cell fragment in the bloodstream.

Polymorph: A type of white blood cell; a granulocyte.

Power (Electrical): See wattage.

Precedent: A previous ruling that serves as a guide in future legal actions.

Pronation: An inward flattening and tilting of the foot, resulting in the lowering of the medial longitudinal arch.

Propagation: Transmission through a medium.

Prostaglandins: A group of substances which are responsible for vasodilation and increased vascular permeability. Prostaglandins are synthesized locally in injured tissues and serve to influence the duration and intensity of the inflammatory process.

Prothrombin: A chemical found in the blood which reacts with an enzyme to produce thrombin.

Proton: A positively charged atomic particle.

Pulsatile Current: See pulsed current.

Pulse Charge: The number of coulombs contained in one electrical pulse.

Pulse Duration: The amount of time from the initial nonzero charge to the return to a zero charge, including the intrapulse interval.

Pulse Frequency: The number of electrical pulses that occur in a 1-second period.

Pulse Period: The period of time between the initiation of a pulse and the initiation of the subsequent pulse, including the intrapulse interval and the interpulse interval.

Pulse Width: See pulse duration.

Pulsed Current: A flow of electrons marked by discrete periods of nonelectron flow.

Quadripolar Stimulation: Electrical stimulation applied with two channels.

Radiant Energy: Heat gained or lost through radiation.

Radiation: The transfer of electromagnetic energy that does not require the presence of a medium.

Range of Motion: The distance, measured in degrees, that a limb moves in one plane (e.g., flexion/extension, adduction/abduction).

Raynaud's Phenomenon: A reaction to cold consisting of bouts of pallor and cyanosis.

Rebound Vasoconstriction: A reflex constriction of blood vessels due to prolonged exposure to extreme temperatures.

Reflection: The return of waves from an object.

Refraction: The bending of a wave as it passes through an object.

Resistance Stage: The second step in the general adaptation syndrome. During this stage the body adapts to the stresses placed on it.

Resistor (Electrical): A material having to oppose the flow of electric currents. Resistors have few free electrons. Within the body, tissues having a low water content are considered to be resistors.

Respondeat Superior: See vicarious liability.

Retinaculum: A fibrous membrane that holds an organ or body part in place.

Root-Mean-Square Value: A conversion of the electrical power delivered by an alternating current into the equivalent direct current power. Calculated by multiplying the peak value by 0.707.

Salicylates: A family of compounds that includes aspirin.

Sclerotome: A portion of bone which is supplied by a spinal nerve root.

Secondary Hypoxic Injury: Cell death resulting from a lack of oxygen.

Sedation: The result of calming nerve endings.

Sedative: An agent which causes sedation.

Sequential Compression: Compression of an extremity characterized by a distal to proximal flow.

Series Circuit: A circuit where the current has only one path it can follow.

Serotonin: A substance which causes local vasodilation and increased permeability of the capillaries.

Silica: A finely ground form of sand capable of holding water.

Slander: Defamation of character via the spoken word.

Somatic: Pertaining to the body.

Specific Heat: The ratio of a substance's thermal capacity to that of water, which has a thermal capacity of 1. The specific heats of the three states of water are: ice 0.50; water 1.0; and steam 0.48.

Spondylolisthesis: Forward slippage of the lower lumbar vertebrae on the sacrum.

Sprain: A stretching or tearing of ligaments.

Stabile Cells: Cells possessing some ability to regenerate.

Stable Cavitation: The gentle expansion and contraction of bubbles formed during ultrasound application.

Standard of Practice: The criteria against which an individual's performance is measured. The National Athletic Trainers' Association Board of Certification establishes the Standards for Direct Service.

Standing Orders: A "blanket prescription" from a physician describing how injuries are to be managed when the physician is not present.

Standing Wave: A single-frequency wave formed by the collision of two waves of equal frequency and speed traveling in opposite directions. The energy within a standing wave cannot be transmitted from one area to another and is focused in a confined area.

States of Matter: Physical matter can take three forms: solid, liquid, and gas. Using H_2O as an example, we see the three phases as ice, water (liquid), and steam.

Statute of Limitations: A legal time limit allowed for the filing of a lawsuit.

Strain: A stretching or tearing of tendons or muscles.

Stratum Corneum: The outermost, nonliving portion of the epidermis.

Stress: A force which disrupts the normal homeostasis of a system.

Subacute: Between the acute and chronic stages of injury response.

Subcutaneous: Beneath the skin.

Substance P: A neurotransmitter thought to be responsible for the transmission of pain-producing impulses.

Summation: An overlap of muscle contractions which are caused by electrical stimulation.

Subsequent contractions begin prior to the muscle fibers' return to their original length.

Synapse: The junction where two nerves communicate.

Synovium: Membrane lining the capsule of a joint.

Systemic: Affecting the body as a whole.

T Cell: A transmission cell that connects sensory nerves to the central nervous system. Not to be confused with T cells found in the immune system.

Temporal Average Intensity: The average amount of power delivered during pulsed ultrasound.

Tetany: Total contraction of a muscle achieved through the recruitment and contraction of all motor units.

Thalamus: Gray matter located at the base of the brain.

Therapeutic: Having healing properties.

Thermal Capacity: The number of heat units required to raise a unit of mass by 1°C.

Thermolysis: Chemical decomposition due to heating.

Thermotherapy: The application of therapeutic heat to living tissues.

Thrombin: An enzyme formed in the blood of a damaged area.

Tissue Hydrostatic Pressure: The pressure that moves fluids from the tissues into the capillaries.

Tonic Contraction: Prolonged contraction of a muscle.

Tort: A civil wrong.

Transcutaneous: Through the skin.

Transducer: A device that converts one form of energy to another.

Translation: Sliding or gliding of opposing articular surfaces.

Trigger Point: A localized area of spasm within a muscle.

Turf Burn: A deep abrasion caused by friction between the skin and artificial playing surfaces.

Turnkey System: A system designed to prevent unauthorized access. Some software packages require that a specially coded floppy disk be inserted before the user can gain access to the program or copy data.

Type I Muscle Fiber: These muscle fibers generate a relatively low level of force, but can sustain contractions for a long period of time. Geared to aerobic activity, these muscle fibers are also referred to as tonic or slow-twitch fibers.

Type II Muscle Fiber: These muscle fibers generate a large amount of force in a short time. Geared to anaerobic activity, they are also referred to as phasic or fast-twitch fibers.

Ultraviolet Light: Energy with a wavelength between 180 and 390 nm. Ultraviolet light is invisible to the human eye.

Universal Precautions: A series of steps, established by OSHA, that individuals should take to avoid accidental exposure to bloodborne pathogens.

Unstable Cavitation: The violent oscillation of bubble during the application of ultrasound at too great of an intensity.

Valence Shell: An imaginary shell in which the electrons responsible for chemical reactivity orbit around the nucleus of an atom.

Vasoconstriction: Reduction in a blood vessel's diameter. This results in a decrease in blood flow.

Vasodilation: Increase in a blood vessel's diameter. This results in an increase in blood flow.

Venostasis: Pooling of blood in a vein.

Venule: A small vein exiting from a capillary.

Vicarious Liability: Employers can be held liable for the acts of their employees.

Viscera: Organs enclosed by the abdominal cavity.

Viscosity: The resistance of a fluid to flow.

Visible Light: Electromagnetic energy possessing a wavelength between 390 and 760 nm. Visible light is a combination of violet, indigo, blue, green, yellow, orange, and red.

Voltage: A measure of the potential for electrons to flow.

Volumetric Measurement: Determination of the size of a body part by measuring the amount of water it displaces.

Watt: A unit of power. For an electrical current: Watts = Voltage × Amperage.

Weaning: Decreasing the dependence on a substance or device by gradually reducing its use.

White Light: See visible light.

Writ: A formal, written legal document.

X-ray: An electromagnetic wave 0.05 to 100 angstroms in length and able to penetrate most solid matter.

Bibliography

· ·

Chapter 1

Allen, RJ: Human Stress: Its Nature and Control. Burgess Publishing, Minneapolis, 1983.

Cailliet, R: Soft Tissue Pain and Disability. FA Davis, Philadelphia, 1977.

Charman, RA: Pain theory and physiology. Physiotherapy 75:247, 1989.

Cohen, MJ, Naliboff, BD, and McArthur, DL: Implications of medical and biopsychosocial models for understanding and treating chronic pain. Physical and Rehabilitation Medicine 1:135, 1989.

Enwemeka, CS: Inflammation, cellularity, and fibrillogenesis in regenerating tendon: Implications for tendon rehabilitation. Phys Ther 69:816, 1989.

Fisher, DB, et al: Ultrastructural events following acute muscle trauma. Med Sci Sports Exerc 22:185, 1990.

French, S: Pain: Some psychological and sociological aspects. Physiotherapy 75:255, 1989.

Kloth, LC, McCulloch, JM, and Feedar, JA (eds): Wound Healing: Alternatives in Management. FA Davis, Philadelphia, 1990.

Kolb, P and Denegar, C: Traumatic edema and the lymphatic system. Athletic Training 18:339, 1983.

Lechner, CT and Dahners, LE: Healing of the medial collateral ligament in unstable rat knees. Am J Sports Med 19:508, 1991.

Lord, RH and Kozar, B: Pain tolerance in the presence of others: Implications for youth sports. Physician and Sportsmedicine 17:71, 1989.

Olavi, A, Kolari, PJ, and Esa, A: Edema and lower leg perfusion in patients with post-traumatic dysfunction. Acupunct Electrother Res 16:7, 1991.

Raithel, KS: Chronic pain and exercise therapy. Physician and Sportsmedicine 17:204, 1989.

Russell, B, et al: Repair of injured skeletal muscle: A molecular approach. Med Sci Sports Exerc 24:189, 1992.

Singer, RN and Johnson, PJ: Strategies to cope with pain associated with sport-related injuries. Athletic Training 22:100, 1987.

Smith, LL: Acute inflammation: The underlying mechanism in delayed onset muscle soreness? Med Sci Sports Exerc 23:542, 1991.

Sorenson, MK: The edematous hand. Phys Ther 69:1059, 1989.

Spence, AP and Mason, EB: Human Anatomy and Physiology, ed 3. Benjamin/Cummings, Menlo Park, CA, 1987.

Spengler, DM, Loeser, JD, and Murphy, TM: Orthopaedic aspects of the chronic pain syndrome. In: The American Academy of Orthopaedic Surgeons Instructional Course Lectures, Vol 29. CV Mosby, St. Louis, 1980.

Stuckey, SJ, Jacobs, A, and Goldfarb, J: EMG biofeedback training, relaxation training, and placebo for the relief of chronic back pain. Percep Mot Skills 63:1023, 1986.

Thorton, JS: Playing in pain: When should an athlete stop? Physician Sportsmedicine 18:138, 1990.

Vander, AJ, Sherman, JH, and Luciano, DS: Human Physiology: The Mechanisms of Body Function, ed 3. McGraw-Hill, New York, 1980.

Vanudevan, SV and Melvin, JL: Upper extremity edema control: Rationale of the techniques. Am J Occup Ther 33:520, 1980.

Walsh, D: Nociceptive pathways—relevance to the physiotherapist. Physiotherapy 77:317, 1991.

Wilkerson, GB: Inflammation in connective tissue: Etiology and management. Athletic Training 20:299, 1985.

Chapter 2

Van Heuvelen, A: Physics: A General Introduction. Little, Brown & Co, Boston, 1982.

Weinberger, A and Lev, A: Temperature elevation of connective tissue by physical modalities. Critical Reviews in Physical and Rehabilitation Medicine 3:121, 1991.

Chapter 3

Baker, RJ and Bell, GW: The effect of therapeutic modalities on blood flow in the human calf. JOSPT 13:23, 1991.

Belitsky, RB, Odam, SJ, and Humbley-Kozey, C: Evaluation of the effectiveness of wet ice, dry ice, and cryogen packs in reducing skin temperature. Phys Ther 67:1080, 1987.

Bocobo, C, et al: The effect of ice on intra-articular temperature in the knee of the dog. Am J Phys Med Rehabil 70:181, 1991.

Brown, M and Baker, RD: Effect of pulsed shortwave diathermy on skeletal muscle injury in rabbits. Phys Ther 67:208, 1987.

Carman, KW and Knight, KL: Sensory perception of the foot and ankle following therapeutic applications of heat and cold. Athletic Training 27:231, 1992.

Cote, DL, et al: Comparison of three treatment procedures for minimizing ankle sprain swelling. Phys Ther 68:1072, 1988.

Denegar, CR and Perrin, DH: Effect of transcutaneous electrical nerve stimulation, cold, and a combination treatment on pain, decreased range of motion, and strength loss associated with delayed onset muscle soreness. Athletic Training 27:200, 1992.

Durst, JW, et al: Effects of ice and recovery time on maximal involuntary isometric torque production using electrical stimulation. JSOPT, 13:240, 1991.

Garrett, WE: Muscle strain injuries: Clinical and basic aspects. Med Sci Sports Exerc 22:436, 1990.

Gerig, BK: The effects of cryotherapy upon ankle proprioception (Abstr) Athletic Training 25:119, 1990.

Green, GA, Zachazewski, JE, and Jordan, SE: A case conference: Peroneal nerve palsy induced by cryotherapy. Physician and Sports Medicine 17:63, 1989.

Halvorson, GA: Therapeutic heat and cold for athletic injuries. Physician and Sportsmedicine 18:87, 1990.

Hocutt, JE, et al: Cryotherapy in ankle sprains. Am J Sports Med 10:316, 1982.

Ingersoll, CD and Mangus, BC: Sensations of cold reexamined: A study using the McGill Pain Questionnaire. Athletic Training 26:240, 1991.

Ingersoll, CD and Mangus, BC: Habituation to the perception of the qualities of cold-induced pain. Athletic Training 27:218, 1992.

Ingersoll, CD, Mangus, BC, and Wolf, S: Cold-induced pain: Habituation to cold immersions (abstr). Athletic Training 25:126, 1990.

Isabell, WK, et al: The effects of ice massage, ice massage with exercise, and exercise on the prevention and treatment of delayed onset muscle soreness. Athletic Training 27:208, 1992.

Kaempffe, KA: Skin surface temperature reduction after cryotherapy to a casted extremity. JOSPT 10:448, 1989.

Kitchen, SS and Partridge, CJ: A review of microwave diathermy. Physiotherapy 77:647, 1991.

Knight, KL and Londeree, BR: Comparison of blood flow in the ankle of uninjured subjects during application of heat, cold, and exercise. Med Sci Sports Exercise 12:76, 1980.

Knight, KL: Cryotherapy: Theory, technique, and physiology. Chattanooga Corporation, Chattanooga, 1985.

Lehmann, J (ed): Therapeutic Heat and Cold, ed 4. Williams & Wilkins, Baltimore, 1990.

Lewis, T: Observations upon the reactions of the vessels of the human skin to cold. Heart 15:177, 1930.

Malone, TR, et al: Nerve injury in athletes caused by cryotherapy. Athletic Training 27:235, 1992.

Michlovitz, S (ed): Thermal agents in rehabilitation, ed 2. FA Davis, Philadelphia, 1990.

Miller, CR and Webers, RL: The effects of ice massage on an individual's pain tolerance level to electrical stimulation. JOSPT 12:105, 1990.

Newton, RA: Effects of vapocoolants on passive hip flexion in healthy subjects. Phys Ther 65:1034, 1985.

Nimchick, PSR and Knight, KL: Effects of wearing a toe cap or a sock on temperature and perceived pain during ice immersion. Athletic Training 18:144, 1983.

Parker, TJ, Small, NC, and Davis, PG: Case report: Cold-induced nerve palsy. Athletic Training 18:76, 1983.

Stopka, CB: Hydrotherapy: Invaluable, and now inexpensive. Athletic Training 22:219, 1987.

Strickler, T, Malone T, and Garrett, WE: The effects of passive warming on muscle injury. Am J Sports Med 18:141, 1990.

Taber, C, et al: Measurement of reactive vasodilation during cold gel pack application to nontraumatized ankles. Phys Ther 72:294, 1992.

Travell, JG and Simons, DG: Myofascial Pain and Dysfunction: The Trigger Point Manual. Williams & Wilkins, Baltimore, 1983.

Vanudevan, SV and Melvin, JL: Upper extremity edema control: Rationale of the techniques. Am J Occup Ther 33:520, 1980.

Waylonis, GW: The physiological effect of ice massage. Arch Phys Med Rehabil 48:37, 1967.

Weinberger, A and Lev, A: Temperature elevation of connective tissue by physical modalities. Critical Reviews in Physical and Rehabilitation Medicine 3:121, 1991.

Weinberger, A, et al: The effect of local deep micro-wave hyperthermia on experimental zymosan-induced arthritis in rabbits. Am J Phys Med Rehabil 69:239, 1990.

Wilkerson, GB: Treatment of ankle sprains with external compression and early mobilization. Phys Sport Med 13:83, 1985.

Wilkerson, GB: Treatment of the inversion ankle sprain through synchronous application of focal compression and cold. Athletic Training 26:220, 1991.

Yackzan, L, Adams, C, and Francis, KT: The effects of ice massage on delayed muscle soreness. Am J Sports Med 12:159, 1984.

Chapter 4

Almekinders, LC: Transcutaneous muscle stimulation for rehabilitation. Phys Sportsmed 12:118, 1984.

Alon, G: High voltage stimulation: Effects of electrode size on basic excitatory responses. Phys Ther 65:890, 1985.

Angulo, DL and Colwell, CW: Use of postoperative TENS and continuous passive motion following total knee replacement. JOSPT 11:599, 1990.

Baker, LL, Bowman, BR, and McNeal, DR: Effects of waveform on comfort during neuromuscular electrical stimulation. Clin Orthop 223:75, 1988.

Barr, JO, Nielsen, DH, and Soderberg, GL: Transcutaneous electrical nerve stimulation characteristics for altering pain perception. Phys Ther 66:1515, 1986.

Bechtel, TB and Fan, PT: When is TENS effective and practical for pain relief? J Musculoskel Med 2:37, 1985.

Berlant, SR: Method of determining optimal stimulation sites for transcutaneous electrical nerve stimulation. Phys Ther 64:924, 1984.

Bettany, JA, Fish, DR, and Mendel FC: Influence of high voltage pulsed direct current on edema formation following impact injury. Phys Ther 70:219, 1990.

Boutelle, D, Smith, B, and Malone, T: A strength study utilizing the electro-stim 180. JOSPT 7:50, 1985.

Bowman, BR and Baker, LL: Effects of waveform parameters on comfort during transcutaneous neuromuscular electrical stimulation. Ann Biomed Eng 13:59, 1985.

Cote, DL, et al: Comparison of three treatment procedures for minimizing ankle sprain swelling. Phys Ther 68:1072, 1988.

Cummings, JP: Conservative management of peripheral nerve injuries utilizing selective electrical stimulation of denervated muscle with exponentially progressive current forms. JOSPT 7:11, 1985.

Currier, DP and Mann, R: Muscular strength development by electrical stimulation in healthy individuals. Phys Ther 63:915, 1983.

Currier, DP, Lehman, J, and Lightfoot, P: Electrical stimulation in exercise of the quadriceps femoris muscle. Phys Ther 59:1508, 1979.

Currier, DP, Petrilli, CR, and Therlkeld, JA: Effect of graded electrical stimulation on blood flow to healthy muscle. Phys Ther 66:937, 1986.

De Domenico, G: Interferential Stimulation [monograph]. Chattanooga Group, Chattanooga, 1988.

Delitto, A and Rose, SJ: Comparative comfort of three waveforms used in electrically eliciting quadriceps femoris muscle contractions. Phys Ther 66:1704, 1986.

Delitto, A and Snyder-Mackler, L: Two theories of muscle strength augmentation using percutaneous electrical stimulation. Phys Ther 70:158, 1990.

Denegar, CR and Huff, CB: High and low frequency TENS in the treatment of induced musculoskeletal pain: A comparison study. Athletic Training 23:235, 1988.

Denegar, CR and Perrin, DH: Effect of transcutaneous electrical nerve stimulation, cold, and a combination treatment on pain, decreased range of motion, and strength loss associated with delayed onset muscle soreness. Athletic Training 27:200, 1992.

Denegar, CR, et al: Influence of transcutaneous electrical nerve stimulation on pain, range of motion, and serum cortisol concentration in females experiencing delayed onset muscle soreness. JOSPT 11:100, 1989.

Durst, JW, et al: Effects of ice and recovery time on maximal involuntary isometric torque production using electrical stimulation. JOSPT 13:240, 1991.

Feedar, JA, Kloth, LC, and Gentzkow, GD: Chronic dermal ulcer healing enhanced with monophasic pulsed electrical stimulation. Phys Ther 71:639, 1991.

Ferguson, JP, et al: Effects of varying electrode site placements on the torque output of an electrically stimulated involuntary quadriceps femoris muscle contraction. JOSPT 11:24, 1989.

Fish, DR, et al: Effect of anodal high voltage pulsed current on edema formation in frog hind limbs. Phys Ther 71:724, 1991.

Fulbright, JS: Electrical stimulation to chronic toe-flexor hypertonicity: A case report. Phys Ther 64:523, 1984.

Gersh, MR (ed): Electrotherapy in Rehabilitation. FA Davis, Philadelphia, 1992.

Gersh, MR and Wolf, SL: Applications of transcutaneous electrical nerve stimulation in the management of patients with pain. Phys Ther 65:314, 1985.

Griffin, JW, et al: Reduction of chronic posttraumatic hand edema: A comparison of high voltage pulsed current, intermittent pneumatic compression, and placebo treatments. Phys Ther 70:279, 1990.

Grim, LC and Morey, SH: Transcutaneous electrical nerve stimulation for relief of parturition pain. Phys Ther 65:337, 1985.

Harris, PR: Iontophoresis: Clinical research in musculoskeletal inflammatory conditions. JOSPT 4:109, 1982.

Hasson, SH, et al: Exercise training and dexamethasone iontophoresis in rheumatoid arthritis: A case study. Physiotherapy Canada 43:11, 1991.

Henley, EJ: Transcutaneous drug delivery: Iontophoresis, phonophoresis. Physical and Rehabilitation Medicine 2:139, 1991.

Hobler, CK: Case Study: Reduction of chronic posttraumatic knee edema using interferential stimulation. Athletic Training 26:364, 1991.

Jensen, JE, et al: The use of transcutaneous neural stimulation and isokinetic testing in arthroscopic knee surgery. Am J Sports Med 13:27, 1985.

Jette, DU: Effect of different forms of transcutaneous electrical nerve stimulation on experimental pain. Phys Ther 66:187, 1986.

Kincaid, CB and Lavoie, KH: Inhibition of bacterial growth in vitro following stimulation with high voltage, monophasic, pulsed current. Phys Ther 69:651, 1989.

Kloth, LC and Cummings, JP: Electrotherapeutic terminology in physical therapy. Section on Clinical Electrophysiology and the American Physical Therapy Association, Alexandria, VA, 1990.

Kramer, JF: Effect of electrical stimulation frequencies on isometric knee extension torque. Phys Ther 67:31, 1987.

Lake, DA: Neuromuscular electrical stimulation: An overview and its application in the treatment of sports injuries. Sports Med 13:320, 1992.

Laughman, RK, et al: Strength changes in the normal quadriceps femoris muscle group as a result of electrical stimulation. Phys Ther 63:494, 1983.

Leo, KC, et al: Effect of transcutaneous electrical nerve stimulation characteristics on clinical pain. Phys Ther 66:200, 1986.

Lewers, D, et al: Transcutaneous electrical nerve stimulation in the relief of primary dysmenorrhea. Phys Ther 69:3, 1989.

Lieber, RL and Kelly, MJ: Factors influencing quadriceps femoris muscle torque using transcutaneous neuromuscular stimulation. Phys Ther 71:715, 1991.

Lilly-Masuda, D and Towne, S: Bioelectricity and bone healing. JOSPT 7:54, 1985.

Liu, H, Currier, DP, and Threlkeld, AJ: Circulatory response of digital arteries associated with electrical stimulation of calf muscle in healthy subjects. Phys Ther 67:340, 1987.

Longobardi, AG, et al: Effects of auricular transcutaneous electrical nerve stimulation on distal extremity pain. Phys Ther 69:10, 1989.

MacLean, K: Physiological rationale of electrotherapy. Physiotherapy 76:738, 1990.

Mannheimer, JS: Optimal Stimulation Sites for TENS Electrodes. La Jolla Technology, San Diego, CA, 1980.

Michlovitz, S, Smith, W, and Watkins, M: Ice and high voltage pulsed stimulation in treatment of lateral ankle sprains. JOSPT 9:301, 1988.

Miller, CR and Webers, RL: The effects of ice massage on an individual's pain tolerance level to electrical stimulation. JOSPT 12:105, 1990.

Mohr, T, et al: Comparison of isometric exercise and high volt galvanic stimulation on quadriceps femoris muscle strength. Phys Ther 65:606, 1985.

Mohr, T, et al: The effect of high volt galvanic stimulation on quadriceps femoris muscle torque. JOSPT 7:314, 1986.

Mohr, TM, Akers, TK, and Landry, RG: Effect of high voltage stimulation on edema reduction in the rat hind limb. Phys Ther 67:1703, 1987.

Nash, HL and Rogers, CC: Does electricity speed the healing of non-union fractures. Physician and Sportsmedicine, 16:155, 1988.

Nelson, RM and Currier, DP (eds): Clinical Electrotherapy. Appleton & Lange, Norwalk, CT, 1987.

Newton, RA and Karselis, TC: Skin pH following high voltage pulsed galvanic stimulation. Phys Ther 63:1593, 1983.

Nolan, MF: Conductive differences in electrodes used with transcutaneous electrical nerve stimulation devices. Phys Ther 71:746, 1991.

Nussbaum, E, Rush, P, and Disenhaus, L: The effects of interferential therapy on peripheral blood flow. Physiotherapy 76:803, 1990.

Ottoson, D and Lundeberg, T: Pain treatment by transcutaneous electrical nerve stimulation: A practical manual. Springer-Verlag, New York, 1988.

Paris, DL, Baynes, F, and Gucker, B: Effects of the neuroprobe in the treatment of second-degree ankle sprains. Phys Ther 63:35, 1983.

Parker, MG, et al: Fatigue response in human quadriceps femoris muscle during high frequency electrical stimulation. JOSPT 7:145, 1986.

Ralston, DJ: High voltage galvanic stimulation: Can there be a "state of the art"? Athletic Training 20:291, 1985.

Robinson, AJ and Snyder-Mackler, L: Clinical application of electrotherapeutic modalities. Phys Ther 68:1235, 1988.

Roeser, WM, et al: The use of transcutaneous nerve stimulation for pain control in athletic medicine. A preliminary report. Am J Sports Med 4:210, 1976.

Selkowitz, DM: Improvement in isometric strength of the quadriceps femoris muscle after training with electrical stimulation. Phys Ther 65:186, 1988.

Sinacore, DR, et al: Type II fiber activation with electrical stimulation: A preliminary report. Phys Ther 70:416, 1990.

Smith, MJ: Electrical stimulation for relief of musculoskeletal pain. Physician and Sportsmedicine 11:47, 1983.

Snyder-Mackler, L and Robinson, AJ (eds): Clinical electrophysiology: Electrotherapy and electrophysiologic testing. Williams & Wilkins, Baltimore, 1989.

Snyder-Mackler, L, Garrett, M, and Roberts, M: A comparison of torque generating capabilities of three different electrical stimulating currents. JOSPT 10:297, 1989.

Stanish, WD, et al: The use of electricity in ligament and tendon repair. The Physician and Sports-Medicine 13:109, 1985.

Taylor, K, et al: Effect of a single 30-minute treatment of high voltage pulsed current on edema formation in frog hind limbs. Phys Ther 72:63, 1992.

Taylor, K, et al: Effect of electrically induced muscle contractions on posttraumatic edema formation in frog hind limbs. Phys Ther 72:127, 1992.

Taylor, K, et al: Effects of interferential current stim-

ulation for treatment of subjects with recurrent jaw pain. Phys Ther 67:346, 1987.

Tracy, JE, Currier, DP, and Threlkeld, AJ: Comparison of selected pulse frequencies from two different electrical stimulators on blood flow in healthy subjects. Phys Ther 68:1526, 1988.

Trimble, MH and Enoka, RM: Mechanisms underlying the training effects associated with neuromuscular electrical stimulation. Phys Ther 71:273, 1991.

Voight, ML: Reduction of post traumatic ankle edema with high voltage pulsed galvanic stimulation. Athletic Training 19:278, 1984.

Walker, DC, Currier, DP, and Threlkeld, AJ: Effects of high voltage pulsed electrical stimulation on blood flow. Phys Ther 68:481, 1988.

Weider, DL: Treatment of traumatic myositis ossificans with acetic acid iontophoresis. Phys Ther 72:133, 1992.

Wolf, SL (ed): Electrotherapy. Churchill Livingstone, New York, 1981.

Wong, RA: High voltage versus low voltage electrical stimulation: Force of induced muscle contraction and perceived discomfort in healthy subjects. Phys Ther 66:1209, 1986.

Chapter 5

Angulo, DL and Colwell, CW: Use of postoperative TENS and continuous passive motion following total knee replacement. JOSPT 11:599, 1990.

Baker, RJ and Bell, GW: The effect of therapeutic modalities on blood flow in the human calf. JOSPT 13:23, 1991.

Bensen, HAE, McElnay, JC, and Harland, R: Use of ultrasound to enhance percutaneous absorption of benzydamine. Phys Ther 69:113, 1989.

Bischko, JJ: Use of the laser beam in acupuncture. Acupuncture and Electro-Therapeutic Research International Journal 5:29, 1980.

Black, KD, et al: Alterations in ankle dorsiflexion torque as a result of continuous ultrasound to the anterior tibial compartment. Phys Ther 64:910, 1984.

Boone, T, Cooper, R, and Thompson, WR: A physiologic evaluation of the sports massage. Athletic Training 26:51, 1991.

Cafarelli, E, et al: Vibratory massage and short-term recovery from muscular fatigue. Int J Sports Med 11:474, 1990.

Cameron, MH and Monroe, LG: Relative transmission of ultrasound by media customarily used for phonophoresis. Phys Ther 72:142, 1992.

Ciccone, CD, Leggin, BG, and Callamaro, JJ: Effects of ultrasound and trolamine salicylate phonophoresis on delayed-onset muscle soreness. Phys Ther 71:666, 1991.

Croce, RV: The effects of EMG biofeedback on strength acquisition. Biofeedback Self Regul 11:299, 1986.

Crosman, LJ, Chateauvert, SR, and Wesiberg, J: The

effects of massage to the hamstring muscle group on range of motion. JOSPT 6:168, 1984.

Cummings, MS, Wilson, VE, and Bird, EI: Flexibility development in sprinters using EMG biofeedback and relaxation training. Biofeedback Self Regul 9:395, 1984.

Davick, JP, Martin, RK, and Albright, JP: Distribution and deposition of tritiated cortisol using phonophoresis. Phys Ther 68:1672, 1988.

Day, JA, Mason, RR, and Chesrown, SE: Effect of massage on serum level of β-endorphin and β-lipotropin in healthy adults. Phys Ther 67:926, 1987.

DeLacerda, FG: Effect of angle of traction pull on upper trapezius muscle activity. JOSPT 1:205, 1980.

DePalma, MT and DePalma, B: The use of instruction and the behavioral approach to facilitate injury rehabilitation. Athletic Training 24:217, 1989.

Diehm, SL: The Power of CPM: Healing through motion. Patient Care 8:34, 1989.

Downing, DS and Weinstein, A: Ultrasound therapy of subacromial bursitis. A double blind trial. Phys Ther 66:194, 1986.

Draper, V and Ballard, L: Electrical stimulation versus electromyographic biofeedback in the recovery of quadriceps femoris muscle function following anterior cruciate ligament surgery. Phys Ther 71:455, 1991.

Draper, V: Electromyographic biofeedback and recovery of quadriceps femoris muscle function following anterior cruciate ligament reconstruction. Phys Ther 70:25, 1990.

Drez, D, et al: In vivo measurement of anterior tibial

translation using continuous passive motion devices. Am J Sports Med 19:381, 1991.

Duffley, HM and Knight KL: Ankle compression variability using the elastic wrap, elastic wrap with a horseshoe, edema II boot, and air-stirrup brace. Athletic Training 24:320, 1989.

Dyson, M: Mechanisms involved in therapeutic ultrasound. Physiotherapy 73:116, 1987.

Enwemeka, CS: The effects of therapeutic ultrasound on tendon healing: A biomechanical study. Am J Phys Med Rehabil 68:283, 1989.

Estwanik, JJ and McAlister, JA: Contusions and the formation of myositis ossificans. Physician and Sportsmedicine 18:53, 1990.

Ferguson, BH: A Practitioners Guide to The Ultrasonic Therapy Equipment Standard. U.S. Department of Health and Human Service - Food and Drug Administration, Washington, DC 1985.

Flor, H, Haag, G, and Turk, DC: Long-term efficacy of EMG biofeedback for chronic rheumatic back pain. Pain 27:195, 1986.

Frieder, S, et al: A pilot study: The therapeutic effect of ultrasound following partial rupture of Achilles tendons in male rats. JOSPT 10:39, 1988.

Fukui, K, et al: Pathomechanism, pathogenesis, and results of treatment in cervical spondylotic myelopathy caused by dynamic canal stenosis. Spine 15:1148, 1990.

Gershuni, DH, Hargens, AR, and Danzig, LA: Regional nutrition and cellularity of the meniscus. Implications for tear and repair. Sports Med 5:322, 1988.

Giudice, ML: Effects of continuous passive motion and elevation on hand edema. Am J Occup Ther 44:914, 1990.

Gomez, MA, et al: The effects of increased tension on healing medial collateral ligaments. Am J Sports Med 19:347, 1991.

Gorkiewicz, R: Ultrasound for subacromial bursitis. Phys Ther 64:46, 1984.

Graham, G and Loomer, RL: Anterior compartment syndrome in a patient with fracture of the tibial plateau treated by continuous passive motion and anticoagulants. Report of a Case. Clin Orthop 220:197, 1985.

Greathouse, DG, Currier, DP, and Gilmore, RL: Effects of clinical infrared laser on superficial radial nerve conduction. Phys Ther 65:1184, 1985.

Griffin, JW, et al: Reduction of chronic posttraumatic hand edema: A comparison of high voltage pulsed current, intermittent pneumatic compression, and placebo treatments. Phys Ther 70:279, 1990.

Harmer, PA: The effect of pre-performance massage on stride frequency in sprinters. Athletic Training 26:55, 1991.

Harris, PR: Cervical traction: Review of literature and treatment guidelines. Phys Ther 57:910, 1977.

Henley, EJ: Transcutaneous drug delivery: Iontophoresis, phonophoresis. Physical and Rehabilitation Medicine 2:139, 1991.

Jackson, BA, Schwane, JA, and Starcher, BC: Effect of ultrasound therapy on the repair of Achilles tendon injuries in rats. Med Sci Sport Exerc 23:171, 1991.

Jette, DU, Falkel, JE, and Trombly, C: Effect of intermittent, supine cervical traction on the myoelectric activity of the upper trapezius muscle in subjects with neck pain. Phys Ther 65:1173, 1985.

Kekosz, VN, Hilbert, L, and Tepperman, PS: Cervical and lumbopelvic traction. To stretch or not to stretch. Postgrad Med 80:187, 1986.

Kim, HK, Moran, ME, and Salter, RB: The potential for regeneration of articular cartilage in defects created by chondral shaving and subchondral abrasion. An experimental investigation in rabbits. J Bone Joint Surg (Am) 73:1301, 1991.

King, CE, et al: Effect of helium-neon laser auriculotherapy on experimental pain threshold. Phys Ther 70:24, 1990.

Kitchen, SS and Partridge, CJ: A review of therapeutic ultrasound, I: Background, physiological effects and hazards. Physiotherapy 76:593, 1990.

Kitchen, SS and Partridge, CJ: A review of therapeutic ultrasound, II: The efficacy of ultrasound. Physiotherapy 76:595, 1990.

Kitchen, SS and Partridge, CJ: A review of low level laser therapy. Part I: Background, Physiological Effects and Hazards. Physiotherapy 77:161, 1991.

Kitchen, SS and Partridge, CJ: A review of low level laser therapy, II: The efficacy of laser therapy. Physiotherapy 77:163, 1991.

LaBan, MM, Macy, JA, and Meerschaert, JR: Intermittent cervical traction: A progenitor of lumbar radicular pain. Arch Phys Med Rehabil 73:295, 1992.

McCarthy, MR et al: The clinical use of continuous passive motion in physical therapy. JOSPT 15:132, 1992.

McDiarmind, T and Burns, PN: Clinical application of therapeutic ultrasound. Physiotherapy 73:155, 1987.

Morelli, M, Seaborne, DE, and Sullivan, J: Changes in H-reflex amplitude during massage of triceps surae in healthy subjects. JOSPT 12:55, 1990.

Morelli, M, Seaborne, DE, and Sullivan, SJ: H-Reflex modulation during manual muscle massage of human triceps surae. Arch Phys Med Rehabil 72:915, 1991.

Muhe, E: Intermittent sequential high-pressure compression of the leg. A new method of preventing deep vein thrombosis. Am J Surg 147:781, 1984.

Mullaji, AB and Shahane, MN: Continuous passive motion for prevention and rehabilitation of knee stiffness: A clinical evaluation. J Postgrad Med 35:204, 1989.

Murphy, MJ: Effects of cervical traction on muscle activity. JOSPT 13:220, 1991.

Naliboff, BD and Tachiki, KH: Autonomic and skeletal muscle response to nonelectrical cutaneous stimulation. Percept Mot Skills 72:575, 1991.

Namba, RS, et al: Continuous passive motion versus immobilization. The effect on posttraumatic joint stiffness. Clin Orthop 266:218, 1991.

O'Donoghue, PC, et al: Clinical use of continuous passive motion in athletic training. Athletic Training 26:200, 1991.

Oziomek, RS, et al: Effect of phonophoresis on serum salicylate levels. Med Sci Sports Exerc 23:397, 1991.

Partridge, CJ: Evaluation of the efficacy of ultrasound. Physiotherapy 73:1987.

Patrick, MK: Application of therapeutic pulsed ultrasound. Physiotherapy 64:103, 1978.

Quillen, WS: Phonophoresis: A review of the literature and technique. Athletic Training 15:109, 1980.

Reed, BV and Held, JM: Effects of sequential connective tissue massage on autonomic nervous system of middle-aged and elderly adults. Phys Ther 68:1231, 1988.

Safety Of Electrotherapy Equipment Working Group, The Chartered Society of Physiotherapy: Guide lines for the safe use of lasers in physiotherapy. Physiotherapy 77:169, 1991.

Salter, RB: The biologic concept of continuous passive motion of synovial joints. The first 18 years of basic research. Clin Orthop 242:12, 1989.

Salter, RB, et al: Clinical application of basic research on continuous passive motion for disorders and injuries of synovial joints: A preliminary report of a feasibility study. J Orthop Res 1:325, 1984.

Sherk, HH (ed): Lasers in Orthopaedics. JB Lippincott, Philadelphia, 1990.

Skyhar, MJ, et al: Nutrition of the anterior cruciate ligament. Effects of continuous passive motion. Am J Sports Med 13:415, 1985.

Snyder-Mackler, L and Bork, CE: Effect of helium-neon laser irradiation on peripheral sensory nerve latency. Phys Ther 68:223, 1988.

Snyder-Mackler, L, et al: Effects of helium-neon laser irradiation on skin resistance and pain in patients with trigger points in the back or neck. Phys Ther 69:336, 1989.

Strap, LJ and Woodfin, PM: Continuous passive motion in the treatment of knee flexion contractures. A case report. Phys Ther 66:1720, 1986.

Stuckey, SJ, Jacobs, A, and Goldfarb, J: EMG biofeedback training, relaxation training, and placebo for the relief of chronic back pain. Percep Mot Skills 63:1023, 1986.

Sullivan, SJ, et al: Effects of massage on alpha motoneuron excitability. Phys Ther 71:555, 1991.

Takai, S, et al: The effects of frequency and duration of controlled passive mobilization on tendon healing. J Orthop Res 9:705, 1991.

ter Haar, G: Basic physics of therapeutic ultrasound. Physiotherapy 73:110, 1987.

Walker, GL: Goodley polyaxial cervical traction. A new approach to a traditional treatment. Phys Ther 66:1255, 1986.

Williams, R: Production and transmission of ultrasound. Physiotherapy 73:113, 1987.

Young, SR and Dyson, M: Macrophage responsiveness to therapeutic ultrasound. Ultrasound Med Biol 16:809, 1990.

Zarnett, R, Velazquez, R, and Salter, RB: The effect of continuous passive motion on knee ligament reconstruction with carbon fibre. An experimental investigation. J Bone Joint Surg (Br) 73:47, 1991.

Chapter 6

Gabriel, AJ: Medical communications—records for the professional athletic trainer. Athletic Training 16:68, 1981.

Gabriel, AJ: The problem-oriented approach to sports injury evaluations. Athletic Training 27:9, 1992.

Kettenbach, G: Writing S.O.A.P. Notes. FA Davis, Philadelphia, 1990.

Chapter 7

Abdenour, T: Computerized training room records. Athletic Training 17:191, 1982.

Baley, JA and Matthews, DL: Law and liability in athletics, physical education, and recreation, ed 2. Wm C Brown, Dubuque, IO, 1988.

Banja, JD and Wolf, SL: Malpractice litigation for uninformed consent: Implications for physical therapists. Phys Ther 67:1226, 1987.

Bloodborne Pathogens: Rules and Regulations. Federal Register 56:64175, 1991.

Drowatzky, JN: Legal duties and liability in athletic training. Athletic Training 20:10, 1985.

Ehrlich, NEP: Reducing a trainer's liability: "A practical approach". Athletic Training 20:256, 1985.

Gieck, J, Lowe, J, and Kenna, K: Trainer malpractice: A sleeping giant. Athletic Training 19:41, 1984.

Graham, LS: Ten ways to dodge the malpractice bullet. Athletic Training 20:117, 1985.

Izumi, HE: AIDS and athletic trainers: Recommendations for athletic training programs. Athletic Training 26:358, 1991.

Leverenz, LJ and Helms, LB: Suing athletic trainers, I: A review of case law involving athletic trainers. Athletic Training 25:212, 1990.

Leverenz, LJ and Helms, LB: Suing athletic trainers, II: Implications for the NATA competencies. Athletic Training 25:219, 1990.

Morin, GE: An overview of selected state licensure athletic training laws. Athletic Training 27:162, 1992.

Payne, SDW: Medicine, Sport and the Law. Blackwell Scientific Publications, Oxford, 1990.

Porter, MM and Porter, JW: Electrical safety in the training room. Athletic Training 16:263, 1981.

Pozgar, GD: Legal aspects of health care administration, ed 3. Aspen Publications, Rockville, MD, 1987.

Ray, R and Shire, TL: An athletic training program in the computer age. Athletic Training 21:212, 1986.

Secor, MR: Designing athletic training facilities or "Where do you want the outlets?" Athletic Training 19:19, 1984.

General Sources

Downer, AH: Physical Therapy Procedures: Selected Techniques, ed 3. Charles C Thomas, Springfield, IL, 1981.

Drez, D (ed): Therapeutic Modalities for Sports Injuries. Year Book Medical Publishers, Chicago, 1989.

Griffin, JE and Karselis, TC: Physical Agents for Physical Therapists, ed 3. Charles C Thomas, Springfield, IL, 1988.

Prentice, WE: Therapeutic Modalities in Sports Medicine. Times Mirror/Mosby College Publishing, St. Louis, 1990.

Index

. . . .

Note: Page numbers followed by an f indicate figures; those followed by a t indicate tables.